EIGHTH EDITION

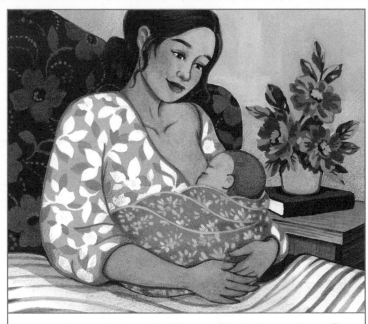

THE NURSING MOTHER'S COMPANION

THE BREASTFEEDING BOOK MOTHERS TRUST, FROM PREGNANCY THROUGH WEANING

KATHLEEN HUGGINS, R.N., M.S., I.B.C.L.C.

WITH **JAN ELLEN BROWN**, B.S., I.B.C.L.C., AND **JENN THORNE**

Foreword by Jessica Martin-W...
Preface by Kelly Bon...
Appendix on Drug Safety by Phil...

HARVARD
COMMON
PRESS

TO THE NURSING MOTHERS OF SAN LUIS OBISPO,
WHO HAVE BEEN MY TEACHERS

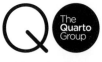

Inspiring | Educating | Creating | Entertaining

Brimming with creative inspiration, how-to projects, and useful information to enrich your everyday life, quarto.com is a favorite destination for those pursuing their interests and passions.

First Published in 2022 by The Harvard Common Press, an imprint of The Quarto Group, 100 Cummings Center, Suite 265-D, Beverly, MA 01915, USA.
T (978) 282-9590 F (978) 283-2742 Quarto.com

The Harvard Common Press titles are also available at discount for retail, wholesale, promotional, and bulk purchase. For details, contact the Special Sales Manager by email at specialsales@quarto.com or by mail at The Quarto Group, Attn: Special Sales Manager, 100 Cummings Center, Suite 265-D, Beverly, MA 01915, USA.

26 25 24 23 22   1 2 3 4 5

ISBN: 978-1-55832-912-6

Digital edition published in 2022
eISBN: 978-1-55832-913-3

Originally found under the following Library of Congress Cataloging-in-Publication Data
Huggins, Kathleen.
The nursing mother's companion : the breastfeeding book mothers trust, from pregnancy through weaning / Kathleen Huggins, R.N., M.S., I.B.C.L.C. ; foreword by Jessica Martin-Weber ; preface by Kelly Bonyata ; appendix on Drug Safety by Philip O. Anderson. — 7th edition.
pages cm
Includes bibliographical references and index.
ISBN 978-1-55832-849-5 (paperback : acid-free paper)
1. Breastfeeding—Popular works. I. Title.
RJ216.H845 2015
649'.33--dc23
2014041988

Cover Illustration: Susie So
Illustrations: Susan Aldridge, Arden Vincent, and Holly Neel
Page Layout: Megan Jones Design
Photography: shutterstock.com; except for pages 131, 171, 194, 351, and 367 Getty Images.

Printed in China

All lactation professionals are upheld to an ethical standard via ILCA and IBLCE to be inclusive and respectful of all parents and families requiring lactation support. In recognition of this, we notice the lack of inclusive language in the birth and lactation world, as well as this publication. You may hear different vernacular regarding lactation and support of families and may wonder what is considered welcoming. In most cases using "p" words are more inclusive. For example, person, parent, and partner can replace commonly used terms in lactation such as woman, mother, or father. In addition, some parents do not choose to use the term "breastfeeding" to describe the act of lactation, instead some parents prefer the term "chest feeding" or simply, "nursing".

Moving forward in this text, you will see the terms mother, breastfeeding, and woman used often. Research and practice in the maternal child health world is still very mother and woman centric and therefore these are the terms used in many studies we are addressing. We recognize the lack of inclusivity with these terms, and therefore wish to preface this text with the caveat that the authors wish to be respectful and inclusive of all families receiving support. The United States Breastfeeding Committee (USBC) compiled specific information pertaining to inclusive lactation practice. To learn more about correct verbiage and why this is important, please visit http://www.usbreastfeeding.org/p/cm/ld/fid=806

—Stephanie Carroll, MBA, BS, IBCLC

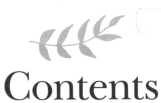

Contents

FOREWORD by Jessica Martin-Weber   v

PREFACE by Kelly Bonyata   vii

ACKNOWLEDGMENTS   ix

INTRODUCTION   1

1. Looking Forward: Preparations during Pregnancy   14

2. Off to a Good Start: The First Week   48
   SURVIVAL GUIDE: THE FIRST WEEK   76

3. Special Situations for Mothers and Babies   131

4. The Learning Period: The First Two Months   171
   SURVIVAL GUIDE: THE FIRST TWO MONTHS   194

5. Expressing, Storing, and Feeding Breast Milk   239

6. Traveling Together, Being Apart   314

7. The Reward Period: From Two through Six Months   332
   SURVIVAL GUIDE: MONTHS TWO THROUGH SIX   344

8. Nursing the Older Baby   351
   SURVIVAL GUIDE: MONTHS SIX THROUGH TWELVE   367

9. Nursing Your Toddler   376

APPENDIX A: Resources for Nursing Mothers   386

APPENDIX B: Determining Babies' Milk Needs
            during the First Six Weeks   396

APPENDIX C: The World Health Organization Growth Standards   399

APPENDIX D: The Safety of Drugs during Breastfeeding   402

REFERENCES & READING   423

INDEX   430

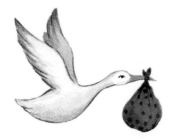

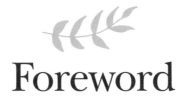

Foreword

N EARLY 21 YEARS AGO, I WAS BREASTFEEDING my first new-born in the middle of the night and in agonizing pain. Both my baby and I were frustrated and in tears. Having already asked for help from various sources, including my mother, a local breastfeeding support group, and healthcare profession-als, I was ready to quit. A friend had given me a few breastfeeding books, but the one I had started just left me feeling even more overwhelmed. I needed answers that were easy to find in my sleep-deprived and emotion-ally spent state. That night, I looked at the basket of books and selected another one to try: *The Nursing Mother's Companion*. After reading the introduction, I flipped through and found the issue I was dealing with. Ten minutes later, I carefully broke off my daughter's painful latch and, following the suggestions I had just read, readjusted my hold—position-ing her differently and paying attention to her chin, lips, and tongue—and latched her again. While there was still some pain initially, I could tell the positioning was an improvement. Within a day, I was healing and my baby was more satisfied. Just like that, a woman I had never met saved my breastfeeding relationship. Throughout my personal breastfeeding journey with six babies, Kathleen Huggins's manual has been my guide and support. More than a dry textbook on human lactation, *The Nursing Mother's Companion* not only put information I could easily understand and apply right at my fingertips at all hours, but it also showed me I wasn't alone. Kathleen's voice of experience blends clinical support with the relatable presence of a friend.

Today, my original copy of *The Nursing Mother's Companion* looks well-loved. This is the only book I give to breastfeeding mothers as a gift— I trust it like a good friend to support moms and help them tap into their own strength and power in mothering their children. It is such a pleasure and an honor to share this revised edition with thousands of other mothers embarking on their breastfeeding journeys and to call Kathleen my personal friend. For those mothers, I wish all the best to you and assure you that you couldn't have a better companion.

—Jessica Martin-Weber
Creator, *The Leaky Boob*, www.theleakyboob.com

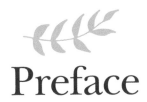

Preface

A T SOME POINT, EVERY MOTHER WILL HAVE QUESTIONS about breastfeeding—this is a new experience, after all, and it changes from week to week and from child to child. More than 75 percent of mothers begin breastfeeding when their child is born, but one-third of them stop within six months, often because of problems they encounter along the way. As a lactation consultant, one of my goals is to help connect mothers with the information they need to combat these problems and have a successful breastfeeding experience.

Our babies and our breasts are biologically hardwired to breastfeed, but that doesn't mean that it always comes easily. If you had been born into an earlier generation when breastfeeding was the norm, you would have seen babies breastfeeding and heard mothers talking about breastfeeding since you were very young; if you had questions, you would be able to look to the women around you for answers. Despite the increase in breastfeeding rates over the last thirty years, many new mothers still have never seen a breastfeeding baby and have never known another woman who had a successful breastfeeding relationship.

The good news is that, in our modern information culture, many good sources of breastfeeding information are available to mothers. This book, written by a board-certified lactation consultant and registered nurse who breastfed her own children, has been a trusted source of breastfeeding information for more than thirty years. It has been newly updated to provide mothers with the most current information on many topics, including:

- latching on and positioning
- safety of medications, tattoos, and milk sharing
- breastfeeding problems and their treatments, including sore or injured nipples, plugged ducts, insufficient glandular tissue, mastitis and MRSA, and low milk supply
- infant issues, such as biting and teething, tongue- or lip-tie, breast refusal and torticollis, high palate, laryngomalacia, and colic
- insurance coverage of pumps and lactation consultant visits
- employer support for breastfeeding mothers under the Fair Labor Standards Act
- breast pumps, "hands-on pumping," and paced bottle-feeding.

This easy-to-use guide's simple format can be read a little at a time as your baby grows. Chapters on pregnancy planning, the first week after birth, and breastfeeding your baby at different ages also contain information on self-care and baby care, in addition to breastfeeding. Each chapter on what to expect at each age ends with a useful "Survival Guide" that describes common problems and possible solutions. Other chapters feature advice on special medical situations, expressing milk, traveling with baby, separations from baby, and breastfeeding after you go back to work. The appendices include a comprehensive list of additional breastfeeding resources, growth standards, and medication safety guidelines.

The information in this book will help you build confidence in yourself as a breastfeeding mother so you can more quickly become an expert on your own baby.

—Kelly Bonyata, B.S., I.B.C.L.C.
Founder and author, www.kellymom.com

Acknowledgments

MORE THAN THIRTY YEARS AGO, a first-time nursing mother came to me about a difficulty she was having breastfeeding her baby. After we successfully resolved it, she suggested I write a book on breastfeeding that included problem-solving techniques. Although I was flattered, such a project seemed monumental. But later, as I recalled her enthusiasm, I began to consider the insights I had gained over years of assisting so many mothers, first as a maternity and newborn nurse and later after founding a breastfeeding clinic (one of the first in the United States) and telephone counseling service. Certainly, I was more than familiar with the common concerns of mothers who are learning to breastfeed, as well as with the occasional problems that can interfere with the development of a successful nursing relationship. The next day, I wrote my rough outline. Without that mother's words to me, this book would never have been written.

During the year I spent writing this book, I received a great deal of encouragement and guidance. I am tremendously indebted to Lynn Moen for her support along the way. I also wish to thank Penny Simkin, R.P.T.

For their thoughtful review of the text I thank Marian Tompson; Andrea Herron, R.N., M.S., C.L.C.; Kathleen Rodriquez Michaelson, B.A., C.L.C.; Vicki McDonald, R.D.; Judith La Vigna; Julie Merrill, R.N.; Tom Robinson; and Kathleen Auerbach, Ph.D.

Jim Litzenburger; Vicki Gadberry, R.N., C.N.M.; Marilynn Schuster, R.N.; Kathleen Long, M.D.; and Dawn Edwards, R.N.C., are most appreciated for their encouragement as well as their friendship.

I am grateful to Donna Janetski for her commitment to this project in preparing the manuscript. My thanks also to Mike Sims for his generosity, and to Susan and Kirk Graves for their efforts.

This book would never have been possible without my husband, Brad, whose love, patience, and faith sustained me. Kate, my beautiful daughter and former nursing companion, was my inspiration throughout.

Note to the Second Edition: For help in preparing this edition I would like to thank Trina Vosti, I.B.C.L.C., and Andrea VanOutryve, I.B.C.L.C. And thanks to John, my current nursing companion.

Note to the Third Edition: For their extensive review of the text I wish to thank Olga Mireles, R.N., C.L.C., and Ellen "Binky" Petok, I.B.C.L.C.

Note to the Fourth Edition: For their generous assistance with revisions, I thank the following women: Dayna Ravalin, R.D.; Sue Petracek, B.S.Ed.; Paula Meier, D.N.Sc., R.N., F.A.A.N.; Lois D. W. Arnold, M.P.H., I.B.C.L.C.; Jan Barger, R.N., I.B.C.L.C.; Darillyn Starr; and Rachel Vireday.

Note to the Fifth Edition: Several years ago, on a parenting website, I was lucky enough to meet "Honeysucklemama," who was nursing her first child. Rarely have I encountered such a thoughtful and supportive counselor assisting other mothers with her insightful writing. Thank you, Tricia Bulger Zack, for your fresh look at this book, as well as your support during my year of recovery from breast cancer.

I would also like to thank perinatal health educator Patricia Donohue-Carey, L.C.C.E., C.L.E.; Nancy Wight, M.D.; Jack Newman, M.D.; Lenore Goldfarb, I.B.C.L.C.; Thomas Hale, Ph.D.; James McKenna, Ph.D.; Cynthia Good Mojab, M.S., I.B.C.L.C., R.L.C.; and Darillyn Starr for reviewing portions of this new edition. My friends Binky Petok, I.B.C.L.C.; Gretta Blythe, R.N., I.B.C.L.C.; and Jan Ellen Brown, I.B.C.L.C., I thank you for your love and support.

Note to the Sixth Edition: Two physicians who specialize in lactation have been particularly helpful with this edition. Dr. Jane Morton has devoted herself to assisting nursing mothers and has shared her experience and research with mothers as well as healthcare providers. Dr. Jack Newman, a Canadian pediatrician, has also graciously shared his vast breastfeeding knowledge with mothers and lactation professionals.

In this edition I have included information about the impact of hospital maternity care on breastfeeding. My friend and co-worker Claudia Goff, R.N., was kind enough to assist me with this.

Penny Simkin, P.T., was helpful in sharing information on mothers who have been sexually abused and the effects of the abuse on breastfeeding.

This edition contains more information on expressing milk, including in-depth reviews of breast pumps. For this, I must thank Catherine Watson Genna and Richard Weston.

There is now a new approach to feeding solid foods to babies. Dawn Wilt, R.D., C.L.E., assisted me greatly to incorporate this information, as did Gill Rapley and Stefan Kleintjes, European experts on breastfeeding.

A surprising resource for me during this past year was my daughter, Kate Gulbransen. After years of working in banking, Kate became a lactation educator. She helped me a great deal with this edition.

Note to the Seventh Edition: First, I thank my husband, Brad, who for the past 30 years has encouraged and supported me. Without him, there never would have been *The Nursing Mother's Companion*.

Although Philip O. Anderson, Pharm.D., is now retired, he kindly agreed to update the drug information in Appendix D for this edition.

I must also thank Maria Lynch, I.B.C.L.C., who was helpful in my understanding of the Affordable Care Act. I appreciate Barbara Wilson-Clay, I.B.C.L.C., and Catherine Watson-Genna, I.B.C.L.C., for their reviews of portions of the text.

Lastly, I must acknowledge Linda Ziedrich, my editor extraordinaire, who has held my hand and polished my words for the past three decades.

Note to the Eighth Edition: I must thank my good friend and fellow lactation consultant Jan Ellen Brown for her help on this edition. No one makes me laugh harder than Jan Ellen. Jenn Thorn, mother of three, kindly went with me to review the incredible number of new pumps on the market. Lastly, I must thank my husband Brad, who carried me over the finish line.

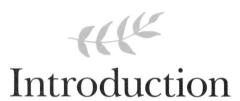

Introduction

- Is Breastfeeding Really Better?
- The Microbiome
- What's in It for Mom?
- Breastfeeding Isn't Always Easy

S INCE THE BEGINNING OF HUMANKIND, women have put their infants to breast. Extending the physical bond that begins at conception, they have nourished and protected their young with their bodies. These tender moments, in return, have brought pleasure and fulfillment to the task of mothering. If you are now pregnant, you are probably looking forward to the time in which you will nourish, comfort, and protect your child in the same way as others before you—at the breast.

Perhaps you already feel committed to the idea of nursing. For you, there is no question that you'll breastfeed your baby. Or perhaps, like many women, you have some uncertainties but still feel it's worth a try. Your outlook depends on many things—the value you place on breastfeeding, how your partner feels about it, how your friends have fed their babies, your lifestyle, and your feelings about yourself and your body.

You probably also have some notions about what nursing will be like. Perhaps you think it will be easy and convenient. Maybe you worry that it might not fit in with your activities and plans. You may have concerns about your ability to nurse. Probably you know of other women who tried to nurse but soon gave up. Whatever your attitudes, expectations, and concerns about breastfeeding, these may become powerful determinants in your ultimate success or failure to nurse your baby happily.

Is Breastfeeding Really Better?

You may be under the impression that the decision to breastfeed or bottle-feed is simply a matter of personal preference. Without a doubt, mother's milk alone promotes optimum health and development for babies. It is uniquely designed to meet the complete nutritional needs of the growing human infant. It also protects the infant against illness throughout the entire first year and beyond, as long as nursing continues. Artificial human milk, whether made from cow's milk or soybeans, will never be able to duplicate nature's formula.

Although they do grow on processed infant formulas, babies, like all young mammals, do best with milk from their own species. Human milk contains proteins that promote brain development. In contrast, cow's milk contains proteins that favor muscular growth. The nutritional properties of breast milk are designed for babies' specific growth and developmental needs. Formula manufacturers are continually challenged to include all of the nutrients in breast milk that scientists are gradually identifying as important to infant growth and development.

> If a multinational company developed a product that was a nutritionally balanced and delicious food, a wonder drug that both prevented and treated disease, cost almost nothing to produce, and could be delivered in quantities controlled by the consumers' needs, the very announcement of their find would send their shares rocketing to the top of the stock market. The scientists who developed the product would win prizes, and the wealth and influence of everyone involved would increase dramatically. Women have been producing such a miraculous substance, breast milk, since the beginning of human existence.
>
> —Gabrielle Palmer, *The Politics of Breastfeeding*

The Microbiome

Recently, the scientific community has come to understand the important role that bacteria have in creating a strong immune system and keeping us healthy. Some bacteria are actually not harmful to our health, but some are actually critical for boosting our immunity keeping our digestive systems running smoothly, our hormone levels balanced, and our brains working properly.

Each of us has a complex ecosystem of microorganisms located within our bodies that is known as the microbiome. The microbiome is a "community of microbes." It has been estimated that the human microbiota consists of the 10–100 trillion microbial cells within each person. The vast majority of the bacterial species that make up our microbiome live in our digestive tract and on our skin.

It has been said by researchers that nearly all diseases can be traced in some way back to the health of the microbiome. Poor gut health is thought to be linked to leaky gut syndrome and diseases like arthritis, dementia, heart disease, cancer, as well as other aspects of our health including obesity and mood disorders.

Throughout our life, we shape our own microbiomes as they adapt to changes in our environment. The foods you eat, the quality of your sleep, the number of bacteria you're exposed to daily, and the amount of stress you live with all help establish and maintain the state of your microbiota.

Newborns receive their microbiomes from passing through their mothers' birth canal during delivery and from the colostrum received from the early feedings.

Caesarean-section deliveries and formula-feeding are commonplace in our modern world today. Both have their place and potential to save lives. However, there is one defining factor that they have in common. They disrupt the development of normal intestinal microbiota, a condition known as *dysbiosis.*

Intestinal dysbiosis makes infants susceptible to gastrointestinal (GI) distress (which can mean dealing with a fussy baby), eczema, and asthma. This early imbalance in bacteria may also play a role in the development of infections, inflammatory bowel diseases, autoimmune conditions, diabetes, and obesity.

Some mothers are asking about "vaginal seeding" following cesarean birth in order to provide the "good bacteria" of those born vaginally. Simply put, the vagina secretions are swabbed and rubbed over the newborn immediately following birth.

Some doctors warn against this practice. But if vaginal birth is considered safe for a newborn, there should be no reason not to consider vaginal seeding. Women can be pre-tested for infectious diseases and potentially pathogenic bacteria, including group B streptococci, herpes simplex virus, chlamydia, and gonorrhea.

Having early "skin-to-skin" contact along with breastfeeding soon after birth is also thought to provide some protection and benefit the child's microbiome. Deciding to breastfeed for as long as possible during the first year of life and beyond, is certainly beneficial to the child's immune system.

In recent years, for example, formula manufacturers have acknowledged that the fatty acids in breast milk are necessary to babies' intellectual, motor, and visual development. Now 90 percent of formula in the United States includes ARA and DHA (arachidonic acid and docosahexaenoic acid) made from fermented microalgae and soil fungus. These lab-produced chemicals are meant to substitute for the omega-3 and omega-6 fatty acids that are naturally found in breast milk. When formula manufacturers started adding ARA and DHA, costs rose by 30 percent, according to Marsha Walker executive director of the National Alliance for Breastfeeding Advocacy. Research has shown little evidence for the companies' claims of beneficial effects on brain and eye development, but we do know that some infants suffer from diarrhea and other side effects after drinking these formulas.

Human milk differs from formula, too, in that it contains specific immunities against human illness. In contrast, cow's milk contains specific immunities against bovine disease. For this and other reasons, babies on a formula diet are at greater risk for illness and hospitalization. Diarrheal infections and respiratory illnesses, including respiratory syncytial virus (RSV), are more frequent and serious among these babies. (RSV is the most common cause of pneumonia and bronchiolitis—inflammation of the small airways in the lung—in children younger than one year of age in the United States.) Formula-fed babies develop many more ear infections, which may lead to later speech and reading problems. Urinary tract infections and bacterial meningitis are also more common among artificially fed infants.

Additionally, powdered formula may be contaminated with bacteria (*Cronobacter spp.,* formerly known as *Enterobacter sakazakii*) that can make infants sick. For this reason, both the World Health Organization and the Food and Agriculture Organization of the United Nations recommend that infants at greatest risk of infection—those younger than two months old, born at a low birth weight, or born prematurely—receive liquid rather than powdered formula. Yet many hospitals routinely give mothers powdered formula samples in gift bags when their newborns are discharged.

Lactoferrin is one of the main proteins found in human milk. It binds to iron making it easier for babies to absorb over 50 percent of it. This binding also makes it unavailable to harmful bacteria that depend on iron to survive. Lactoferrin can help prevent common viral infections such as the common cold, Hepatitis B and C, poliovirus, diarrheal viruses, cytomegalovirus, respiratory syncytial virus, and others. Lastly, the protein has anti-cancer effects and can inhibit the growth of some cancerous cells.

The hormone leptin tells your baby when he is full. Oxytocin, another hormone that causes contractions during labor and stimulates the milk to letdown during nursing, relaxes both you and the baby while nursing.

Recently, formula companies have added probiotics, live intestinal bacteria, to their powdered infant formulas to help prevent diarrheal infections. This poses a dilemma for parents, as the instructions say to mix the powdered formula with cool water so these beneficial bacteria will not be destroyed. But the World Health Organization advises always mixing powdered formula with boiling water, to kill any dangerous bacteria that may be present in the formula.

Infant formula may contain other toxins besides bacteria. High levels of aluminum have been identified in most formulas. In 2008 some formulas were found to contain another toxic chemical as well. After Chinese manufacturers poisoned thousands of infants in China by adding melamine to formula to fake higher protein levels, the U.S. Food and Drug Administration (FDA) announced that it could not establish any safe level of melamine in formula. The FDA then tested the most popular brands of formula sold in the United States to be sure they were free of melamine. Apparently because the chemical is used in some plastic food packaging and in a cleaning solution used on food processing equipment, some of the U.S. formulas were found to have trace amounts of melamine. The agency then changed its view and declared that the amounts of melamine found in U.S. formulas were acceptable.

From time to time, manufacturing errors in the production of infant formula have had serious consequences. More commonly, though, contaminants are introduced at home. Babies have suffered lead poisoning when their formulas have been mixed with tap water high in lead content. Water pollution is a potential problem even if water is purchased in a sealed bottle. And older feeding bottles can contain toxins such as the chemical bisphenol-A (BPA) that can leach into the baby's formula.

Formula-feeding has other risks for babies:

- Formula-fed infants have higher incidences of colic, constipation, and allergic disorders. In fact, a significant number of babies are allergic to formulas, both those based on cow's milk and those based on soy.

- Formula-feeding appears to be one of several factors implicated in sudden infant death syndrome (SIDS). Babies who have received formula, in any amount, have a doubled risk of SIDS at one month of age compared with babies who are exclusively breastfed.
- Tooth decay, malocclusion (improper meeting of the upper and lower teeth), and distortion of the facial muscles may also directly result from sucking on bottles.

Some studies suggest that the benefits of breastfeeding extend into later childhood, adolescence, and adulthood. Breastfed babies have lower cholesterol levels and less coronary artery disease, on average, when they become adults. Breastfeeding is protective against chronic digestive disorders, such as Crohn's disease and ulcerative colitis. Although asthma rates are not significantly different between breastfed and non-breastfed babies, adults who were breastfed have a lower rate of asthma. Breastfed babies have a smaller chance of developing obesity, which can start with overfeeding in infancy, and both type 1 (juvenile-onset insulin-dependent) and type 2 (late-onset) diabetes. Cancers, including leukemia and cancer of the lymph glands, are also less common in children who were breastfed.

There is mounting evidence that artificially fed infants more often develop learning disorders and generally experience lower levels of intellectual functioning. Recent large-scale, international studies confirm previous studies' findings that breastfed babies have higher IQs and perform better in reading, writing, mathematics, and other school subjects. Studies also reveal that it is breast milk, not the act of breastfeeding, that is responsible for this.

Breastfeeding helps, of course, in establishing a close bond and meeting the emotional needs of a child. Nursing women produce hormones that promote a physiologic bonding between mother and child. And in what better way can a baby be nurtured, comforted, and made to feel secure than snuggled within his mother's loving arms, against the warmth of her breast?

Dispelling Common Fears about Breastfeeding

Breastfeeding will be inconvenient. In fact, experienced nursing mothers boast about the ease and convenience of breastfeeding.

Breastfeeding will be painful. Normally, women find nursing comfortable and pleasurable. Some women develop sore nipples during the early days of nursing, but most soreness can be avoided by correctly positioning the baby at the breast (see page 52, Positioning at the Breast). You may have heard that babies sometimes bite their mothers while nursing. When a baby is sucking, his tongue covers his lower gums and teeth so he cannot bite. Still, some babies do occasionally bite at the end of feeding, usually during a period of teething. Most babies learn very quickly not to do this.

Breastfeeding will be embarrassing. Although we all know that making milk is the natural function of our breasts, many of us feel embarrassed about exposing them. At first you may be more comfortable nursing in private, but most women find that, with a little time and experience, nursing in the presence of others can be discreet and comfortable.

Breastfeeding will tie you down. In fact, you can take your nursing baby anywhere with as little equipment as a spare diaper.

You'll have to stop breastfeeding when you go back to work. Today, a growing number of women are combining motherhood, nursing, and working, and doing it quite successfully, thanks to recent advances in milk collection and storage equipment. Having a healthy baby is especially important to a working mother, and breastfed babies are sick less often. And thanks to the Affordable Care Act, insured mothers can usually get a breast pump through their insurance. Low-income mothers who are enrolled in the Women, Infants, and Children (WIC) program may also be eligible for a pump while they are nursing and working or attending school.

Breastfeeding will ruin the shape of your breasts. Pregnancy typically causes the breasts to enlarge and sometimes to develop stretch marks. During the first few months of nursing, women whose breasts are normally small or medium-size generally find them to be bigger. As the baby gets older and begins nursing less often, most women notice their breasts reduce in size. At weaning, the breasts typically appear smaller still and somewhat droopy, but within six months they often resume their usual size and shape. A recent U.S. study found that increased maternal age, more pregnancies, higher body-mass index, larger pre-pregnancy bra size, and smoking were all independent risk factors for sagging breasts. But women who nursed generally had no more sagging than women who bottle-fed.

Your milk may be inadequate for your baby. Some mothers wonder if their diet, breast size, or temperament will keep their milk from being rich or abundant enough. None of these factors affect the amount of breast milk produced, which depends on the frequency of feedings and the baby's effectiveness at the breast. And the quality of a mother's milk is rarely an issue.

Additionally, mothers who have a poor body image may have a difficult time with the idea of breastfeeding or may decide to stop nursing very early after giving birth. These mothers feel that their newborns are not getting enough milk, that the baby feeds too often, or that the baby was simply not satisfied. Mothers without support will often turn to bottles of formula early in the breastfeeding relationship. On the other hand, having a good support system in place from partners, friends, family, and healthcare providers can make all the difference in successfully nursing while also increasing the mothers' self-esteem.

When it comes to bottle-fed babies, many argue that the relationship is different—partly because bottle-feeding doesn't require much human contact. The bottle-fed baby generally receives less stroking, caressing, and rocking than the breastfed baby. He is talked to less often, and he spends more time in his crib away from his parents. Although no one knows how prevalent the practice of propping bottles for young infants is, probably the overwhelming majority of babies who are able to hold their own bottles become almost entirely responsible for feeding themselves.

For all of these reasons, the American Academy of Pediatrics recommends that infants be offered only breast milk for the first six months after birth, and that breastfeeding continue throughout the first year and then as long as mutually desired.

What's in It for Mom?

Although the health of an infant and the emotional benefits of breast-feeding are reasons enough to nurse, women frequently have additional motives. Some nursing mothers like the ease and convenience of breastfeeding. They are often quick to add that information, guidance, support, and reassurance were essential at the start. After the first few weeks, however, nursing a baby simplifies life considerably.

Nursing saves money. Feeding your baby on 8-ounce cans of ready-to-feed formula would cost about $4,000 for the first year of life. Using 32-ounce cans instead would cut the cost to about $1,800. Concentrated formula, which must be reconstituted with water, would cost about $1,500 for the year, and using powdered formula would cut the price a little more, to about $1,200 (keep in mind that powdered formula is not recommended in the first two months of life). Formula is now so expensive that in many stores it is kept behind lock and key!

Most nursing mothers are also glad that they don't have to prepare bottles. Instead up getting up at night to fix a bottle, you can simply pull the baby to your breast and doze off again. You can go on outings with your baby without carting around formula, bottles, and nipples. (But just because the breastfed baby is easy to take along doesn't mean she can't be left behind. When you and your infant must be apart, you can leave your own milk for her. See Chapter 6 for more information.) Many mothers have been grateful that they could nurse their babies through natural disasters such as storms, flooding, and fires when formula and clean feeding supplies were unavailable.

Many women worry about how they will look after they have had a baby. The fat you accumulate during pregnancy is intended for caloric reserves while nursing. Most mothers find that they gradually lose weight while they are breastfeeding so long as they are not overeating.

Breastfeeding has other beneficial effects on a woman's body. Recent studies have found that women reduce their risk of type 2 diabetes by as much as 12 percent for each year they breastfeed. Swedish researchers have determined that mothers who nurse for at least 13 months cut their risk of developing rheumatoid arthritis in half. Mothers who have multiple sclerosis may find that breastfeeding reduces the number of relapses while they are nursing.

Many studies report lower rates of ovarian cancer and breast cancer among women who have breastfed, and it appears that the risk of cancer decreases the longer a woman nurses. New studies also reveal that breastfeeding has a significant impact on reducing the risk of developing heart problems in women. While it is well known that obesity, high cholesterol, and diabetes all lead to heart disease, it is less known that breastfeeding reduces the risk of all these. There is some evidence, too, that nursing offers protection against developing osteoporosis (brittle bones) later in life. And breastfeeding generally lengthens the time before menstrual periods resume after childbirth; most nursing women have no menstrual cycle for several months to two years after delivery, so long as they are nursing frequently. Recent studies comparing breastfeeding and bottle-feeding mothers suggest a lower rate of postpartum depression among nursing mothers as well.

Breastfeeding Isn't Always Easy

If breastfeeding is natural, it must be easy, right? Sometimes it isn't. Today, close to half of all mothers who start out nursing their babies give it up within the first six weeks. The reason for this is rarely that the mother is unable to produce enough milk. Typically, it is because she is alone in her efforts to nurse.

All too many new mothers know little about the nursing process and the breastfed infant, have little or no guidance, and lack support while they are learning. Today many mothers reach out to online support groups but may not receive the thorough evaluation and care offered by an experienced lactation professional. Although breastfeeding is natural, it is not instinctive—it must be learned. The chapters that follow will tell you what you need to know.

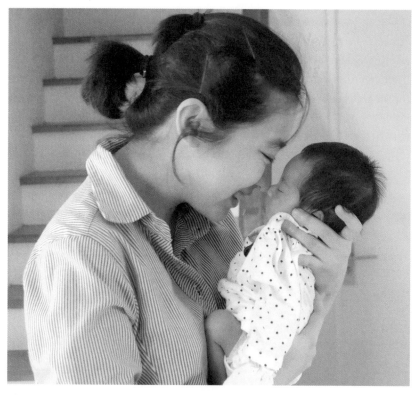

There's no pleasure to equal watching your baby grow from the nourishment of your own body.

Many excellent books have already been written on the benefits of nursing over artificial feeding methods. I set out, however, to provide mothers with a practical guide for easy reference throughout the nursing period. The first part of the book provides basic information about the breast, preparation for nursing, and nursing during the first week; the remainder of the book is intended for reading as the baby and the nursing relationship grow and develop. There are chapters on each of the three later phases of nursing—from the first week through the second month, from the second month through the sixth, and after the sixth month. Following each of these chapters is a Survival Guide—a quick yet thorough reference for almost any problem you or your baby may encounter during the phase covered. Although you may rarely need to consult the Survival Guides, I have included them to ensure that, when you do, you will be able to identify and resolve your problem as quickly as possible. Because many nursing women occasionally find themselves in need of medication, Dr. Philip O. Anderson has provided an appendix on drugs and their safety for the breastfed baby.

Mothers who nurse do so not only because they want the very best nourishment and protection for their babies and because they personally derive many practical benefits from breastfeeding, but simply because they enjoy the experience. The loving relationship established between mother and infant at the breast is emotionally fulfilling and pleasurable. You'll know no greater reward as a mother than witnessing your child grow from your body—first in the womb, and then at the breast.

All that said, keep in mind that, even with all of the best information and support, things sometimes don't turn out as we hope. If after giving breastfeeding your best effort you end up having to feed formula, you have not failed as a mother. Be proud of your efforts to nurse, and concentrate on providing your baby with all of the cuddling and loving that you can.

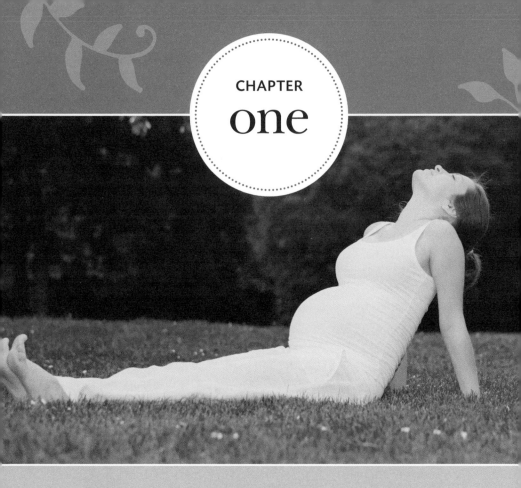

LOOKING FORWARD: PREPARATIONS DURING PREGNANCY

- Learning about Breastfeeding
- Your Breasts
- Ensuring the Purest Milk
- Planning for a Natural Birth
- Planning for the First Days
- Planning for the First Weeks

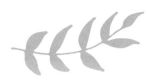

YOU MAY HAVE DECIDED TO NURSE your baby long before you became pregnant. Or perhaps you have just begun to consider breastfeeding. Although nourishing a baby at the breast is natural, many new mothers are surprised to find it is a learned skill—one that usually takes several weeks to master.

Success at nursing often depends upon a woman's confidence and commitment. You can develop your confidence by learning as much as possible about breastfeeding ahead of time. You can strengthen your commitment to nurse by developing a strong support system for yourself.

Learning about Breastfeeding

Generations ago, most new mothers turned to their own mothers for support and guidance on breastfeeding. Happily, many women today can do so, too. But many can't.

If your mother didn't breastfeed, or if she gave it up quickly, there are several ways you can learn about nursing ahead of time. Reading about it is certainly beneficial. In some communities, breastfeeding classes are offered. Expectant mothers are also most welcome to attend La Leche League meetings, which are held monthly in most areas. La Leche League is the organization of nursing mothers whose purpose is to support breastfeeding worldwide. In some areas, other groups, such as the Nursing Mothers Counsel, provide classes and telephone counseling for pregnant and nursing women. These groups are listed in Appendix A (see page 386). In addition, hospitals, county health departments, and WIC (the Special Supplemental Nutrition Program for Women, Infants, and Children) programs may sponsor prenatal breastfeeding classes. See Appendix A, page 386, for more information about WIC.

Another excellent way to learn about breastfeeding is to spend time with women who are nursing their babies. It may be that you have never seen, close-up, a mother and baby breastfeeding. Most nursing mothers will delight in your interest, and one or two may become good sources of information and support for you in the days to come. Be sure to ask them about their first weeks of nursing. Most likely you will hear of a variety of experiences, and perhaps you will develop a sense of what the early period of breastfeeding can be like.

Your Breasts

During pregnancy, many changes occur in your breasts in preparation for nourishing your baby. In early pregnancy, you probably noticed they were more full and tender than usual. Their increasing size during the first few months of pregnancy is caused by the development of the milk-making structures within them. Most women prefer to wear a supportive bra throughout pregnancy, although a few women are just as comfortable without one. From early or mid-pregnancy on, your rib cage expands. You will probably find that your bra band feels tighter, and this may require you to purchase new bras or bra extenders, inexpensive fabric pieces that make a bra band longer.

As your breasts grow in size, the blood flow to them increases, and veins in the breasts may become clearly visible. Some women develop stretch marks on their breasts, like the ones that can occur on the abdomen during pregnancy.

The nipple and the area around the nipple, the areola, may double in size and deepen in color; this darkening may serve as a visual cue to the newborn. Also during this time, small glands located in the areola, known as Montgomery's tubercles, become pronounced. Their function is to secrete an antibacterial lubricant that keeps the nipple moist and protected during pregnancy and breastfeeding. This is why soaps and special creams are unnecessary in caring for your breasts, and may even be harmful: soaps remove the breast's natural lubricant, and creams may interfere with its antibacterial action.

The nipples often become more sensitive during pregnancy. Some women find that their nipples even hurt when touched. This sensitivity diminishes as pregnancy advances; it should not make breastfeeding uncomfortable. Other women enjoy the sensitivity and feel great pleasure when their breasts are fondled during lovemaking.

By the fifth or sixth month of pregnancy, the breasts are fully capable of producing milk. Some women begin to notice drops of fluid on the nipple at this time. This fluid, known as colostrum, comes from several tiny openings in the nipple and is the food your baby will receive during the first few days after birth. Some women do not leak colostrum, but it is there in the breasts just the same.

As women, we all receive messages about our bodies and what they "ought" to look like. These messages affect our self-image, including our feelings about our breasts and how they look. You can probably remember how you felt about your breasts as they developed in early adolescence. You may have felt proud as they grew larger and you began wearing a bra. Perhaps you were embarrassed if they developed earlier or grew larger than the other girls' breasts. You may have felt anxious if they took a long time to grow or self-conscious if they were small.

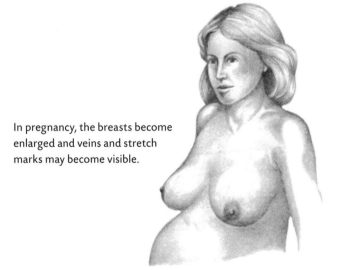

In pregnancy, the breasts become enlarged and veins and stretch marks may become visible.

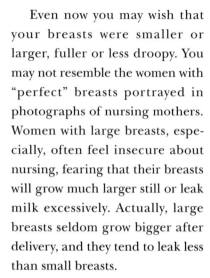

Caring for Your Breasts

During the last months of pregnancy, avoid soaping your breasts; just rinse them during your bath or shower. Soaps tend to dry the nipples and the areola. If your breasts are dry or itchy, a mild cream or lotion may feel soothing, but avoid getting it on the nipple or areola.

Even now you may wish that your breasts were smaller or larger, fuller or less droopy. You may not resemble the women with "perfect" breasts portrayed in photographs of nursing mothers. Women with large breasts, especially, often feel insecure about nursing, fearing that their breasts will grow much larger still or leak milk excessively. Actually, large breasts seldom grow bigger after delivery, and they tend to leak less than small breasts.

Each woman's breasts are different from all others, but most breasts, regardless of size, are perfectly designed for their ultimate purpose—to nourish and nurture our children. The breasts not only provide an infant with superb nutrients for growth and development but offer the warmth, the comfort, and the security that every growing baby needs. In this respect, they are most beautiful.

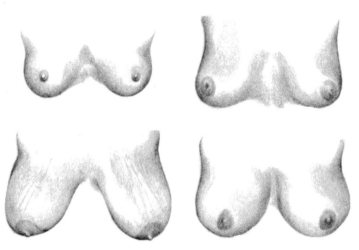

Breasts come in all shapes and sizes.

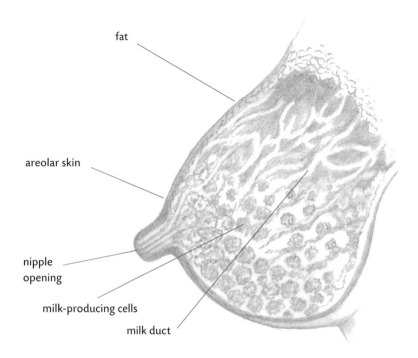

fat

areolar skin

nipple
opening

milk-producing cells

milk duct

Cross-section of a lactating breast.

The Making and Giving of Milk

After the birth of your baby, colostrum is readily available for her first nursings. Colostrum is the ideal food for her first days; it is both perfect nutritionally and important for protection against infection. Mature milk generally appears by the second or third day, but occasionally not until the fourth or fifth day or even later. The late onset of milk production, which is becoming a common problem, may be related to events that occur during birth (see page 23, Planning for a Natural Birth).

A woman's body is signaled to initiate milk production with the delivery of the placenta. This causes the hormone prolactin to activate the milk-producing cells of the breast. The initial manufacture of milk occurs whether the baby nurses or not. Continued milk production is another matter. This depends on frequent and regular stimulation of the breast and the drainage of milk. The baby's sucking stimulates the nerve endings in the breast, which in turn trigger the release of the two hormones essential to milk production and release—prolactin and oxytocin.

Prolactin, as mentioned previously, activates the milk-producing cells in the breast to manufacture milk. Oxytocin is responsible for the release of the milk from the tiny sacs where the milk is made. This release is referred to as the ejection or letdown reflex. As the baby nurses, the milk is propelled forward toward the nipple. It is the baby's job to get the milk out by compressing the areola with her tongue and gums as she nurses. During the early months of her life, your baby will receive plenty of milk as long as you nurse her frequently (at least eight times in twenty-four hours), she latches on and sucks properly, and you allow her a sufficient amount of time to complete each feeding. This is because breastfeeding works by supply and demand. The more your breasts are stimulated and emptied by the baby's sucking, the more milk you will produce.

Ensuring the Purest Milk

A mother may occasionally wonder if her milk is entirely safe for her child. Most frequently, this concern arises because she needs to take medication. Although most medications pass into the breast milk, the vast majority pass in only small amounts and are considered safe for the nursing infant. A comprehensive guide to drugs in breast milk, by Dr. Philip O. Anderson, can be found in Appendix D (see page 402). Another source of such information is LactMed, an online database developed by Dr. Anderson for the National Library of Medicine (www.toxnet.nlm.nih.gov). See Appendix A (see page 386) for more. You can also find information about medications at The Infant Risk Center at Texas Tech University. Contact information for The Infant Risk Center can be found in Appendix A (see page 386).

More and more questions have arisen about the environmental pollutants we are exposed to, such as insecticides and other toxic chemicals. Many of these substances are stored in fatty tissues of the body; as a result, small amounts may be detected in breast milk. Experts on the subject, however, have been unable to identify any risks to the baby from such amounts, and most believe that the nutritional and immunological benefits of breast milk far outweigh the possible risks of environmental pollutants. Sadly, our children receive even greater exposure to some of these chemicals in the womb than they do at the breast.

If you want to minimize your baby's exposure to toxic chemicals, follow these guidelines during pregnancy and as long as you are breastfeeding:

- Stop using pesticides in the home, in the garden, and on pets.
- Avoid exposure to organic solvents, which are in paints, furniture strippers, gasoline fumes, non-water-based glues, nail polish, and dry-cleaning fluids. Air dry-cleaned and mothballed clothes outdoors before wearing them, and avoid permanently mothproofed garments.

Seafood, Safe and Not

The U.S. Food and Drug Administration says that pregnant women should avoid eating shark, swordfish, marlin, king mackerel (which is among the species known as *saba* in Japanese restaurants), orange roughy, big eye tuna, tilefish from the Gulf of Mexico (also known as golden or white snapper), and big eye tuna, but can safely eat 12 ounces (340 g) per week of any other types of cooked fish. The Environmental Working Group is even more conservative; this nonprofit organization suggests also avoiding fresh tuna (including varieties sold in sushi restaurants as *ahi, maguro, meji, shiro,* and *toro*), sea bass, Gulf Coast oysters, marlin (*makjiki*), halibut, pike, walleye, white croaker, and large-mouth bass, and eating no more than 3 to 6 ounces (85 to 170 g) per month of canned tuna, mahi-mahi, blue mussels, Eastern oysters, cod, pollock, Great Lakes salmon, Gulf Coast blue crab, wild channel catfish, yellowtail (known in sushi restaurants as *hamachi, kanpachi, inada,* or *buri*), bonito (*katsuo*), wild trout, and lake whitefish. Lastly, avoid fish caught in contaminated waters, especially the Great Lakes.

Safe fish and shellfish, with mercury levels lower than 0.2 parts per million, include farmed trout, farmed catfish, fish sticks, shrimp, pollock, wild Pacific salmon, haddock, summer-caught flounder, croaker, clams, flatfish, mid-Atlantic blue crab, freshwater sport fish, and scallops. Check with your state or local health department about the safety of local species.

Tattoos

Some nursing mothers consider getting a tattoo and wonder if it is safe. Many tattoo artists will not knowingly perform work on a pregnant or nursing mother, as it is recommended that women wait a year after giving birth before getting one. However, there is no evidence that getting a tattoo has any effect on breast milk.

It is very important to screen tattoo artists to verify that they follow adequate safety measures, as local or even systemic infections can occur otherwise. Some local health departments have specific laws and regulations in place, so you might begin your search there. The tattooist should follow universal precautions, such as sterilizing the tattoo machine with an autoclave, using single-use needles, ensuring that the inks are not contaminated, and wearing gloves. When these precautions are not followed, diseases such as hepatitis, tetanus, and HIV can be transmitted.

If you do get a tattoo, be sure to guard against a local infection by washing the tattooed area with mild soap and water. Avoid picking at the scabs and keep the area covered when in the sun.

Laser removal of tattoos can safely be done while nursing. The laser causes the pigments of the tattoo to break up into small particles and then be filtered out by the body. There is no bleeding, and the procedure has minimal side effects.

- Avoid eating fish species that have been found to have high levels of mercury or PCBs (see sidebar for more information), and for more advice go to https://www.fda.gov/fishadvice.

- Adopt a diet low in animal fat by choosing lean meats and low-fat dairy products.

- Avoid smoking and the company of those who smoke around you.

- Carefully wash or peel fresh fruit and vegetables. Avoid crash diets, which can increase the excretion of toxic substances into breast milk.

- If you work with chemicals, ask your doctor to refer you to a specialist who can advise you about their safety.

Planning for a Natural Birth

Over the past two decades, the number of mothers who have their labor induced, who have epidural anesthesia, and who deliver by cesarean section have skyrocketed. It is now known that these high-tech interventions often affect breastfeeding.

A complicated birth often ends with the separation of mother and baby following the birth. This may make the start of breastfeeding more difficult. All too often, a complicated birth also means the late onset of milk production. Several factors may be responsible: a long labor, epidural anesthesia, the use of synthetic oxytocin (Pitocin) to augment or induce labor, and the administration of large volumes of intravenous fluids. When milk production is delayed beyond seventy-two hours after birth, the newborn may become jaundiced, lose too much weight, and require supplemental feedings. A mother in this situation becomes more likely to abandon nursing.

Nature begins preparing for birth during the last weeks of pregnancy. The baby drops down into the pelvis; the cervix tilts forward and begins to soften. The baby's lungs mature, he receives maternal antibodies that will protect him against infection in the early weeks of life, and he puts on a layer of fat. His body stores more iron, and he develops a coordinated sucking and swallowing ability. When the baby is ready to be born, he releases a small amount of a hormone that in turn stimulates the mother's body to secrete the hormones that initiate labor. When the baby, maternal hormones, uterus, cervix, and placenta are ready, labor begins. When labor begins on its own in this way, the labor tends to be easier, and the baby is usually born ready to breastfeed.

The March of Dimes is an organization whose purpose is to fight for the health of mothers and infants. One of their missions is to prevent prematurity and the number of premature births. Over the past thirty years, the March of Dimes has followed the number of elective deliveries in the U.S. In 2006, they reported that the number of induced labors in the U.S. had more than doubled from 1990. Induced births had increased to more than one out of every five pregnancies.

Much of this increase in inductions occurred without a medical reason. And inducing deliveries before 39 weeks' gestation comes with a significant risk for the newborn and with no benefits to the mother.

A doctor may persuade a mother by describing induction as a routine procedure to avoid a middle-of-the-night rush to the hospital, to guarantee that certain family members can be in attendance, or by voicing concern about the baby's size. Some mothers may request induction simply because they are tired of being pregnant. None of these are good reasons for induction. Studies of thousands of cases have shown that inductions increase the incidence of labor complications and surgical delivery without improving newborn outcomes.

A mother who has agreed to an induction usually finds herself admitted to the hospital before labor is well established or even begun. If her due date was incorrectly estimated, the baby may be born weeks early. A developmentally immature newborn is at increased risk for complications such as temperature instability, low blood sugar, respiratory problems, and jaundice. Babies born three weeks or more early often don't learn to nurse well until near the time that they were meant to be born.

If breaking the water bag fails to bring on effective contractions, artificial oxytocin (Pitocin) may be used to strengthen them. During a natural labor, the mother produces her own oxytocin, which leads her body to also manufacture endorphins, natural pain reducers. Artificial oxytocin, given intravenously, does not reach the brain and so does not stimulate the release of natural endorphins. Besides feeling more painful, Pitocin-induced contractions are often longer, and Pitocin may prevent the uterus from fully relaxing between contractions. Because Pitocin can increase the stress to both the uterine muscle and the baby, the mother will need continuous electronic monitoring. As a result, she may be confined to a bed instead of helping her labor along by moving freely, and she may be unable to take relaxing baths or showers to ease her labor pains.

A study of thousands of first-time mothers revealed that those whose labors were induced—by rupture of the membranes, Pitocin, or both—were four to ten times more likely to undergo cesarean surgery. Many of these women will deliver their future children by cesarean as well.

But sometimes complications during pregnancy make induction a good choice. It may be risky for the baby to remain in the uterus when pregnancy has lasted 42 weeks or longer, when the mother has high blood pressure or an infection of the uterus, or when she has another health problem such as diabetes. Induction may also be the best option if the baby stops growing or if the amount of amniotic fluid is very low.

Whether or not their labors are induced, most women today choose to have epidurals. An epidural is an injection of a narcotic and an anesthetic into the space around the spinal cord. The drugs block the nerve impulses from the lower spinal segments, and this results in decreased sensation in the lower half of the body.

For 80 percent of laboring women, an epidural provides good pain relief. But it may also cause undesirable complications. Labor is usually longer. Contractions become weaker and less frequent, because an epidural lowers the mother's own production of oxytocin, the substance that causes the uterus to contract. This means that a mother is more likely to need artificial oxytocin.

Epidurals have other side effects. Because the drugs block the nerves that regulate blood pressure, one-third of women who have epidurals experience low blood pressure, and in 12 percent of these cases the drop is low enough to seriously deprive the baby of oxygen. In an attempt to prevent a blood pressure decrease, the mother may be given large amounts of intravenous fluids before the epidural. These fluids may be a factor in the delayed onset of milk production.

Having both an epidural and Pitocin can affect the baby's heart rate. A survey of first-time mothers who experienced both of these interventions found that half required cesarean births for fetal distress.

Epidural anesthesia also often causes relaxation of the pelvic-floor muscles, which can interfere with the normal flexion and rotation of the baby's head as it passes through the birth canal. This interference can lead to an abnormal presentation (that is, the baby descends facing the mother's front or side), which makes delivery difficult, or to the baby's failure to descend, an indication for a cesarean. An epidural also reduces a mother's ability to push (and occasionally makes it impossible for her to move her lower body at all), so delivery by forceps or vacuum extractor may be necessary. The incidence of cesarean section increases by three times when epidurals are given. Mothers having an epidural are also at greater risk for excessive bleeding after birth.

About 24 percent of women who have an epidural will develop a fever. Any elevation in temperature could mean that the mother has an infection, so the newborn will need to be checked. If the baby also has a fever, he will be further tested and treated with antibiotics. In one large-scale study, mothers who had fevers during delivery more often had babies with low Apgar scores, poor muscle tone, and seizures than did babies of mothers without fever. And a baby who is being tested and treated for fever is separated from his mother during the hours when breastfeeding ideally begins.

Not only do mothers whose labors are lengthened and complicated by medical interventions tend to get their milk in later, but their babies tend to be less able at the breast. In general, a baby's breastfeeding ability is highest when the mother has given birth with neither intravenous narcotics nor an epidural. The baby's breastfeeding ability is lowest when the mother has used both intravenous and epidural drugs during labor.

If you're sure you need medication in labor, you might ask for patient-controlled epidural anesthesia (PCEA). Available in many hospitals and birth centers, PCEA allows a mother to give herself a bolus of narcotic and anesthetic when she feels the need. The dose is low, so it blocks the pain sensors but allows more movement in bed. Once the cervix is totally dilated, the epidural is turned off so the mother can respond to her desire to push. The mother's recovery tends to be better after PCEA; she can walk about sooner, and walking may help prevent her bladder from becoming distended and may also prevent excessive bleeding. Because the baby has taken in less narcotic with PCEA, he tends to show a more normal interest in and ability at the breast.

Prepare for a Vaginal Birth

- Attend childbirth classes, preferably ones taught by certified Lamaze or Bradley instructors, to learn more about a traditional birth.
- Recognize that your due date is approximate. Let your caregiver know that you prefer to wait until labor begins on its own.
- If your caregiver is concerned about the well-being of the baby as the due date approaches, discuss having a non-stress test (electronic fetal monitoring) every two to four days for reassurance that the baby is well.
- Stay at home during early labor until your water breaks or your contractions are coming every three to four minutes and are lasting for 1 minute.
- Consider hiring a doula to assist you in coping with the discomforts of labor and birth.
- When you begin to push, try to rest between contractions. Push only when the urge comes or when your caregiver or nurse directs. Short pushes, of no more than four to six seconds each, will help conserve your energy.
- Take advantage of a water tub or shower to lessen the intensity of contractions.
- Try to delay an epidural until after labor is well established and your cervix is dilated 5 centimeters.
- If you feel you need pain medication, ask about PCEA.
- Once your cervix is completely dilated, use upright positions to assist gravity and to increase the diameter of your pelvis, so as to help the baby descend through the birth canal.
- When you begin to push, try to rest between contractions. Push only when the urge comes or when your caregiver or nurse directs. Short pushes, of no more than 4 to 6 seconds each, will help conserve your energy.

If You Must Schedule a Cesarean Birth

As many surveys have shown, babies born more than seven days before their due date tend to have complications. Respiratory problems, infections, low blood sugar, and the need for intensive care are especially common in babies born at thirty-seven weeks' gestation or earlier. These problems usually result in separation of mother and baby and a delay in the start of breastfeeding. In addition, babies born at thirty-seven weeks or earlier are often poor feeders (see page 153, The Late Preterm Baby and the Near-Term Baby).

In spite of these risks, one-third of cesareans are performed before 39 weeks' gestation. If you must have a cesarean, request that it be scheduled for 39 weeks or after, or when tests show that the baby's lungs are mature.

For advice on breastfeeding after a cesarean birth, see page 59.

Planning for the First Days

Nipple Preparation

Often, mothers who plan to breastfeed are advised to prepare their nipples during pregnancy. In fact, studies have shown that nipple "toughening" maneuvers, such as brisk rubbing or twisting, do little to prevent soreness during early breastfeeding. Whether or not they have especially sensitive skin, blondes and redheads do not generally experience any more nipple soreness than other women. Sore nipples are usually prevented by correct attachment of the baby at the breast (see page 52, Positioning at the Breast).

If you have had one or both nipples pierced, remove the jewelry before giving birth and leave it out as long as your baby is nursing. You'll probably be able to nurse without complication, but you may find that you leak milk from the site of the piercing.

One preparation is very important during pregnancy: You should make sure your nipples can extend outward. Your baby may have difficulty grasping the breast if the nipples do not protrude enough on their own or cannot be made to protrude. Even if you had a breast exam

USUAL NIPPLE APPEARANCE	APPEARANCE WHEN PINCHED	
	SATISFACTORY	NEEDS CORRECTION
Protruding	Nipple stays protruded	
Flat	Nipple can be pinched outward	Nipple moves inward or cannot be pinched outward
Dimpled or folded	Entire nipple extends outward	Nipple moves inward or flattens
Inverted	Entire nipple extends outward	Nipple extends out only slightly, remains inverted, or inverts further

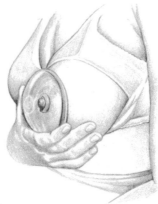

Breast shells can improve nipple shape.

earlier in your pregnancy, your nipples may not have been fully checked. Take the time to perform your own assessment.

First, look at both your nipples. They may protrude, or one or both may be flat, dimpled, folded in the center, or inverted. Next, do the "pinch test": Gently squeeze just behind the nipple with your thumb and forefinger. This imitates the motion your baby will make while nursing. See how both nipples respond. If your nipples are flat, pull them outward to determine if they can lift away from the inner mass of the breast. The chart on page 29 will help you determine whether you need to take further steps to minimize initial nursing difficulties.

When nipples need correction. The flat nipple that cannot be pinched outward, or the nipple that moves inward or flattens when compressed, is said to be "tied" to the inner breast tissue by tiny adhesions. The physical changes of pregnancy help the nipples to stand out, but one or both may still need correction. In this case, special plastic breast shells may solve the problem before breastfeeding begins.

Worn inside the bra, breast shells exert a steady but gentle pressure on the areola and cause the nipple to extend outward through the opening in the shell. This may help to loosen adhesions beneath the nipple. Breast shells should be worn as soon as you have determined that improvement is needed, ideally from about mid-pregnancy on. They can be purchased in most maternity shops or ordered through Medela (see Appendix A, page 386). Gradually work up to wearing the shells most of the day, letting comfort be your guide. Also consider purchasing Supple Cups to help bring out flat or inverted nipples. See Appendix A for purchasing information.

The Postpartum Setting

Too few mothers realize ahead of time the tremendous effect the immediate postpartum experience—in a hospital, in a birth center, or at home—can have on their breastfeeding success. It is most worthwhile to evaluate the situation you will be in after delivery to make any necessary arrangements for early nursing.

> Studies show that mothers who nurse during the first two hours after giving birth are much more likely to be successfully nursing weeks and months later.

The maternity unit's policies should encourage mothers and babies to remain together for the first few hours after birth, or at least assure that nursing takes place within the first two hours, when the baby is likely to be alert and eager to suck. Ideally, the baby isn't swaddled, weighed, bathed, and placed in a crib after birth but simply dried and placed naked against his mother's bare chest; then they are both covered. Newborns treated this way tend to have more respiratory stability and higher blood-sugar levels and to cry much less than other babies. If the birth was un-medicated, the baby will generally be quiet but alert and able to "crawl" to the breast and latch on unaided in thirty to sixty minutes (you can see a video of a newborn crawling to the breast on YouTube; search for the title "The Crawl: Baby's First Crawl - Initiation of Breastfeeding"). Weighing, bathing, eye treatment, and other baby care procedures are best postponed until after the first feeding.

Breastfeeding goes best when nursing is frequent, every one to three hours, during both day and night. "Rooming in" with the baby, at least during the day and evening, is conducive to frequent nursing, and allows the mother and baby to become better acquainted before going home. Preferably, the nursing staff does not routinely give the babies water or formula supplements, as this lessens their interest in nursing and sometimes interferes with their ability to breastfeed. It can be an added bonus if the nurses enjoy assisting breastfeeding mothers, if one nurse is specifically responsible for breastfeeding counseling, or there is a lactation consultant on the staff.

Some women have the opportunity to select among several hospitals or birth centers for their delivery. If you are making such a choice, be sure to get a recommendation from your childbirth educator or a local breastfeeding counselor. She will probably know which places are most supportive of nursing mothers and infants. Even if only one hospital is available to you—and many birth attendees practice at only one—it is well worth your time to ask about the policies of the maternity unit. This will help assure that your nursing gets off to the best possible start.

Take advantage of the maternity tours, teas, and classes that most hospitals and birth centers offer, or call the postpartum unit to learn about policies and routines. Be sure to inquire:

- How soon after delivery will I be able to nurse? What if I have a cesarean birth?
- Will I be able to hold the baby skin-to-skin right after the birth?
- How often is nursing encouraged during the day and at night?
- Can the baby stay in the room with me? If not, how often and for how long will we be together?
- What assistance with breastfeeding does the staff offer?
- Does the staff avoid supplemental bottle-feeding?
- Is there a lactation professional on staff?

In 1990, the United Nations Children's Fund and the World Health Organization created an award of recognition for those hospitals worldwide that have enacted ten policies to support breastfeeding mothers and babies. Hospitals that have implemented the "Ten Steps" are awarded the designation "Baby-Friendly." As of this writing, over 600 U.S. hospitals and birthing centers in all fifty states and the District of Columbia are considered baby-friendly, while many others are working toward the designation. Over one million babies, or nearly 30 percent of all newborns in the U.S., are born each year in Baby-Friendly facilities. When inquiring about a hospital's breastfeeding policies, ask if it has earned or applied for the Baby-Friendly certificate. If it has, you can be assured that the nurses are committed to your breastfeeding success. If it hasn't, perhaps your inquiry will inspire the hospital to enact baby-friendly policies. You can find all "Baby-Friendly" hospitals in the United States listed at www.babyfriendlyusa.org.

If the nurse is friendly and receptive to your questions, you might also ask which pediatricians she feels are particularly knowledgeable about breastfeeding and supportive of it.

If you are planning an early discharge from a hospital or birth center, or will be delivering at home, you may also want to inquire about home visits by a nurse, lactation professional, or midwife during the first few days.

The Baby's Doctor

Your breastfeeding experience can be greatly influenced by your choice of physician for your child. You may want a pediatrician for your baby, or you may prefer to use a family practitioner, perhaps the one who may attend your baby's birth. In selecting a doctor, start by getting the names of some who are said to have a positive attitude about breastfeeding. Ask your obstetrician, midwife, childbirth educator, or a lactation professional for recommendations. You might also inquire about physicians in your area who work with nurse practitioners. These nurses have training in well-baby care, and they usually provide mothers with extra attention and counseling on a variety of parental concerns, including breastfeeding.

Most doctors and nurse practitioners will set aside time for a preliminary visit with expectant parents. Usually this visit is free of charge. Be sure to visit at least two before making a final decision, even if the first one seems satisfactory. At each office, meet the nurse. She will often be the one who will answer your questions or concerns when you call during office hours. She can be a good resource for you, especially if she has breastfed successfully herself or has a special interest in breastfeeding.

Let the doctor or nurse practitioner know that you are going to breastfeed your baby. To gauge his or her overall support of nursing mothers, ask what the recommendations would be should you experience difficulty in breastfeeding. The best pediatric practitioners offer practical assistance with breastfeeding or referrals to lactation professionals. Other practitioners provide reassuring words about feeding infant formula. Take time to discuss your preferences for feeding the baby in the hospital. If the maternity unit's policies are not ideal, ask about written orders to allow early nursing and rooming-in and to prevent the feeding of supplements to your baby. A few pediatric practices have lactation consultants on their staff or can refer you to experienced lactation consultants in your area.

There may be other questions you will want to ask about the hospital or birth center, or about well-baby care. Bring a list with you so you don't forget any of them. Be sure to inquire about any necessary procedures for notifying the doctor or nurse practitioner when the baby is born. It is often said that the pediatrician takes care of the parents perhaps even more than the child. Trust your intuition when making your final choice about which pediatrician, family doctor, or nurse practitioner is right for you.

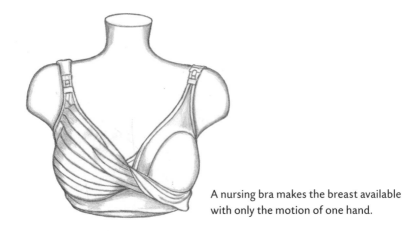

A nursing bra makes the breast available with only the motion of one hand.

Nursing Bras and Pads

During the early weeks of breastfeeding, the average breast weighs three to four times as much as it did before pregnancy. Although a bra isn't an absolute necessity in this period, you'll probably be more comfortable in one, at least if it fits well. If you leak milk and want to use breast pads, you'll definitely need a bra to hold them in place. A stretch bra that can be pulled out of the way may work fine if you're small-breasted, but otherwise you may prefer a nursing bra with removable cup flaps.

After you give birth, both your cup size and band size will most likely change. If you buy a nursing bra in early pregnancy, it may not fit when milk production begins. A better time to shop for nursing bras is during the last couple of weeks of pregnancy or after your baby is born. To be on the safe side, limit your purchase to two or three bras; you'll be more sure of the size and style that suits you after a few weeks of nursing.

The salesperson in the maternity shop or department may be able to help you choose a bra that will fit well while you are nursing. If she doesn't know a lot about bras, though, you can figure out your size yourself by following these guidelines: While standing, wearing an unpadded bra and breathing normally, measure your chest just under your arms with a tape measure. Round up to an even number of inches; this number is your band size. Now measure around your body at the fullest part of your bust. As shown in the chart on page 36, the difference between the bust measurement and band size determines your cup size.

Since finding larger bra sizes can be difficult, you may have to use a mail-order supplier. To locate one, see Appendix A, page 386.

To check a bra for fit, fasten it on the outside row of hooks. Before raising the straps over your shoulders, bend forward, allowing your breasts to fill the cups. Now stand straight and adjust the straps.

Check the cup fit. When the flaps of a nursing bra are hooked at their highest points, the cups should have just a little extra room at the top for when milk production begins. If the cups are roomier than this, try a smaller cup size. If your breasts are overflowing at the top, outsides, or center, you need a larger cup size.

Next check the bottom band. While fastened on the outside row of hooks, the band should be snug; an inner row of hooks will allow you to tighten the band as your rib cage contracts after birth. Check to see that the band is level all around or slightly lower in the back. If the bra rides up in the back, the shoulder straps may be too tight. Otherwise, try a larger cup size.

Aside from a good fit, other valuable features of a bra for breastfeeding include all-cotton or microfiber cups to absorb moisture, non-elastic straps for better support, and front-flap fasteners that are manageable with one hand.

A word about underwire bras: Poorly fitted ones are associated with plugged milk ducts and breast infections. If you want to wear an underwire bra while nursing, it is very important to get one that fits properly. The bend of the wire must be wide enough to fall where there are no milk ducts—that is, well behind the breast tissue. If you have a lot of breast tissue below the armpits, as many women do, a soft-cup bra is definitely preferable. If you do use an underwire bra while nursing, alternate it with a soft-cup bra, and never wear the underwire bra during sleep.

You may also wish to purchase breast pads before delivery, to keep your bra and clothing dry during the early weeks of nursing (not all women leak, so you may want to start with just one

> The arms of an adult are never a safe place for an infant or small child riding in an automobile. If you use a car, buy an infant restraining seat; every U.S. state now requires the use of one.

pack). Breast pads are sold in two varieties, disposable and reusable. Whichever you select, be sure the pads do not contain plastic or water-proof liners, as these can contribute to nipple soreness. If you prefer, you can use handkerchiefs or cut-up cloth diapers instead of commercially made pads.

Sometimes mothers consider using plastic breast shells instead of pads to keep dry. The primary purpose of these shells is to improve nipple shape. When they are routinely worn in place of pads, milk may leak excessively.

See chart for cup size.

DIFFERENCE BETWEEN BUST MEASUREMENT AND BAND SIZE	CUP SIZE
Up to 1 inch	A
1 to 2 inches	B
2 to 3 inches	C
3 to 4 inches	D
4 to 5 inches	DD or E
5 to 6 inches	F
6 to 7 inches	G
7 to 8 inches	H

Other Purchases You May Be Considering

Although all infant car seats sold today must meet federal safety standards, the seats vary considerably in both features and price. The best car seats for infants are rear-facing, semi-reclined, and labeled for use with babies up to 30 or 35 pounds (13.6 to 15.8 kg) in weight or, depending on the seat, up to 32 inches (81 cm) in height. These seats cradle young infants more securely than do convertible infant-toddler seats. In choosing a model, look for latches you can operate easily. You may also prefer a washable cover.

Some parents use car seats both in and out of the car to carry their babies outside the home and to contain them within the home, whether the babies are awake or asleep. A baby who spends many hours each day in a car seat may experience delayed muscular and sensorimotor development because the lower brain is not stimulated by normal movement. In addition, many newborns have trouble keeping their airways open when they are placed in car seats because their chins rest on their chests.

Because a newborn can't control her head well, she needs special support to allow her to breathe freely while riding in a car seat. A study of car seat models (Tonkin et al., 2006) found that all newborns need blanket rolls at either side of the body and another across the top of the head. Many also require a blanket roll between the crotch belt and the legs to keep from sliding down in the seat. This is particularly important for infants born early.

Unless it's from a rental or loan program sponsored by a hospital or other agency, think twice about getting a used car seat. The seat may not meet current standards or may have been recalled, as many are. If you decide to use a secondhand seat, be certain that it is not more than two years old, that the model is still in production and has not been recalled, and that you have the instructions for installation and use. In addition, the National Highway Traffic Safety Administration recommends that you never use a car seat that has been involved in a moderate to severe car accident, as its integrity may have been compromised.

Infant car seats are often improperly installed. Install yours according to the manufacturer's directions, and then shake it hard. It should not move more than 1 inch (2.5 cm) in any direction. You might also have the installation checked by a child passenger safety technician. Your local health department or highway police department can help you find

> Babies need to spend most of their time in a horizontal position, whether in someone's arms or on a safe, level surface. A crib, bassinet, cradle, or blanket on the floor is a better place than an infant seat to leave your baby for any period of time. Or carry your baby in a pouch or sling, keeping your arms free for other things. Holding, rocking, and carrying your baby against your body will stimulate his physical and mental development while strengthening the loving bond between you.

one for a free inspection. See page 37 for further information on car seat safety.

You'll want to either buy diapers or arrange for a diaper service for the first few weeks. Besides being more environmentally responsible than disposable diapers, cloth diapers are more economical as well, if you have access to a washer and dryer. A diaper service is usually no more expensive than disposable diapers and is a luxury all new parents deserve.

Some mothers buy breast pumps before delivery. Although a pump is not a necessity for everyone, you may at some time want to use one. Under the Affordable Care Act, most health insurance providers are required to cover the cost of breastfeeding equipment including a breast pump. Or you may prefer to learn the technique of hand expression, which is described on page 240. If you decide to purchase or rent a pump ahead of time, see pages 275 to 313 for reviews of various models and information on obtaining them. While your insurance provider may be required to provide you with a breast pump, some brands that they offer may not be very effective. See Chapter 5, page 246, about ordering a pump through your insurance. You might also speak with a lactation consultant, who will have experience with high-quality breast pumps and may even have them available for sale if your insurance carrier does not offer breastfeeding equipment to nursing mothers. Many mothers end up disappointed with pumps they buy at discount, baby, online, and big-box stores, so try and get recommendations of high-quality pumps before purchasing one. See my reviews of the many breast pumps on the market today in Chapter Five.

Some mothers need a clinical-grade (also known as a rental-grade or multi-user) electric pump in the first few days after delivery. Whether you buy another sort of pump or not, find out where you can rent a clinical-grade pump should the need arise. If your baby isn't nursing well upon leaving the hospital or is at risk of underfeeding for another reason (see page 233), you should go home with a clinical-grade electric pump, ideally with a double collection kit. You can locate a rental station by calling the toll-free numbers provided in Appendix A, page 386.

A Place to Nurse

A comfortable armchair can make positioning your newborn at the breast much easier and provide more support for you while nursing. An upholstered living-room, dining-room, or office chair with arms, or a wooden rocking chair, may make a great place for nursing your baby. Consider borrowing an appropriate chair or buying one secondhand if you can't afford a new one.

You can get by without an armchair, of course. Most couches are too deep to sit up straight on, and propping yourself upright against the headboard of your bed makes it hard to position the baby and may contribute to poor posture and muscle fatigue. But a couch or bed can work well if you can prop yourself up as straight as possible, using pillows behind you until the baby is a bit older and latching is simple for you both.

Although ordinary bed pillows can work well in helping to position a baby for nursing, a variety of "nursing" pillows are marketed specifically for this purpose, and they are becoming very popular for the early weeks of nursing. If you'd like to try one of these pillows, choose one with flat surfaces rather than one that is shaped like a croissant. The latter type creates a gap between the top of the pillow and the mother's body, and the baby tends to slip down in between. See Appendix A, page 386, for information about my favorite nursing pillow.

Many mothers have found that a footstool specially designed for nursing is very helpful in reducing the strain of holding the baby at the breast. The angled stool raises the mother's feet and legs, lifting her lap. This relaxes her abdomen and supports her lower back, preventing arm and shoulder strain. Nursing stools are available from "big-box stores" and some nursing supply retailers; see Appendix A, page 386.

In the first weeks after giving birth, many mothers find it helpful to keep a log of their nursing times and their babies' stools and urine output. One study has suggested that women who keep such logs tend to breastfeed longer than those who don't. You might consider purchasing *The Nursing Mother's Companion Breastfeeding Diary* (see page 423, References & Reading) as a handy record book and keepsake for the early weeks. Breastfeeding apps are also helpful in keeping track of feeds and diapers, especially for first-time mothers.

A Place to Sleep

Although mothers and babies have slept together as long as mammals have roamed the earth, recent warnings about the dangers of bed sharing are worrying new parents. The American Academy of Pediatrics (AAP) has stated that bed sharing can be hazardous under certain conditions, and in 1999 the Consumer Product Safety Commission recommended against parents and babies sleeping together at all. But many physicians, scientists, and sudden infant death syndrome (SIDS) researchers—including one of the Safety Commission members—disagree with this recommendation.

SIDS, or crib death—that is, sleep apnea resulting in a baby's death—has many risk factors. The most common factor is placing a baby to sleep on her stomach. The second most common is the mother's smoking, either before or after the baby's birth. Formula feeding and overheating are other risk factors, and another is putting the baby to sleep alone in a room. The largest SIDS study to date has shown that infants who sleep alone in a room are more than twice as likely to die from crib death as are infants who share a room with parents. In countries where bed sharing is common, where smoking is not, and where breastfeeding is the norm, SIDS is rare.

Anthropological and developmental studies suggest that mothers and infants are biologically and psychologically designed to sleep next to each other. Parents who sleep with their infants report that they enjoy this closeness and find it makes nighttime parenting easier. Being close to the baby in the night means being more aware of her cues and therefore more responsive to her needs. Even though bed-sharing mothers and babies wake more frequently, they go back to sleep sooner and so get more sleep overall than mothers and babies who sleep separately. Babies who sleep with their parents also cry significantly less than babies who sleep alone.

Because bed-sharing mothers nurse more frequently, they produce more milk than they would otherwise. This can be especially important to women who must spend time apart from their babies during the day. Women who work outside the home also often find that bed sharing helps them feel more connected to their infants.

The AAP recommends that babies sleep in the parents' room for the first six months. James McKenna, an anthropologist at the University of Notre Dame and an expert on infant sleep, also urges parents to sleep in the same room with the baby, if not the same bed, for at least the first six months of life. Dr. McKenna believes that a parent's close breathing may help regulate an infant's own breathing pattern, and that bed sharing may thus reduce instances of SIDS. His review of studies suggests that when a mother and her baby are close enough during nighttime sleep to sense each other in at least two of four ways—sight, scent, sound, and touch—the baby's risk of succumbing to SIDS is significantly decreased. As Dr. McKenna points out, the sharpest recent decline in rates of SIDS and other infant deaths has occurred among middle-class whites, the very group that has most increased its rate of parent-child bed sharing over the same period.

In his sleep laboratory at Notre Dame, Dr. McKenna has found that bed-sharing mothers and their infants are extremely sensitive to each other's movements and physical condition throughout the night, across all sleep stages. For instance, healthy, full-term babies whose air passages become blocked alert their bed-sharing mothers and, under normal circumstances, maneuver out of danger. Babies who sleep alone, Dr. McKenna has found, spend more time in deeper stages of sleep, which may be harmful for babies with inherent arousal deficiencies. He also has a helpful website, including an 18-minute video devoted to infant sleep that parents may want to see (https://cosleeping.nd.edu).

Other researchers have suggested that babies who sleep with their mothers develop into children who are independent, sociable, confident, and well able to handle stress. Children who have never slept in their parents' beds are, according to their parents, harder to control, less happy, more prone to tantrums, more fearful, and more dependent.

There are certainly hazards to avoid in bed sharing, but there are hazards in laying the baby to sleep anywhere. Wherever the baby sleeps, the dangers are mostly the same: pillows, toys, and quilts that could suffocate; cords and ties that could strangle; gaps in which a baby could become wedged; heights from which she could fall; and overheating. Bed sharing poses the additional risk of "overlying"—accidental smothering—but this is generally a concern only when other children are sleeping in the same bed or a parent is intoxicated, under the influence of drugs, or extremely exhausted. Generally, adults have a sense of their own boundaries even when asleep; this is why you don't fall out of bed.

For most of the benefits of bed sharing, you can also consider placing your baby's bassinet very close to your own bed. You can even buy a bassinette (Arms Reach Bedside Co-Sleeper) that attaches to an adult bed so you can reach your baby without getting up even though she is sleeping on a separate surface (see Appendix A, page 386). The Halo BassiNest is a stand-alone bed that swings over your bed for an easier reach (see Appendix A, page 386). There are also stand-alone beds that can be placed next to you on top of your bed (see the Snuggle Nest at www.babydelight.com).

Recently, there have been many infant deaths that occurred in rocking "hammock" shaped bassinets with soft padded sides and a safety belt. The deaths happened when the infants in these hammocks rolled from their back to their side or stomach. Keeping the baby on their back and on a flat surface is always a safer choice for where your baby sleeps.

The following are some guidelines for safe infant sleep:

- Put the baby on her back to sleep. Putting babies to sleep on their stomach is a risk factor for Sudden Infant Death.
- Use a firm mattress that fits the bed or crib frame well, without gaps in which a baby could become wedged.
- Stretch the sheet tightly around the mattress.
- Avoid nightclothes with strings or ties, both for the baby and, if you're sharing the bed, for yourself and your partner.
- Keep the baby's face uncovered.
- Leave off the comforters, bumper pads, feather beds, stuffed animals, lamb skins, and other soft things that could pose a risk of suffocation. The baby doesn't need a pillow.
- Don't smoke, and don't let other people smoke in the house.
- Avoid overheating the room in which the baby sleeps, and avoid overdressing the baby. If you share a bed, keep the room cool so that the warmth of your body combined with the warmth of the covers does not overheat the baby, or have the baby sleep outside the covers.

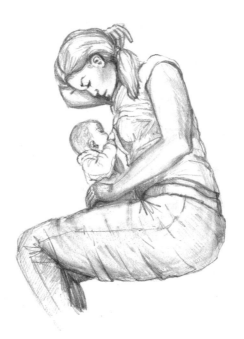

- Don't leave a young baby, especially one born prematurely, to sleep in a car seat or infant seat. If the baby's upper body is inadequately supported, her airway may become blocked. A study reported hundreds of infant deaths that occur every year when babies sleep in sitting devices such as car seats, strollers, bouncers, swings, and other infant seats. None of these devices should ever be used as a substitute for cribs or bassinets. The average age at death in this large study was just two months of age.

If your baby sleeps in a crib, follow these guidelines:

- Make sure the rails are no farther than 2⅜ inches (6 cm) apart.
- When the baby learns to sit, lower the mattress so that she can't fall out or climb over the side rail.
- Hang any crib mobile well out of the baby's reach, and remove it when the baby starts to sit up or reaches five months of age, whichever comes first.
- When she learns to stand, set the mattress at its lowest level.

- When she reaches a height of 35 inches (89 cm), or when the side rail is less than three-quarters of her height, move her to a toddler bed.
- Remove any "crib gym" when a baby can get up on all fours.
- Avoid laying the baby to sleep near dangling cords or sashes.
- Dress the baby in a blanket sleeper (often referred to as a "sleep sack") instead of using a blanket.
- Consider using a baby monitor with the speaker turned toward the baby during naps. Background noise from the monitor may protect the baby as well as bed sharing.

If your baby sleeps with you, follow these guidelines:
- Don't place the bed against the wall or against other furniture, since the baby could become trapped in between.
- Don't leave the baby to sleep alone in your bed.
- Fasten back your hair, if it is very long.
- After drinking or taking drugs that may cause you to sleep too soundly, and at any time that you are extremely exhausted, put the baby to sleep in a separate bed.
- Don't use bed rails in the baby's first year, since she could become wedged between the mattress and the rail.
- Don't let an older sibling share a bed with an infant younger than one year old.
- Don't share a waterbed with your baby, since the surface could hamper breathing if your baby were to turn face down.
- Consider bed sharing carefully if you or your partner is obese. Your weight might create a depression in the mattress that the baby could roll into. Sleeping on a very firm mattress might be safer in this case.
- Don't sleep with the baby on a sofa or overstuffed chair. Suffocation is more common on these types of furniture.

Different sleeping arrangements may work best for you at different times. You might place your baby in a bassinet at bedtime but move her into your bed later for night feedings. You might instead nurse the baby to sleep in your bed and then move her to her own bed afterward. Or you might put the baby to sleep in the nursery but then sometimes end up sleeping there all night yourself. It is normal to either follow a certain pattern for many months or to change more often as your baby grows and your own needs change.

Planning for the First Weeks

During your first few weeks of motherhood, caring for the baby and yourself will take just about all of your time and energy. Most new mothers find they are often tired and have emotional highs and lows. Planning ahead can make these important first weeks go much more smoothly for both you and your family.

If your partner can possibly manage to take time off from work, by all means encourage them to do so. Not only can they fix meals, manage the household, and care for any other children at home, but they also need and deserve time to get to know the baby. And they can be a great source of support and encouragement while you are learning to breastfeed.

Other family members can also make these weeks easier, but invite them to stay with you only if you feel they will make a positive contribution and be supportive of your nursing.

Perhaps some of your friends in the area have already offered to help when the baby arrives. There are many things they can do, like fixing a meal, washing a load or two of laundry, running errands, minding any older children, or spending an hour or so straightening up your house.

It's also a good idea to stock up on groceries before the birth. Include foods that are easy to prepare and plenty of things to drink. You may also want to plan some simple menus or freeze a few dinners ahead of time.

Your Support System

About half of American women who start out breastfeeding give up and begin bottle-feeding within the first three months after birth. As medical anthropologist Dana Raphael wrote more than forty years ago, "The odds in our culture today are stacked heavily against successful breastfeeding, and the emotional price for failure is high." Although more breastfeeding help is available now, those words still hold true. Mothers frequently give up breastfeeding in the learning stage because they have too little information, guidance, and support.

When a nursing mother is encouraged and cared for by others, her motivation can carry her through almost any difficult situation. When she feels alone and unsupported, however, the nursing relationship seems to fall apart at the slightest provocation.

As enthusiastic as you may feel now, you probably have difficulty imagining that during the early weeks, you may sometimes doubt your ability to nurse. In fact, many new mothers experience periods of anxiety while they are learning to breastfeed. If you are lucky, you can turn to your own mother for advice and reassurance about nursing. Many of today's grandmothers, however, nursed for only a few weeks. You may hear them say, "The baby was never able to take the breast" or "I just didn't make enough milk" or "Nursing hurt too much." Comments such as these reflect an era when women received little encouragement and support in their efforts to nurse, and the lactation consulting profession was in its infancy. Consider for a moment the idea of giving birth all alone. Awful, right? It is probably important to you that someone you love and trust will be with you, encouraging you each step of the way. During your early weeks of breastfeeding, you need the same kind of support—the presence of someone who provides reassurance, guidance, and encouragement.

You may be fortunate enough to have friends who have nursed—or are nursing—their babies, and a partner who believes with you that breastfeeding is healthy and

You can find the names of International Board Certified Lactation Consultants in your area by going to www.ILCA.org and clicking on "Find a Lactation Consultant."

natural. Even so, you may discover in time that not everyone in your life shares your feelings about breastfeeding. In fact, many people feel indifferent, and some downright opposed, to this way of feeding and nurturing a baby. Your partner, mother, or best friend may not be entirely enthusiastic about your decision. Some people may even try to discourage you along the way. Perhaps they feel a bit threatened, fearful, or even jealous of the intimate relationship you will be establishing with the baby. The sad fact of the matter is that despite the renewed enthusiasm of young women today toward breastfeeding, many new mothers still get too little support—from family, friends, health professionals, and society in general.

Develop a support system for yourself ahead of time. Let your partner and other family members know how much breastfeeding means to you and how important they will be to your success. If they have concerns or fears about nursing, find out what they are and provide them with the information they need to correct any misconceptions. If you have older children, talk with them about nursing so they know what to expect.

Be sure to identify sources of guidance. Perhaps you are close to women who have successfully nursed their babies. Many WIC (the Special Supplemental Nutrition Program for Women, Infants, and Children) offices provide breastfeeding support and guidance to moderate- to low-income mothers (see Appendix A, page 386). Take time to find the names of lactation professionals in your community. Your childbirth educator, your hospital's maternity unit, or your obstetrician's or pediatrician's nurse may know of some. In addition, your insurance carrier may be required under the Affordable Care Act to cover the cost of consulting a lactation professional with no cost sharing. When you have gathered these supports, you will have stacked the odds in your favor.

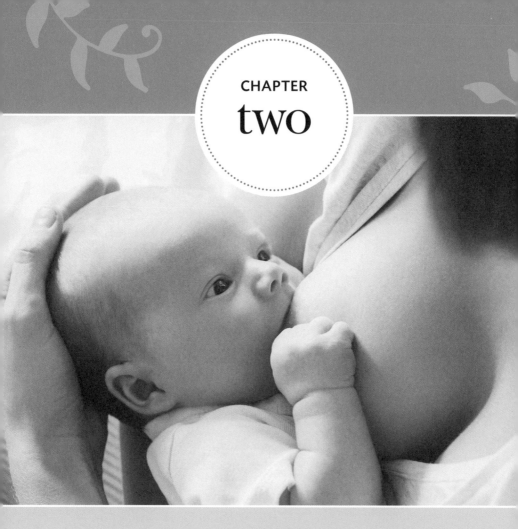

OFF TO A GOOD START: THE FIRST WEEK

- In the Beginning
- Ensuring Your Milk Supply
- The First Week of Nursing

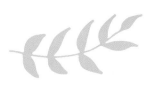

YOU MIGHT EXPECT THAT AFTER THE WORK of labor and birth, a mother and her newborn infant would be too exhausted to greet each other. But no matter how fatigued birth may have left her, the mother usually brightens with renewed energy to explore her baby. Some mothers seem to meet their infants for the first time with puzzlement, as if searching for some sign of familiarity. Others react as if they have always known this tiny being and are overjoyed to meet him at long last.

After several minutes of adjustment to breathing, the temperature change, and lights and sounds, the unmedicated infant likewise becomes alert, opening his eyes and moving his mouth. The newborn who is placed skin-to-skin with his mother is soon crawling toward the breast and is actively rooting about. With his fists to his mouth, or perhaps his lips against someone's arm, he seeks out the comfort of the breast. Ideally, the mother and baby should be left skin-to-skin until the first nursing takes place.

In the Beginning

Colostrum

Throughout the first two hours after birth, the infant is usually alert and eager to suck. At this time he is most ready for his first nursing.

It is not unusual to hear a first-time mother tell a nurse, "I don't think I have anything yet to feed the baby." Although small in amount, colostrum is available in the breast in quantities close to the stomach capacity of the newborn. This "liquid gold," which is often yellow but may be colorless, is more like blood than milk in that it contains protective white blood cells capable of attacking harmful bacteria. Colostrum also acts to "seal" the inside of the baby's intestines, preventing the invasion of bacteria, and provides the baby with high levels of anti-bodies from the mother. Newborns receive many of their microbiomes, the critical bacteria, from the colostrum in these important early feedings.

Not only does colostrum thus offer protection from sickness, it is also the ideal food for the newborn's first few days of life. It is high in protein and low in sugar and fat, making it easy to digest. Colostrum is also beneficial in stimulating the baby's early bowel movements. The black, tarry first stools, called meconium, contain bilirubin, the substance that causes newborn jaundice. Colostrum in frequent doses helps eliminate bilirubin from the body and may lessen the incidence and severity of jaundice.

In the hospital the first nursing may take place in the delivery room, the birthing room, or the recovery area. With minimal assistance from your nurse or partner, the baby will probably seek out your breasts and suck within the first hour or so. It is ideal for the baby to be naked against your bare chest (see page 30).

Many specialists believe that when the first nursing is delayed much beyond the first two hours, the infant may be somewhat reluctant to take the breast in the hours thereafter. Most babies fall asleep about two hours after birth, and they become more difficult to rouse over the next few hours. Nursing without delay also boosts the confidence of the mother and stimulates the action of hormones that cause the uterus to contract and remain firm after delivery. These contractions may help speed delivery of the placenta and minimize blood loss afterward (breastfeeding alone is insufficient, however, in the case of postpartum hemorrhage, when prompt intervention by the medical staff is essential). During the first few days after birth, some mothers feel these contractions, or "after pains," while nursing. Mothers who have had other children may be quite uncomfortable with after pains. If you experience these contractions during breastfeeding, you can ask for a mild pain reliever like acetaminophen (Tylenol) or ibuprofen (Motrin, Advil) an hour or so before nursing.

Should you not have the opportunity to nurse right after delivery, or if you can't persuade your baby to take the breast, don't get discouraged.

Many mothers have established successful nursing hours or even days after giving birth.

Just the Breast

When you have finished your first nursing in the hospital, let the nurses know (if you have not done so previously) that you prefer your baby be given no supplementary bottles of water or formula and no pacifiers. Water or formula is unnecessary, and artificial nipples may cause your baby to have difficulty recognizing your nipple while she is learning to breastfeed. (If you deliver at a "Baby Friendly" facility [see page 32], you won't need to be concerned about this.) A study reveals that mothers whose babies received supplements or pacifiers in the hospital were far less likely to achieve exclusive breastfeeding.

Newborns do not normally require any fluids other than colostrum (the exception is the baby who has low blood sugar—because her mother is diabetic, her birth weight was low, she was very large, or she underwent unusual stress during labor or delivery). Supplemental feedings, moreover, can be harmful: They may cause the baby to lose interest in the breast and to nurse less frequently than needed. This is because bottle nipples may lessen the baby's instinctive efforts to open her mouth wide, as she needs to do to grasp the breast, and condition her to wait to suck until she feels the firm bottle nipple in her mouth. The baby who has sucked on bottle nipples may also become frustrated while nursing, since milk does not flow as rapidly from the breast as it does from the bottle.

Giving newborns large amounts of water can be dangerous. Because young babies can't excrete water quickly, large amounts can lower sodium levels in their bodies, causing complications that include low body temperature and, sometimes, seizures.

A newborn given a pacifier may fail to recognize her mother's soft, short nipple and therefore have trouble latching on to the breast. Introducing a pacifier early on could lead to later problems, too. Recent studies associate the use of pacifiers with early weaning, and older babies who use pacifiers are more likely than others to have frequent ear infections.

If you are not giving birth in a Baby Friendly facility, be sure all the nurses know of your preference not to give a bottle or pacifier to your nursing newborn. Ask them to place a sign on the baby's crib like this one:

To all my nurses:

While I'm here and learning to breastfeed, PLEASE, no bottles or pacifiers. My mom will be happy to nurse me whenever I fuss.

Thanks!! Baby Reynolds

Time at the Breast

Some healthcare providers tell mothers that, to prevent sore nipples, they should limit their nursing time during the first several days. Probably nothing else about breastfeeding is as poorly understood as the causes of sore nipples. It may be explained that keeping feedings short will prevent soreness and will help "toughen" the nipples. Actually, sore nipples usually result from improper positioning of the baby on the breast, not from long nursing. Another myth often heard by new mothers is that the breast "empties" in a prescribed number of minutes. Most newborns require 10 to 40 minutes to complete a feeding. As long as your positioning is correct and nursing is comfortable, there is no need to restrict your nursing time. Besides being unnecessary, limiting nursing time may frustrate the baby and lead to increased engorgement when milk production begins.

Positioning at the Breast

A baby is correctly positioned at the breast when he has latched on to it with a wide-open mouth so that his lower gum is well below the base of the nipple on the areola, the dark area around the nipples. In this off-center or "asymmetrical" position he will compress the sinuses located beneath the areola to draw out milk. If he instead latches on to the nipple only, or latches on with the nipple centered in his mouth, and starts sucking, the nipple will probably become sore and cracked and

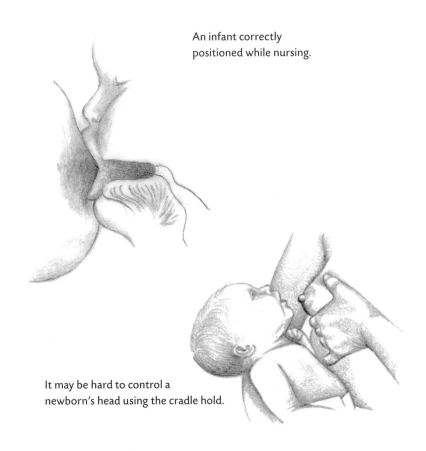

An infant correctly positioned while nursing.

It may be hard to control a newborn's head using the cradle hold.

may even bleed. The baby will also be unable to compress the sinuses beneath the areola well and may therefore get less milk.

Probably the most important skill for you to master, initially, is that of getting the baby on the breast correctly. Some mothers can do this easily, but many need guidance and practice.

The cradle hold, or cuddle hold, in which the baby's head is held in the crook of the mother's arm, is considered the classic breastfeeding position. I have come to believe that for most new mothers and babies, this position is neither the easiest nor the most effective for getting a baby well latched on to the breast. In the first few weeks after birth, a baby hasn't developed enough muscular coordination of the head and neck to easily latch on without help; she needs a good deal of direction from her mother. But it is difficult to direct a newborn's head accurately with the inside of one's forearm. Also, it is usually not possible to get an off-centered latch using this position. Although most mothers sooner or later begin using the cradle hold for most of their daytime nursings, in the early days of breastfeeding the crossover and football holds are generally more useful.

The crossover hold. Take time to position yourself comfortably. If you are nursing in a hospital bed, sit up as straight as possible with a pillow behind you. As soon as you are able, sit in a chair with arms (most couches are too deep, unless there is a pillow supporting your back to help you sit up straight and more forward). Unwrap your baby; this will encourage his interest in latching on and make it easier for you to check his position. Place one or two pillows on your lap so that the baby is at the level of your breast. Lay him on his side with his chest and abdomen against your body.

Instead of placing the baby's head in the bend of your elbow, as in the cradle hold, hold him with the opposite arm so that your hand rests between his shoulder blades and supports the back of his neck and head. Place your thumb behind and below one ear and your other fingers behind and below the other ear. Tip his head back slightly so that when you pull him onto the breast, his chin will reach it first. Now shift the baby, if necessary, so that the area just above the upper lip—not his mouth—is right in front of your nipple. In this position he is most likely to latch on asymmetrically, with his lower jaw far below the base of the nipple.

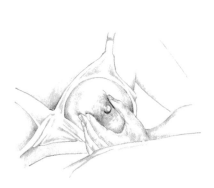

Hand position for the crossover hold.

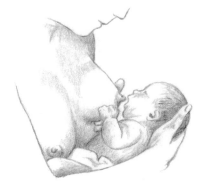

Crossover hold.

If you're starting on the left breast, hold it with your left hand so that your thumb is positioned at the margin of the areola, about 1½ inches (3.8 cm) from the nipple, at the spot where the baby's upper lip will touch the breast (or at about two o'clock, if you imagine a clock face printed on your breast). Place your index finger the same distance from the nipple at the spot where the baby's chin will touch the breast (or at about eight o'clock). Gently compress the breast to match the shape of your baby's open mouth.

Before you bring the baby onto the breast, you must stimulate him to "root." With the baby's forehead tipped back, touch the baby just under the nose with your nipple, and wait until he opens his mouth wide. When his lower jaw is dropped all the way down, quickly bring his shoulders and head together to the breast. With his head tipped slightly back, his chin should reach the breast first. Don't lean into the baby or move your breast. Keep the areola compressed until he begins sucking. You'll know that he is well latched on if his lips are far apart and flared, if he has more of the bottom of the areola in his mouth than the top, and if you feel comfortable.

You may need to repeat this process a few times before the baby latches on correctly. Common mistakes include lining up the baby's mouth rather than the upper lip area with the nipple, pulling the baby on before his mouth is wide open, not pulling him on quickly enough or far enough, and letting go of the breast before he is well latched on.

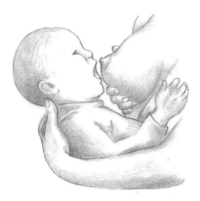

Just before latch-on: Tip the baby's head back a bit, and aim your nipple at his upper lip.

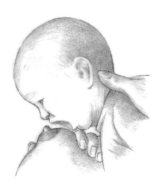

Just before latch-on, from your point of view.

When you're first learning to get a baby latched on, it helps to see someone else do it. Dr. Jane Morton—a pediatrician in general practice, a clinical professor at Stanford University, an executive board member of the APP's Section on Breastfeeding, and a fellow of the American Academy of Breastfeeding Medicine—has produced wonderful videos about breastfeeding (see Appendix A, page 386). "A Perfect Latch" is intended for physicians but is also helpful for mothers who are learning to get a baby latched on. This video is available for viewing online if you search for "A Perfect Latch" at the Stanford School of Medicine website (http://med.stanford.edu).

Once the baby is actively nursing, you'll probably need to support the breast for him by gently pressing your fingers against the underside. If your breasts are small, though, you may be able to let go of the breast or even switch arms and continue nursing using the cradle hold.

Football hold. The football hold is a great position to use in the following circumstances:

- You have had a cesarean birth and want to avoid placing the baby against your abdomen.
- You need more visibility while getting the baby to latch on.
- Your breasts are large.
- You are nursing a small baby, especially if he is premature.
- You are nursing twins at the same time.

Sit in a comfortable armchair with a pillow at your side to help support your arm and lift the baby. Support the baby in a semi-sitting position facing you, with her bottom at the back of the chair. Your arm closest to your baby should support her back, with your hand holding her neck and head. Place your thumb behind and below one ear and your other fingers behind the other ear. Position the baby with her head just below the breast and her nose in front of the nipple. This way she'll latch on to the areola off-center, with her lower jaw well below the base of the nipple.

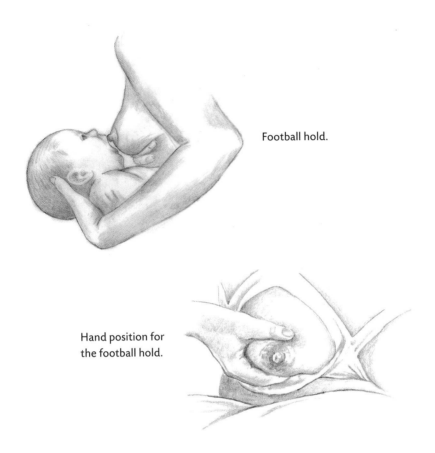

Football hold.

Hand position for
the football hold.

Support your breast with your free hand so that your thumb is about
1½ inches (3.8 cm) above the nipple, at twelve o'clock, and your index
finger is the same distance below the nipple, at six o'clock. Compress
the areola with your thumb and index finger so that your hand forms a
C-shape. This will more closely match your breast to the shape of your
baby's mouth so she can take in more of the breast. As with the crossover
hold, stimulate the baby to open her mouth wide, and bring her up onto
the breast.

Side-lying position. The side-lying position is an especially good choice for nursing in these cases:

- You must lie flat after a cesarean birth.
- You are uncomfortable sitting up.
- You need help from someone else to get the baby latched on.
- The baby is sleepy and reluctant to begin nursing or stay awake very long.
- You are nursing during the night.

You and your baby lie on your sides, tummy to tummy as with the cuddle hold. Place your fingers beneath the breast and lift upward, wait for the baby to root with a wide-open mouth, and then pull him in close.

The side-lying position becomes much easier after four to six weeks, when the baby has better head control and can come onto the breast without much assistance.

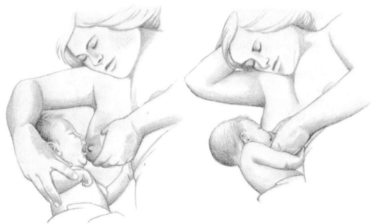

Side-lying position.

Ending the Feeding

Waiting until your baby lets go of the nipple is the ideal way to end a feeding. If the baby does not come off the breast by himself after twenty or so minutes on a side, and you want to switch breasts or rest awhile, you can take him off by first breaking the suction. Even if he is not actively sucking, his hold on the nipple is tremendously strong. To release the suction, place your finger at the corner of the baby's mouth, pulling the skin gently toward his ear, until you hear or feel the release.

After taking the baby off the breast, leave your bra flaps down so that the air can dry your nipples. If your nipples are tender or damaged and you want to soothe them, you may be offered a modified lanolin preparation. If your nipples are tender or injured and you are using a nipple ointment, be sure to wash your hands frequently and especially right before nursing. I also suggest some other measures and products for treating tender or injured nipples on page 76, Survival Guide: The First Week.

After a Cesarean Birth

If you are awake for your delivery, let the staff and the baby's physician know that you wish to nurse as soon as possible. While some hospitals, mostly those who are "Baby Friendly" (see page 32), assist mothers in holding their baby skin to skin in the operating room, not every mother feels well enough to enjoy this experience.

As long as neither you nor the baby is having difficulties, however, there is no reason to delay nursing for long. One option is to have a nurse or your partner bring your baby to you in the recovery room. If you were not fully conscious during the delivery, or if the doctor orders that the baby be kept in the nursery, you can still begin nursing after your initial separation.

When the baby arrives, place him against your skin, and cover him. Enjoy his attempts to crawl to the breast and nurse. If he doesn't latch on even with your help, have your partner or the nurse help you feed him in the side-lying position. Leave the side rails of the bed up so that turning will be easier. A pillow behind your back and one between your legs may be helpful.

Because you will be recovering from surgery, you will face some discomfort and possibly some difficulty in maneuvering the baby to your breast. The pain medication you'll receive, probably a narcotic, is important for your comfort during the first few days, and it will not hurt the baby. If you take the medication right after you nurse, moreover, only a minimal amount will be in your milk at the next feeding. After the first couple of days, a non-narcotic pain reliever, like acetaminophen (Tylenol) or ibuprofen (Motrin, Advil), may be adequate to control your pain most of the time.

When you begin sitting up to nurse, a pillow or two on your lap will make you more comfortable. If you want to keep the baby off your abdomen, the football hold may work well for you.

After a day or so, you may want to keep the baby in the room with you. Remember to ask for help whenever you need it. Sometimes the staff may forget you gave birth by cesarean.

Whether or not your cesarean was planned, your milk should come in just as if you had delivered vaginally, although it may be delayed if you had a long or complicated labor and received large amounts of intravenous fluids (see page 25).

Ensuring Your Milk Supply

Frequent Nursing

Most babies nurse infrequently during the first twenty-four hours of life. But thereafter your baby should be nursing often, at least eight times in twenty-four hours. Studies show that the numbers of daily nursings on the second, third, and fourth days of life are directly related to how much milk is produced on days five and fourteen. Until your milk comes in, your baby needs frequent feedings of colostrum. After your milk comes in, probably about seventy-two hours after the birth, a good feeding every few hours will help ensure a plentiful milk supply. If for some reason you and your baby(ies) are separated after birth and the baby needs to be kept in the nursery/NICU for several hours, pumping at around one to two hours following birth is recommended to help bring in an abundant milk supply in the days that follow.

During the first few days after birth, many babies are sleepy. If your newborn has not nursed after two to three hours (counted from the start of the last feeding), unwrap her from her blankets. Rub her back and talk to her, or place her, dressed in only her diaper, against your bare chest. She will probably then become interested in nursing.

In the hospital, keeping the baby with you in your room helps ensure frequent nursing. If you are not sharing a room with your baby, ask the nurses to bring her to you at least every three hours (more often if she fusses), including whenever she wakens in the night.

Encourage the baby to have a good feeding each time you nurse her. Until your milk is in, you can probably persuade her to take both breasts at each feeding. Listen for the sound of your baby swallowing; when you hear it, you will know that she is taking colostrum or milk.

Dr. Jack Newman, of the Newman Breastfeeding Clinic and Institute in Canada, has produced some excellent videos that show both babies who are latched on and swallowing well and others who are taking very little milk. You can find links to these videos at www.ibconline.ca/breastfeeding-videos-english. The clip entitled "Really Good Drinking" shows a baby who is a few days old. The mother's milk has come in, and the baby is vigorously sucking and swallowing. Not only can you see the baby drinking and occasionally hear him swallowing milk, but you can see that he has taken the breast deeply into his wide-open mouth. (Before the milk has come in, a baby may not swallow quite as much.) For contrast, you can see a baby who is only nibbling at the breast, with little if any swallowing, in the video clip entitled "Nibbling."

In the video entitled "Baby 28 Hours Old, Baby-Led Mother-Guided Latching," a lactation consultant and Dr. Newman show a mother how to compress her breast to stimulate milk flow to the baby. With the help of breast compression, this one-day-old baby begins swallowing colostrum. Breast compression is easy to do: When the baby is sucking but is not swallowing, gently squeeze the breast until the baby begins taking long sucks with pauses for swallowing.

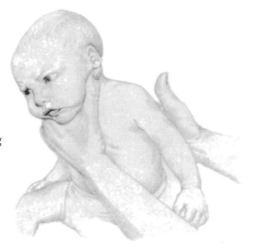

You can burp the baby by sitting her up, one hand under her jaw. Firmly pat her lower back with the other hand.

When your baby has released the nipple, or when you have nursed her for 20 to 25 minutes and she is no longer swallowing, burp her. Hold her up over your shoulder and pat her back, or sit her upright, bent slightly forward with your hand supporting her lower jaw, and firmly pat her lower back. After burping, she will probably regain interest in nursing and take the second breast. If she doesn't burp within a few minutes, just switch sides. If she refuses to nurse on the second breast or nurses for only a short time, be sure to start her on that side at the next feeding.

The first few days of colostrum and milk removal is a critical period for determining whether a mother ends up with a generous milk supply or an inadequate one. Infrequent and/or inadequate feedings may also delay the onset of milk production.

At any time, if mature milk removal is infrequent, the resulting pressure often leads to low production. If no milk is removed, milk production stops entirely (this is how women who don't nurse stop producing milk).

So ensuring a good milk supply depends on having a vigorous nursing baby from early on, or using an effective breast pump, that drain the breasts every few hours around the clock.

Avoiding Unnecessary Supplements

Another way to help ensure your milk supply is to avoid unnecessary supplemental feedings. Some babies develop a strong preference for an artificial nipple when a bottle is introduced during the first few days (see page 51, Just the Breast). Glucose (sugar) water offers few calories and may discourage the baby's interest in nursing. Also, babies fed glucose water more frequently develop jaundice in the first few days after birth. After taking formula, a baby frequently may not want to nurse for four hours or longer, since formula takes more time to digest than breast milk. The decrease in breast stimulation may delay the onset of milk production as well as decrease the amount of milk produced. Again, the exception are newborns who have low blood sugar in the early hours following birth.

Putting Your Fears to Rest

In the early days of breastfeeding, you may be surprised at how often your baby wants to nurse. He may be especially fussy on the second night following birth, before milk production begins; most babies want to nurse nearly hourly during this period. Even after your milk comes in, your newborn may seem fussy and hungry much of the time. This may make you wonder if you have enough milk, and if you should pump your milk and feed it by bottle to see how much the baby is getting. Well-meaning friends and family members may even suggest you supplement your milk with formula.

Most newborns want to nurse eight to twelve times in each twenty-four-hour period after the first day or two of life. This frequent nursing is normal; it seldom reflects a poor milk supply, and it never reflects "weak milk." Unless you or your baby fall into one of the categories described on page 65, Babies Who May Not Get Enough, your baby is probably getting plenty of milk.

Without introducing a bottle, though, how can you know your baby is getting enough? You can look for these signs of adequate milk intake:

- *Your milk has come in by the third day after birth (or at about seventy-two hours postpartum).* When milk production begins, the breasts become firmer and heavier. The firmness may be less apparent with large breasts, but the breasts should still feel heavier.

- **Your baby is nursing at least eight times in a twenty-four-hour period after the first twenty-four hours.** This means your baby is nursing every two to three hours (measured from the start of one feeding to the start of the next) during the day, with a sleep stretch of up to five hours at night. If your baby isn't nursing this often, you may have to wake her for feedings.

- **Your baby is nursing for ten to forty-five minutes at each feeding and seems content after feedings.** Babies vary in the length of time they nurse, but they typically need ten to forty-five minutes to complete a feeding. Although babies don't always fall asleep after nursing, they should usually seem satisfied after feedings.

- **Your baby has several periods of swallowing during each feeding.** When babies are getting milk, they take long, drawing sucks and can be heard swallowing or gulping (see page 61).

- **Your breasts feel softer or lighter after the baby has nursed.** Once milk production has begun, you should be able to feel a decrease in fullness or heaviness after feeding your baby.

- **Your baby is having bowel movements every day, and by the fifth day they have turned yellow.** This is the clearest sign that a baby is getting enough colostrum at first, and then later enough breast milk. Most newborns have at least two to three bowel movements each day during the first month. Only after the first month is it normal for breastfed babies to go several days without a bowel movement.

- **Your baby is wetting more diapers by the fifth day after birth.** Before your milk comes in, your baby will urinate infrequently, but by the fifth day you should notice more frequent and wetter diapers. Be aware that most disposable diapers today are so absorbent that they can make wetness difficult to detect.

If not all of the points just listed hold true for you and your baby, you should have him weighed and examined. In the first four to five days after birth, a baby loses weight. After the fifth day, a baby should gain an ounce (or more) every day. An initial loss of 10 percent or more of a baby's birth weight suggests the baby is underfed (see Appendix B, page 396). Even if your baby has lost less than 10 percent of his birth weight, have him weighed again in a couple of days to see if he has started gaining an ounce per day.

Babies Who May Not Get Enough

Some mothers are at risk for delayed and/or limited milk production, and some babies are at risk for underfeeding. Many of these can be identified even before milk production begins.

Often, conditions and complications that occur during pregnancy, labor, delivery, and postpartum lead to the late onset of milk production (see page 79, Late Onset of Milk Production).

- Maternal obesity. For unknown reasons, mothers who are obese may have delayed milk production.
- Mothers with nipples as large as or larger in diameter than a quarter (see page 114, Sucking Problems).
- Mothers who have polycystic ovary syndrome, (PCOS) or other endocrine issues (see page 138).
- Mothers who have had previous breast surgery involving an incision around the nipple or areola, such as in some breast augmentation and reduction procedures (see page 138, Nursing after Breast Surgery).
- Mothers who have widely spaced, long, thin breasts that did not get larger in pregnancy and that may differ markedly from each other in size (see page 134, Insufficient Glandular Tissue).
- This group also includes those mothers having long labors, especially with several bags of IV fluids, and those ending up with unplanned cesarean births following long labors, or long labors with epidural anesthesia.
- Mothers whose ankles, feet, and even fingers and hands are swollen with edema following birth.
- Mothers with high blood pressure (preeclampsia) and HELLP syndrome. HELLP Syndrome is somewhat similar to preeclampsia, but more severe. This syndrome also affects the liver and blood and can be life-threatening (see page 80).

- Mothers with diabetes (including gestational diabetes) (see page 146).

- Mothers who may have placental fragments still in their uterus This also includes mothers with excessive blood loss (see page 79, Late Onset of Milk Production).

- Mothers who have very soft breasts with no noticeable change in fullness and no other signs of milk production at seventy-two hours following birth and after (see page 79, Lake Onset of Milk Production).

- Babies who are born at 37 weeks' gestation or earlier (see page 153, The Late Preterm Baby, and the Near-Term Baby).

- Babies weighing less than 6 pounds (2.7 kg) at birth (see page 153, The Late Preterm Baby, and the Near-Term Baby).

- Babies who may have poor muscle tone, such as those with Down syndrome (see page 169, Developmental and Neurological Problems).

- Babies who have unusual conformations in their mouths, such as a short frenulum (the string of tissue on the underside of the tongue) (see page 119, Tongue-tie), a high palate (see page 115), or a cleft lip or palate (see page 111, The Baby Who Has Not Yet Nursed, and page 167, Cleft Lip and Palate).

- Babies who aren't yet latching on or sustaining sucking twenty-four hours after birth (see page 114, Sucking Problems).

If you or your baby falls into one of these risk groups, a few days of sluggish nursing and limited milk removal can have a devastating effect on your milk production, even if breastfeeding seems to be getting off to a good start. (For help, see page 79, Survival Guide, The First Week, Late Onset of Milk Production and Concerns about the Baby, and Underfeeding and Weight Loss.) Consider renting a clinical-grade breast pump, preferably with a double collection kit, which may be more reliable than your baby in stimulating continued milk production. Starting on the third day after birth, or sooner, pump for ten to fifteen minutes with a double collection kit right after each nursing. If you don't have a double collection kit, pump each side twice, for a total pumping time of twenty to thirty minutes. If your baby isn't able to latch on or clearly isn't sucking effectively, start pumping earlier than the third day, and pump for fifteen to twenty minutes with a double collection kit or ten to fifteen minutes per side without one. This should assure that you'll have an abundant milk supply even if your baby's sucking is sluggish. You can refrigerate, or freeze, the pumped milk for later use.

If your baby is latching on and sucking, watch her closely for the reassuring signs of adequate milk intake listed on pages 63 and 125. Weigh her at three to four days of age and approximately every two days thereafter until she is clearly gaining an ounce a day. If she loses 10 percent or more of her birth weight or does not gain an ounce a day after five days of age, she needs your pumped breast milk or formula as a supplement. If she has regained her birth weight, you can gradually stop pumping over a few days. Before returning the pump, though, make sure the baby has gained an ounce a day since the last weighing. See page 126, Treatment Measures for Underfeeding.

The First Week of Nursing

Although most unmedicated babies are alert and eager to nurse during the first two hours after birth, during the next few days they may sleep much of the time. The average baby, after the first couple of days, begins to wake up to nurse about every one to three hours. At night, he will sleep from one to five hours at a stretch. If your baby is not waking on his own to nurse at least eight times in each twenty-four-hour period, including at least once in the night, awaken him for feedings.

The typical length of a feeding varies greatly from baby to baby. A baby who is "all business"—who sucks and swallows with few pauses—may complete a feeding in as little as ten minutes. At the other extreme is the baby who sucks and swallows five or six times and then pauses. This pattern of frequent pausing may extend a feeding beyond forty minutes. Most babies' feedings fall between these extremes; the average is twenty to thirty minutes. Although your baby may not fall asleep after feeding, he should seem content.

A baby who takes longer than forty-five minutes to complete most of his feedings may not be getting sufficient amounts of milk and should be weighed to make sure that he has not lost too much weight or, after the fifth day of life, that he is gaining weight.

After your milk comes in, you should hear a lot of swallowing while nursing the baby. Swallowing sounds something like "eh, eh, eh." Some babies gulp noisily, whereas others swallow more quietly. Between swallows, babies take long, drawing sucks. (They take short, choppy sucks when they are not swallowing milk.) These long, drawing sucks usually occur in bursts, that is, five to ten continuous sucks followed by a resting pause. Babies who are taking enough milk usually have several bursts of continuous sucking and swallowing during a feeding.

You should not hear clicking noises while your baby nurses. Clicking often means that the baby is not sucking adequately and therefore may not be receiving enough milk. Some babies make clicking sounds if they have a very high palate (roof of the mouth) or they are tongue-tied (see page 119). The baby may not be able to press the nipple up against it if it is very high, deeper than the underside of a teaspoon. Some babies have such high palates that you will need to place your cheek on their chest to be able to see the top of it. The baby should have such a strong hold on the breast that the nipple does not easily slip from his mouth when you pull him slightly away. His cheeks should remain smooth with each suck; dimples on the cheek while nursing are a sign of inadequate suction and faulty sucking (see page 114, Sucking Problems, if your baby's cheeks are dimpling or if you don't hear much swallowing). One exception to clicking being abnormal can occur when a baby is getting so much milk and is swallowing so much that she momentarily unlatches without coming off the breast, which may also causes a clicking sound.

During the first day after birth, babies sometimes spit up mucus they have swallowed during delivery. Occasionally a baby will gag on this mucus. After the first twenty-four hours, this is usually no longer a problem.

Some babies also spit up colostrum or milk. The amounts are usually smaller than they seem, though you may wonder if your baby is keeping anything down. Spitting up a teaspoon or two after feedings is normal for some babies.

Babies also get hiccups, often after a feeding. Hiccups are the result of the baby's full tummy. You may remember the baby hiccuping in utero after drinking amniotic fluid. If the baby starts hiccuping after nursing at the first breast, it may be difficult to interest him in the other. You don't need to give him water or anything else. The hiccups are painless for him; just wait until they go away.

The baby's first stools, called meconium, are black and sticky. Having bowel movements every day and yellow stools by the fifth day usually indicates an adequate intake of colostrum, first, and then breast milk. Frequent yellow stools are one of the surest signs that a newborn is getting enough to eat. Most newborns have at least two bowel movements each day during the first month. (This rule may not hold true if the baby is receiving water or formula supplements.)

The yellow stools of a breastfed baby are soft, loose, or even watery, and sometimes they look seedy. Babies normally strain and grunt when passing their stools. This does not mean they are constipated.

Wet diapers are usually infrequent in the first few days, but they should be more frequent and wetter by the fifth day. Eight or more diapers wet with pale urine each day, along with daily yellow stools, are usually a sign of sufficient milk intake. (This rule may not hold true if the baby is receiving water or formula supplements.)

All newborns lose weight after birth. Expect your baby to lose 5 to 9 percent of his birth weight. He should begin gaining weight by the fifth day, about an ounce a day. (See Appendix B, page 396) to determine if your baby has lost too much weight.

Caring For Your Breasts

Your daily bath or shower is sufficient for cleaning your breasts. Avoid getting soap or shampoo on the nipple and areola; this would counteract the naturally occurring oils that cleanse this area. Antiseptic applications to the nipples are also unnecessary, but do take care to wash your hands before nursing.

You will probably want to wear a nursing bra for convenience and comfort, especially after your milk comes in. Again, bras with cotton or microfiber rather than synthetic cups allow for better air circulation to the nipples.

If the baby does not come off the breast by herself when the nursing session is over, take care to release the suction by pulling with your finger at the corner of the baby's mouth, toward her ear. Leave your breasts exposed to the air for five to ten minutes before covering up.

In the past, nursing mothers were discouraged from using nipple creams, since some women develop sore nipples in reaction to preparations containing lanolin, vitamin E, or cocoa butter. Some lanolin preparations were also discovered to be contaminated with pesticide residues. However, a purified form of lanolin has been developed; it rarely causes allergic reactions. Other options for soothing tender or injured nipples are discussed in "Survival Guide: The First Week," page 76.

If you are using plastic breast shells to improve the shape of your nipples, you may find during the first few weeks that they cause your milk to leak excessively and keep your nipples damp. You might try placing the shells in your bra just ten to twenty minutes before the feeding (milk collected this way should be discarded if it has been in the cups longer than a half hour or so). Don't routinely use breast shells in place of nursing pads; this usually causes more leakage. Breast shells should be washed after each nursing in hot soapy water and rinsed thoroughly.

When Your Mature Milk Comes In

Mature milk production generally begins on the second or third day after birth, but occasionally not until the fourth day or later (if your milk hasn't come in by the third day, see page 79, Late Onset of Milk Production). At first the milk will be mixed with colostrum, and so will be pale orange in color. After a few days the milk will become whiter. This mature milk will look more watery than cow's milk; it may resemble skim milk.

Most women notice that their breasts become larger, fuller, and more tender as the mature milk comes in. Large-breasted women may notice only a change in heaviness. This change, known as engorgement, is caused by increased blood flow to the breasts as well as beginning milk production. Fullness may be more apparent if your breasts are normally small or medium-size. They may feel lumpy, and the lumpiness may extend all the way to your armpits, since milk glands are also located there. After nursing, your breasts should feel softer or lighter.

Engorgement normally lasts twenty-four to seventy-two hours. During this time a nursing bra will provide support and comfort.

Frequent nursing, at least every two to three hours, is the best treatment. Heat treatments such as warm showers, hot packs, and heating pads may worsen the swelling. You may get relief, though, with cool applications to the breast and by gentle massaging or compressing the breast while the baby is nursing. This will encourage more milk to letdown. It is important to pay careful attention to the way the baby latches on while the breast is engorged. When latch-on is incorrect, because the baby isn't positioned well or the areola is overly full, soreness often follows. If the areola is hard, you can express some milk, by hand or with a pump. (For further advice on managing engorgement, see page 77, Engorged Breasts.)

When you put your baby to breast, you may feel any of these normal sensations: warmth, relaxation, sleepiness, thirst, and even hunger.

It is normal for milk to leak from the breasts. When the baby nurses at one breast, milk may drip or even spray from the other. This leaking may continue for several weeks, or it may never happen at all.

For women who leak milk, nursing pads are usually necessary to prevent wet or spotted clothing. You can buy the pads in two varieties: reusable and disposable. A new type that helps lessen leaking is called LilyPadz. Made of gas-permeable silicone, these pads apply a gentle pressure on the nipple to stop milk leakage (see Appendix A, page 386, for ordering information).

From Hospital to Home

In many hospitals, it is customary at the time of discharge to give new mothers an array of sample products that manufacturers would like them to try. You might conclude that the staff endorses these products, but this is not necessarily so. One of the gifts is usually something that may be labeled a "breastfeeding kit"—infant formula (often powdered, although powdered formula isn't safe for newborns—see page 10), bottle nipples, and a pamphlet on breastfeeding, which may contain misleading information. Since you have chosen to breastfeed, it is best to leave the kit behind. You won't be needing it.

Well worth taking home, however, are the names and telephone numbers of people who have a good reputation for helping nursing mothers and infants. Ask any nurse who has been encouraging or helpful with your early breastfeeding for this information. She may know of volunteers in La Leche League or the Nursing Mothers Counsel, and most certainly local lactation consultants (IBCLCs, board certified lactation consultants) in your community.

When you're getting ready to leave the hospital by car, have ready some small blankets to support your baby in her car seat, even if you'll have a short drive home. Because a newborn can't control her head well, she needs special support to allow her to breathe freely while riding in a car seat. A study of car seat models (Tonkin et al., 2006) found that all newborns need blanket rolls at either side of the body and another across the top of the head. Many also require a blanket roll between the crotch belt and the legs to keep from sliding down in the seat. This is particularly important for infants born early.

If a baby has been born before 37 weeks' gestation, the AAP recommends that the hospital staff observe her while she reclines in a car seat to be sure her breathing, heart rate, and oxygen levels remain normal. Nurseries that care mainly for full-term babies may not be aware of this recommendation, so you may need to ask for your baby to be monitored before she is discharged.

At home. As any experienced nursing mother can tell you, the first few days at home with a baby are exhausting and, at times, emotional. These days are best spent caring for only yourself and the baby. Besides recovering from the birth, you are doing the important work of getting to know your baby and learning to breastfeed. Rest and a quiet, pleasant environment are important in preventing anxiety and "baby blues." Try to eat well, but don't worry if your appetite has lessened; this can be normal during the first couple of weeks after delivery. Do be sure to drink enough water in order to stay hydrated. Ideally, you should spend the first several days nursing and resting with the baby, while a supportive partner or helper (or both) manages your home, meals, and callers.

If you have another child or children, you'll want help with them, too. Otherwise you may find yourself feeling suddenly, unexpectedly impatient or irritable with a beloved older child. When my second child was born, I found myself wishing someone could take away my nine-year-old for a while. Such feelings may arise from a natural protective urge that allows a mother to focus her total attention on the vulnerable newborn; shifting hormones and lack of sleep may contribute, too. Other species also defend their babies aggressively. For instance, picking up the new babies of a household pet may make the new mama growl, though in a few weeks she may not care at all when someone handles them.

In women, as in cats and dogs, such feelings usually lessen over time. In the meantime, they present a fine opportunity for your older child to strengthen a relationship with their other parent, Grandma or Grandpa, or another adult. This is also a great chance for your older child to learn patience and responsibility. You can encourage him to accept the big-kid role by saying outright that "the baby comes first." Your child may feel proud to help by fetching a diaper or glass of water, and he may later be able to apply the baby-comes-first principle with other helpless creatures, such as pets.

Some parents find it helpful to keep a log of the baby's feedings and urine and stool output during the early days of breastfeeding. This information may reassure them that the feedings are going well and help a doctor or lactation professional analyze any problem that may arise. If you don't have a copy of *The Nursing Mother's Breastfeeding Diary* (see page 423, References & Reading), your caregiver may give you a blank log, you can find one on the Internet (for example, at www.kellymom.com), or you can create your own. For each twenty-four-hour period, include the number of nursings, the number and color of stools, and, perhaps, the number of wet diapers. There are also now smartphone apps to keep track of infant feedings.

Because all newborns are susceptible to declining oxygen levels when they remain in a seated position, researchers recommend minimizing car travel and avoiding the use of car seats as carriers and other seating devices, such as swings and bouncer seats, in which the baby is at an incline, and sits up, in the early months of life.

Regardless of how you gave birth, you may continue to require pain medication for the first week or so at home. Use over-the-counter pain relievers such as acetaminophen (Tylenol) or ibuprofen (Motrin, Advil) as often as you need for afterpains or pain from an episiotomy or cesarean incision. Use narcotic pain relievers only when the over-the-counter medications are not enough.

Taking narcotic pain relievers often and for more than a few days after birth can, in some instances, make a baby sleepy and in rare cases lead mothers to experience withdrawal symptoms when the medication is stopped. Withdrawal symptoms may include depression, anxiety, crying, difficulty sleeping, nausea, vomiting, diarrhea, excessive sweating, and dilated pupils. Some of these symptoms mimic a normal postpartum emotional upset, but others do not.

It is not uncommon for things to suddenly "fall apart" shortly after a new mother comes home from the hospital. Suddenly responsible for a new baby, you may feel shaky, and at times your confidence may vanish. The dramatic hormonal shift that begins immediately after birth may also affect your emotional state for a while. You may find yourself exhausted and upset—especially if you've been taking responsibility for more than the baby and yourself.

Many new mothers have times when they feel that nursing "isn't working" and think about giving it up. Combined with the mood swings that follow birth, fears that the baby may not be getting enough milk, struggles with getting the baby to latch on, or problems like sore nipples, nursing can be overwhelming. A non-birth parent may become very concerned when witnessing these struggles and emotional episodes, and may become anxious to find a solution. If your partner can't "fix" your breastfeeding problems, they may encourage you to give up on nursing.

Your partner will be more supportive if they feel they play an important role in helping the family adjust after childbirth. So encourage them to help—even if they put the diaper on backward. They might tend to the baby while you nap, put meals together, tidy the house, care for other children, and even track down a lactation consultant for you (see Appendix A, page 386).

Despite tearful moments, rest assured that most early nursing difficulties can be overcome with patience and help. Don't hesitate to seek assistance. Just a phone conversation with a knowledgeable person may be enough to get you and your baby back on track.

The postpartum period is a time of physical and emotional adjustment. As with most of life's great transitions, this one is usually accompanied by some turmoil. It will take several weeks, and most of your time and energy, to get to know your baby and learn how to care for her. So don't do more than you must, and accept offers for help. Adjusting to motherhood is always easier when you are supported and cared for by others.

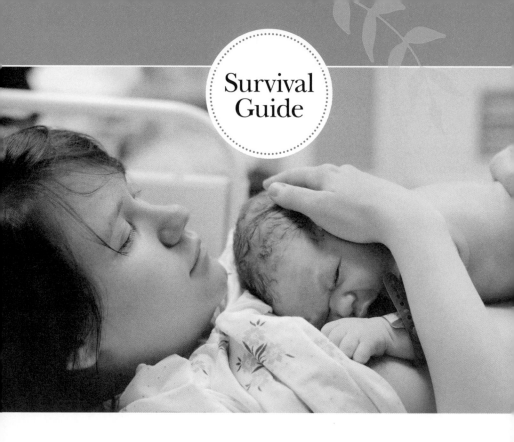

THE FIRST WEEK

CONCERNS ABOUT YOURSELF

- Engorged Breasts
- Late Onset of Milk Production
- Sore Nipples
- Breast Pain
- Leaking Milk
- Letdown Difficulty
- Milk Appearance
- Difficult Latch-on: Flat, Dimpled, or Inverted Nipples
- Fatigue and Depression

CONCERNS ABOUT THE BABY

- Sleepy Baby
- Bowel Movements
- Jaundice
- Difficult Latch-on: Refusal to Nurse
- Sucking Problems
- Tongue-tie
- Fussiness and Excessive Night Waking
- Underfeeding and Weight Loss

I n the early days following childbirth, mothers are not only physically recovering from childbirth but are working to get to know their newborn and get breastfeeding established. Occasionally, first-time nursing mothers may feel overwhelmed. Several common breastfeeding issues arise during these early days. Seeing a lactation professional as soon as problems arise can make all the difference between a successful nursing relationship and abandoning breastfeeding during this critical first week.

CONCERNS ABOUT YOURSELF

Engorged Breasts

Two to four days after a woman gives birth, her breasts usually become engorged, or temporarily swollen with milk. The breasts typically feel fuller, although large-breasted women may notice only more heaviness. Engorgement is caused by the increased flow of blood to the breasts and the start of milk production. For some women the breasts become only slightly full, but for others they feel very swollen, tender, throbbing, and lumpy. Sometimes the swelling extends all the way to the armpit.

Engorgement may sometimes cause the nipples to flatten, making it difficult for the baby to latch on. The problem usually lessens within twenty-four to seventy-two hours, but the swelling and discomfort may worsen if nursing is too brief or infrequent or if the baby sucks ineffectively. If engorgement is unrelieved by nursing or pumping, milk production declines and ultimately stops altogether.

Although many healthcare providers recommend applying direct heat (warm washcloths, heating pads, hot water bottles, or hot showers) to engorged breasts, this may actually aggravate engorgement.

Treatment Measures for Engorged Breasts

1. Wear a supportive nursing bra, even during the night. Be sure your bra is not too tight.

2. Nurse frequently, every one and a half to three hours. This may mean waking the baby (see page 103, Sleepy Baby).

3. Avoid having the baby latch on when the areola is very firm. To help keep the baby's mouth from sliding down onto the nipple and injuring it, use a technique developed by Jean Cotterman (2004): Just before nursing, soften the areola by placing two or three fingers at the base of the nipple and pressing firmly against the areola. Hold this position for at least one minute, and then move your fingers to a different spot at the base of the nipple and repeat the pressure. Or soften the areola and extend the nipple by manually expressing or pumping a little milk (see Chapter 5). Wearing plastic breast shells for half an hour before nursing may also help to soften the areola.

4. Encourage the baby to nurse for at least ten minutes or longer. It is preferable to nurse on just one side until the breast is soft, even if the baby goes to sleep, than to limit the baby's nursing time on the first side so you can nurse from both sides in one feeding.

5. Gently massage or compress the breast by squeezing it gently as the baby nurses. This will encourage the milk to flow and will help relieve some of the tightness and discomfort you feel (see Chapter 2, page 82, to learn more about the videos you can watch about breast compression).

6. To relieve the pain and swelling, apply a cold pack to the breast for a short

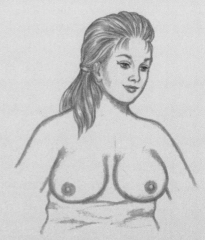

The breasts may grow astonishingly big and hard as milk production begins.

period after nursing. You can use ice in a plastic bag or, better, soak a disposable diaper in water, shape it, and then freeze it. Lay a thin cloth over your breast before applying the cold pack or diaper.

7. If you need to, take a mild pain reliever such as acetaminophen (Tylenol) or ibuprofen (Motrin, Advil).

8. If, forty-eight hours after your milk has come in, you still find yourself overly full right after nursing, use a pump to drain both breasts as completely as possible. In this first week, habitual pumping along with nursing can lead to more engorgement and chronic overproduction, but pumping after nursing once every twenty-four hours or so should relieve your engorgement, not prolong it.

9. If the baby is not nursing well enough to soften at least one breast every few hours, use a clinical-grade pump as necessary (see Chapter 5, page 245).

Late Onset of Milk Production

For some mothers, milk production is delayed beyond the typical seventy-two hours after giving birth. Sometimes it begins hours or even days later. In the meantime, the breasts remain soft, and the baby sucks but gets little milk. In these circumstances, some babies may seem sleepy and content, but most act dissatisfied. They may spend a long time sucking at the breast only to act hungry when they stop feeding. They have infrequent bowel movements, many become jaundiced, and they lose more weight than expected.

Most all breastfed newborns lose weight following birth during the first few days. While some healthcare providers consider a weight loss of up to 8 percent to be normal, others are comfortable with a weight loss of up to 10 percent. Losing more than 10 percent of birth weight is a red flag that the baby has lost too much weight, which can lead to dehydration, jaundice, poor feeding, and even more serious complications (see the "Ten Percent Weight Loss" chart in Appendix B, page 396).

Some babies lose an excessive amount of weight due to the late onset of milk production while others lose too much weight because of ineffective nursing (see page 125, Underfeeding and Weight Loss, regarding information on ineffective nursing). Certain woman are at risk for the late onset of milk production. These mothers include:

- Mothers who are obese. For unknown reasons, obesity is a risk factor for delayed milk production.

- Mothers with PCOS or other endocrine issues (see page 138, Polycystic Ovarian Syndrome).

- Mothers with Insufficient Glandular Tissue (IGT). These mothers have widely spaced, long, thin breasts that do not grow much larger in pregnancy. They may differ markedly from each other in size. Mothers with IGT also may have a delay in the onset of milk production (see page 134, Insufficient Glandular Tissue).

- Mothers with diabetes (including gestational diabetes) are also at risk for delayed milk production.

- Mothers with high blood pressure (preeclampsia) and HELLP syndrome. HELLP Syndrome is somewhat similar to preeclampsia but more severe. This syndrome also affects the liver and blood and can be life-threatening.

- Events during labor and birth can also delay the onset of milk production. Over hydration with intravenous fluids during labor is a frequent finding with delayed milk production (see Chapter 1). Mothers having labor induced using medications such as Pitocin ("Pit") along with bags of IV fluids may lead to delayed onset of milk production. This group also includes those mothers having long labors, following epidural anesthesia especially with several bags of IV fluids, and those ending up with unplanned cesarean births following long labors.

- Mothers whose ankles, feet, and even fingers and hands are swollen with edema following birth.

- Mothers who may have placental fragments still in their uterus. This also includes mothers with excessive blood loss. It is thought that the hormones secreted by even small placental parts still attached to the uterine wall can keep the milk from coming in.

Suspect retained placental fragments if you experienced postpartum hemorrhage or if, since the birth, you've had some of these symptoms: cramping, heavy bleeding, passing of tissue, foul-smelling lochia, and fever. Even some women who have delivered by cesarean have had retained placental fragments. When a doctor removes the fragments, milk production usually begins.

If your milk is late coming in, you may need to supplement with whatever colostrum you can express and/or formula until it does. But you should continue to nurse frequently in the meantime.

Treatment Measures for Late Onset of Milk Production

1. If within seventy-two hours after the birth you suspect that your milk is not in, have your baby weighed. If he has lost 10 percent or more of his birth weight (see the chart in Appendix B, page 396), nurse frequently, every two to two and a half hours during the day or evening, or more often if the baby seems hungry, and every three hours in the night, or more often if the baby wakes sooner.

2. While the baby is at the breast, listen for swallowing. When he drifts off to sleep and is no longer swallowing, massage or compress your breast (see Chapter 2, page 61). You can also switch breasts as the swallowing slows, to help the baby wake and begin swallowing again. Massaging, compressing, and switching back and forth for twenty to thirty minutes will help stimulate the breast and maximize the amount that the baby takes.

3. On the third day, as soon as you realize that your breasts are not becoming heavier or firmer with milk, find out where you can rent a clinical (or rental grade) pump (see page 245). Upon your discharge from the hospital, it is preferable to secure this type of pump and use it along with a double collection kit. This should assure that you will bring in an abundant milk supply even if your baby's sucking is sluggish or nonexistent. NOTE: A pump that you purchase, borrow, or receive from your insurance carrier is generally not effective enough to bring in a full milk supply for your baby. These "personal use" pumps are not always the same quality as "rental-grade" pumps.

4. After each nursing, pump your breasts for five to ten minutes or longer if milk is still coming out. After each pumping, take a few more minutes to hand express colostrum or breast milk to stimulate even more milk. Some mothers may find they get even more milk by performing manual expression after pumping. You can read about manual expression and pumping in Chapter 5. You can learn the technique of hand expression from a lactation consultant or by viewing a helpful video made by Dr. Jane Morton of Stanford University at http://newborns.stanford.edu/ Breastfeeding/ HandExpression.html. Another great video from lactation consultant Mya Bolman can be seen at http:// bfmedneo.com/resources/videos/.

5. Feed your baby the colostrum you collect along with any necessary formula (see Appendix B, page 396, to determine how much milk or formula your baby needs). Keep in mind that a newborn that has lost an excessive amount of weight, 10 percent or more of his birth weight, may be sluggish and ineffective at the breast. If you want to avoid using a bottle, you can offer your colostrum or milk using a plastic spoon, syringe, or dropper. Some mothers may be given or sold a "supplementer" by a lactation consultant for feeding the baby additional milk with a small tube while the baby nurses at the breast (see Appendix A, page 386).

6. Check the baby's weight every day or two.

7. Seek advice from a lactation professional, if at all possible. She can check the baby's weight and determine how much the baby is getting at a feeding and let you know when to discontinue pumping and supplementing.

8. If your milk is late coming in, also see page 125, Underfeeding and Weight Loss. You may need to supplement with whatever colostrum or breast milk you can express and/or supplement with formula until it does. You should continue to nurse (and pump) frequently in the meantime. Pumping may be much more effective at stimulating milk production than a newborn who may be sluggish at the breast.

9. Consider using herbs known to stimulate milk production (see box on page 84).

10. If you have possible symptoms of retained placenta (see page 81), call your doctor or midwife.

11. When your milk comes in, see page 125, Underfeeding and Weight Loss, for guidance in estimating your production and weaning your baby off expressed milk or formula. Have the baby weighed often as you gradually stop using formula and pumping. After the fifth day of life, all babies should be gaining at least an ounce per day.

12. If milk production is slow to come in, and other measures such as frequent nursing, pumping, and herbs are not increasing milk production, you may want to consider using medications to increase your supply.

Herbs for More Milk

Various herbs are known to stimulate milk production. One of the best-known herbs is fenugreek, whose fragrant seed is used as the flavoring ingredient in artificial maple syrup. You can make a tea from the seeds, but more convenient and effective are 580- or 610-milligram capsules containing the seeds. Mothers who take three capsules three times a day typically notice an increase in the milk supply within forty-eight to seventy-two hours. Some mothers find that fenugreek causes gassiness in their babies. Mothers may also notice the distinct odor of maple in their sweat and urine. A few mothers can get diarrhea that does end when discontinuing the herb. Although fenugreek capsules are usually taken for several days, some mothers continue to use them for weeks or months without any difficulties. Fenugreek costs just a few dollars for a bottle of one hundred capsules. There is a faster acting fenugreek tincture available through Motherlove Herbal Company that costs about $20.00.

NOTE: Fenugreek should never be taken during pregnancy, and two sources of fenugreek should not be taken together due to intestinal disturbance. Fenugreek is also not recommended for mothers who are insulin dependent or have hypothyroidism. Lastly, fenugreek should not be taken by mothers who are allergic to legumes or chickpeas.

Blessed thistle (*Cnicus benedictus*) is also an herb helpful in stimulating milk production. Like fenugreek, this herb is available in most health-food stores in capsule form. The typical dosage is three 390-milligram capsules three times a day. Consider using fenugreek and blessed thistle together to stimulate greater milk production.

Other herbs known to increase milk include nettle leaf and fennel. Motherlove Herbal makes a few preparations to increase milk production: More Milk, More Milk Plus, and More Milk Special Blend. More Milk contains blessed thistle, nettle, and fennel, without fenugreek and is designed to increase milk production quickly. More Milk Plus is More Milk with fenugreek. More Milk Special Blend, with the same herbs as More Milk Plus and goat's rue, is designed to stimulate the development of breast tissue, as well as increase the milk supply in women who have polycystic ovary syndrome (PCOS), or who have a history of breast surgery involving an incision around the areola, or who have underdeveloped breasts (see page 134, Insufficient Glandular Tissue). It is often used by mothers who are adopting.

All of these preparations are offered in either capsule and tincture form. Tinctures are stronger and faster acting than capsules. The large capsules may be hard to swallow for some women. The tinctures are unpleasant tasting but the amount is just a full dropper.

Another herbal preparation is made from the leaves of the Malunggay tree and has been shown to increase milk production in one study. Malunggay is also sold by Motherlove and can be taken with other herbal supplements, like More Milk, More Milk Plus, or More Milk Special Blend. Mothers who are sensitive to fenugreek or whose babies are gassy from the use of fenugreek may prefer Malunggay.

Motherlove's latest and best-selling product is More Milk Moringa. This preparation includes the addition of moringa, also known as malunggay, a known super food herb. Without the inclusion of fenugreek, this formulation has been very popular for mothers wanting to increase their milk production. Mothers who are sensitive to fenugreek or whose babies are gassy from the use of fenugreek may prefer malunggay. Also including blessed thistle, nettle, and fennel, this concentrated extract has shown to be a potent galactagogue in capsule form. A bottle of 60 capsules costs $25.95 and a bottle of 120 capsules is $43.95.

Motherlove products generally need to be ordered through their website (www.motherlove.com), though they are also available in some health food stores, baby supply stores, and lactation practices. (For information, see Appendix A, page 386.)

Another herbal company that produces Mulunggay to increase milk production is Natolac. After just 24 hours of starting Natolac, mothers notice breast engorgement and those with high blood pressure also notice increased milk production.

Last, but not least, is Shatavari or "wild asparagus root" that is well-known in India and China for increasing milk production by probably increasing the hormone prolactin. Available by capsule or powder, Shatavari should not be used during pregnancy.

For information on sources and ordering Motherlove products, see Appendix A, page 386. Motherlove's best-selling More Milk Plus (either capsules or tinctures) is available at many health food stores and often at Target. You can use Motherlove's "Store Locator" to find a store near you or order products on line. It still may be best to call the stores ahead of time before venturing out. Other herbs to increase milk production are available from Legendairy Milk (www.legendairymilk.com).

Sore Nipples

There is no doubt about it: Sore nipples can make a trial of what ought to be a joyous experience. For a few days after giving birth, you may feel slight tenderness during the first minute or two of nursing, when the baby latches on and the nipple stretches into her mouth. Such tenderness is normal at this time.

If your nipples become really sore, however, they are probably injured or irritated and require treatment beyond simple comfort measures. It is important for you to identify the cause of the problem so that you can help your nipples heal. At any time that you are unable to tolerate the pain, and the position changes recommended do not help, consult a lactation professional. If none is available, you may want to temporarily stop nursing; pump your milk with a clinical-grade rental pump using a double collection kit for twenty-four to seventy-two hours, or until the nipples heal (see Chapter 5 for information on expressing milk).

There are two basic types of sore nipples: the traumatized nipple and the irritated nipple. The traumatized nipple may be blistered, scabbed, or cracked. The irritated nipple is very pink and often burns. Occasionally a mother may have both types of soreness at once.

In addition to the specific treatments listed for each category of sore nipples, the tips below will help speed healing and provide comfort.

Drugs that Stimulate Milk Production

Two pharmaceutical drugs used to help build the milk supply are
Metoclopramide (Reglan) and Domperidone.

Metoclopramide is prescribed in the United States primarily for gastric
reflux. But several studies have shown it to be effective and safe for increasing
a mother's milk supply, although the U.S. Food and Drug Administration (FDA)
has not approved the drug for this use. Metoclopramide has not been shown
to cause any problems for a nursing baby; in fact, it is occasionally prescribed
for infants. It may, however, make the mother sleepy. More worrisome side
effects, such as agitation and uncontrolled muscle movements, are uncommon; if they occur, the drug should be discontinued. The typical dosage is
10 milligrams every six to eight hours for fourteen days. If taken for longer
than a few weeks, metoclopramide can lead to depression and other problems
that may not resolve simply by discontinuing the medication. It should therefore never be taken for more than two to four weeks.

Although Domperidone is marketed only for gastrointestinal disorders, studies show that it safely increases milk production, and the AAP has
approved this drug, as well as metoclopramide, as safe to take while nursing.
Domperidone apparently works by stimulating production of prolactin, the
hormone that stimulates the breast to produce milk.

Because Domperidone does not enter the brain tissue in significant
amounts, it has far less frequent and serious side effects in the nursing mother
than does metoclopramide. The side effects that can occur—headache, abdominal cramps, and dry mouth—are extremely uncommon when the drug is taken
orally in normal doses for stimulating milk production, no higher than 40 milligrams four times per day. (The FDA issued a warning about Domperidone after
reports of sickness when the drug was administered in high intravenous doses
as treatment for gastrointestinal disturbances. According to Thomas Hale, a
professor of pediatrics and pharmacology at Texas Tech University School of
Medicine, this use of the drug caused blood levels eighty to 150 times higher
than that of women who take Domperidone orally in normal doses.)

Domperidone is not manufactured in the United States, and it cannot
legally be made here in compounding pharmacies. It is available without a
prescription—and inexpensively—when ordered through InHouse Pharmacy
in Vanuatu and CanUSAmeds in Canada (see Appendix A, page 386).

General Comfort Measures for Sore Nipples

1. A half hour before nursing, take acetaminophen (Tylenol), ibuprofen (Motrin, Advil), or a pain reliever prescribed by your doctor.

2. Avoid using nipple shields (see page 100) for nursing, unless you are under the care of a lactation consultant. These thin, soft silicone nipple covers are designed to help infants who are having difficulty latching on to the breast. Nipple shields can make soreness worse, and they can sometimes decrease milk production. Nipple shields come in different sizes; a wrong fit may not allow adequate breast compression and can cause the baby to get too little milk.

3. Do not delay nursings. Shorter, more frequent nursings (every one and a half to two hours) may be easier on the nipples than longer, infrequent nursings.

4. While nursing, massage or compress your breasts (see page 61) to encourage the milk to flow and to speed emptying.

5. If you are sore during the entire feeding, you can restrict nursing to one breast only per feeding. This may not necessarily mean nursing more often. If nursing is still too painful, rent a clinical-grade pump with a double collection kit until your nipples are feeling better.

6. Release the baby's suction carefully (see page 59) before removing him from the breast.

7. After nursing, wash your hands and then apply a thin coating of modified lanolin (see page 70) or other ointment to your nipples to soothe them and promote healing.

8. Other soothing ointments are Motherlove Nipple Cream, which contains three herbal remedies for healing, sore, or injured nipples. Medical-grade Manuka honey is well known for its healing and antibacterial properties; see Appendix A, page 386, for help locating a source. Note: Manuka honey has been irradiated so that there are no botulism spores present.

9. Between nursings, you might wear vented, hard plastic breast shells (see page 30) to keep your bra off your sensitive nipples. If you use plastic breast shells, wash them daily.

10. Change disposable or cloth nursing pads after each nursing and when they become wet.

11. Wear cotton or microfiber bras. Other fabrics do not allow adequate air circulation.

12. Suds and rinse your nipples in your daily shower and rinse them in warm water after each nursing. Take care to wash your hands before handling your breasts.

13. If you are using a breast pump instead of nursing during a period of soreness, pump your milk often—at least eight times a day—to keep up your supply. Again, anything other than a clinical-grade rental pump with a double collection kit may not be effective enough to maintain your milk supply. (See Chapter 5 for more information on expressing milk.)

Traumatized nipples. Cracks, blisters, and abrasions usually result because a baby is improperly positioned for nursing; her gums close on the nipple instead of the areola. This often occurs when a baby fails to open her mouth wide enough or when her gums slide off the areola onto the nipple, commonly because the breast is engorged or unsupported.

Babies who have a faulty suck or who are "tongue-tied" (see page 119) can also cause cracks, blisters, and abrasions. Cracking of the nipples may also occur with irritated nipples (see page 92) and thrush nipples (see page 195).

Bacteria in an open nipple wound from the surrounding skin and unclean hands can delay healing. One study by two Canadian physicians found that 75 percent of mothers with injured nipples at five days postpartum or beyond, usually from a faulty latch, develop mastitis in the coming weeks (Livingstone and Stringer, 1999). Because so many mothers develop wounded nipples during the early days of nursing, I often recommend oral antibiotics to help the wound heal and prevent getting a breast infection later.

If you have an injured nipple(s) at or after five days postpartum or beyond, call your midwife or obstetrician for a prescription of oral anti-biotics to quickly heal infected nipples and prevent mastitis. If they are reluctant to prescribe an oral antibiotic, they may be willing to call in a prescription of Dr. Jack Newman's all-purpose nipple ointment "APNO" (all-purpose nipple ointment, see the ingredients on page 198). If they are unwilling to call in either one for you, consider purchasing Manuka honey (see opposite).

Treatment Measures for Traumatized Nipples

1. Carefully review page 52, Positioning at the Breast, so that you clearly understand the details of correct latch-on technique. Review the video recommended on page 53.

2. If your breast is so full that the areola cannot be easily com-pressed, soften it by pressing with your finger, as described on page 78, or by manually expressing (see page 240) or pumping a little milk. This will allow the baby to get more of the areola into her mouth and help stimulate the milk to letdown.

3. If your baby is reluctant to open her mouth wide, don't let her chew her way onto the breast. Patiently wait until she opens her mouth wide. Letting the baby suck on your finger for a few sec-onds may stimulate her sucking reflex and encourage her to open wider.

4. If your nipples are creased when the baby releases her latch, consider the possibility of "tongue-tie" as the underlying cause of traumatized nipples (see page 119).

5. Do not hesitate to take the baby off the breast as soon as you real-ize that she is not in the right position. You may need to help her latch on a couple of times before you succeed at getting her far enough onto the breast. Ask your partner or a lactation consul-tant to observe your latch-on technique. A helper can also guide your arm when the baby opens wide so that she is pulled in as quickly and as close as possible.

6. Don't turn to a nipple shield when dealing with traumatized nipples. You may not find the correct size shield, which can

make nipple pain worse or may not allow the baby to empty the breast well.

7. With clean hands right after feedings, apply a thin coating of modified lanolin (see page 70, Motherlove Nipple Cream, Appendix A, page 386) or Manuka honey.

8. Medical-grade Manuka honey is a well-known honey in New Zealand made from the pollination of the Manuka bush. This honey has antibacterial and healing properties. Manuka also has anti-inflammatory properties that can quickly reduce pain and inflammation. The higher the "UMF" (Unique Manuka Factor) number, the higher the healing strength. A UMF number of sixteen or higher is ideal. The honey has been irradiated to destroy any botulism spores and therefore is safe to use while nursing an infant. You can use a nursing pad to keep your nipple from sticking to your bra. Manuka honey can be found in health food stores and online. Manuka is also helpful for the quick healing of scrapes and cuts on the entire family—without the "stinging" during application. See Appendix A, page 386, for ordering information.

9. Ask your midwife or physician about trying Dr. Jack Newman's APNO (all-purpose nipple ointment), an ointment recipe for healing sore nipples. It was developed to treat nipple soreness or injury stemming from any number of underlying causes including bacteria, yeast, and inflammation. This ointment needs to be ordered by a doctor or midwife and mixed by a pharmacist, usually in a compounding pharmacy. It is well absorbed into the skin and the baby will not take in very much at all. The mixture is to be used sparingly after each feeding and not wiped or washed off prior to nursings, although rinsing both nipples after nursing and before applying the ointment is still recommended by lactation consultants. (See the entire prescription written out for your doctor on page 198.)

Irritated nipples. Irritated nipples are reddened and sometimes slightly swollen, and generally they burn. Some mothers may feel burning between, as well as during, feedings. In severe cases, the nipples may be cracked, peeling, or oozing. Nipple irritation may be caused by yeast (thrush), bacteria, a chemical sensitivity or allergy, or a skin condition such as eczema or impetigo. See Nipple Dermatitis on page 198, under Survival Guide for the First Two Months.

Thrush nipples. When a mother's nipples become sore after weeks or months of comfortable nursing, thrush (or yeast) (also see page 195) is the usual cause. But a thrush infection can also occur in the early weeks after delivery, and when it does, it may be overlooked as the cause of the nipple soreness. A newborn with thrush may have picked up a yeast infection in the birth canal during delivery; this often happens if the mother is diabetic. A thrush infection may also result if a mother or her baby is given antibiotics. (After a cesarean, antibiotics are often given in intravenous fluids.)

If you suspect a case of thrush, carefully inspect the baby's mouth. You may see a white film or patches on the inside of the cheeks, inside the lips, and possibly on the tongue. Sometimes a baby will have no symptoms in the mouth but will have a diaper rash caused by yeast. This rash, usually in the genital area, will be very defined, very red, and a bit raised. It may also appear in the folds of the baby's diaper area. There may be "satellite" areas apart from the main rash, and the rash may appear scaly. Another difference is that a yeast rash will not respond to typical remedies like frequent cleaning and the usual diaper rash creams. For treatment, see page 196.

Nipple dermatitis. A slight reddening and a burning feeling in the nipples, in the absence of thrush or another underlying skin condition, may indicate dermatitis. Nipple dermatitis can result from bacterial growth on the nipples or an allergy or sensitivity to a nipple cream or oil, laundry detergent, or fabric softener.

Common offenders are vitamin E preparations—oils, creams, or capsules. Mothers allergic to chocolate may develop an allergic reaction to preparations with cocoa butter, such as Balm Barr. Unmodified lanolin can also cause an allergic response, usually in a mother who is allergic to wool (from which lanolin comes) or very sensitive to it. Lanolin is found in pure hydrous and anhydrous forms and in many commercial creams, such as Massé breast cream, Mammol ointment, Eucerin, and A+D ointment. Modified lanolin, which has had the allergenic component removed, seldom causes allergic reactions.

Simply discontinuing use of the cream or oil, or switching to hypoallergenic detergents (free of perfumes and dyes), may bring relief, but usually additional measures are necessary.

Treatment Measures for Nipple Dermatitis

1. You might try using Dr. Jack Newman's APNO on your nipples for several days (see page 198). If that doesn't help or you can't get your doctor to prescribe for you, try to locate a dermatologist.

2. If you don't know a local dermatologist you may be able to find one by contacting a lactation consultant. Usually, a moderate- or high-strength anti-inflammatory cream and an antibiotic cream are prescribed.

3. Apply the medication to the irritated areas after every other nursing with clean hands, making sure your nipples are completely dry first. Apply the cream sparingly so that all of it is absorbed. If you see traces on your nipples when you are ready to nurse again, you are using too much. Dab the area with a tissue to absorb the excess.

4. Use the medication for as long as advised by your doctor. Although the pain may be gone in a day or two, the dermatitis may take from one to two weeks to completely heal.

5. Should you find that the medication aggravates your soreness, stop using it immediately. This may indicate that yeast is present and should be treated (see page 195, Thrush Nipple).

6. Place cool, wet compresses on the nipples after nursing.

7. Review page 88, General Comfort Measures for Sore Nipples.

Breast Pain

Occasionally mothers complain of pain inside the breasts while nursing. You may feel pain in your breasts if you become engorged, which usually happens two to four days after delivery (see page 77, Engorged Breasts). If your nipples are burning and pinker than normal, see page 92, Irritated Nipples. If you feel a mild aching at the start of nursing, it may be related to the beginning of letdown.

Deep breast pains, sometimes described as "shooting," that occur soon after nursing may be related to the sudden refilling of the breast. These pains usually disappear after the first weeks of nursing. Shooting pain in the breast can also accompany plugged milk ducts (see page 201) and nipple irritation from yeast or dermatitis (see page 92).

Leaking Milk

During the early weeks of nursing, milk may drip, leak, or spray from the breasts. This is a normal sign of letdown. While the baby nurses at one breast, milk often drips or sprays from the other. Letdown, and leaking, may occur frequently and unexpectedly between nursings as well. Milk may leak during sleep. It may be stimulated by the baby's sounds, by thoughts about nursing, or by any routines associated with feeding time. A shower may stimulate letdown. Dripping, leaking, and spraying usually lessen considerably after a few weeks of nursing.

Some mothers' breasts do not leak and many don't feel letdown sensations. Women who have nursed previously may notice that their breasts leak less with subsequent children. Both of these situations are usually normal.

Coping Measures for Leaking Milk

1. While nursing, open both bra flaps and let the milk drip onto a small towel or diaper.

2. Change cloth or disposable nursing pads as soon as they become wet.

3. Try silicone LilyPadz (see Appendix A, page 386), which don't absorb milk but instead apply a gentle pressure on the nipple to help prevent leakage.

4. Avoid routine use of plastic breast shells if you do not need them to improve the shape of your nipples. They may keep your clothes dry, but they can cause excessive leaking and keep your nipples moist. Milk collected in the shells between nursings may be unsafe for feeding unless if the shells are washed just prior to nursing and put in place during nursing can the milk be stored for later feedings.

5. There are some products that can be worn on one side while the baby nurses from the other for the purpose of collecting this "drip" milk. See page 251, Milkies On-the-Go Milk Savers.

6. If you want to collect milk, the soft, pliable and inexpensive "Haakaa" breast pump when squeezed is another way to get "drip milk" on the side not being nursed on or pumped. See page 312.

7. Don't try to control leaking by habitually pumping your breasts in addition to nursing. Frequent pumping actually stimulates greater milk production and could make your breasts fuller and more prone to leaking.

8. If your breasts leak during the night, place extra cloth or disposable pads in your bra or use silicone pads. Or simply spread a bath towel over the bed sheet to keep it and your mattress dry.

Letdown Difficulty

During the early weeks of breastfeeding, the letdown response is developing. Sometimes mothers are told that they must be happy, relaxed, and carefree for the letdown of milk to occur. If this were the case, few women would ever succeed at nursing. Although many mothers worry that their milk won't be available as needed, letdown failure is extremely rare among women who nurse regularly and often.

For the establishment and maximal functioning of the letdown reflex, nurse the baby every two to three hours around the clock during the first week. Make sure that she is positioned correctly and is compressing the ducts beneath the areola, and that her feeding time is not limited. Ideally, the baby should be allowed—encouraged, if necessary—to drain one or both breasts well at each feeding.

It is important to try to make yourself as comfortable as possible for feedings. The milk may not release completely if you are experiencing much pain—whether from sore nipples or from the trauma of delivery. Taking a mild pain reliever such as acetaminophen (Tylenol) or ibuprofen (Motrin, Advil) a half hour or so prior to nursing may help.

The signs of milk release (letdown) during the first week will vary for each woman. They may include:

- mild uterine cramping during nursing;
- increased vaginal flow during nursing;
- dripping, leaking, or spraying of milk, especially during nursing;
- occasional sensations in the breast during nursing;
- softening of the breasts after nursing; and
- increased thirst.

The most reliable indicator of milk letdown is the baby's swallowing. As the milk releases, the baby will swallow after every one or two sucks. Most women, particularly first-time mothers, do not feel the letdown reflex during the first few weeks after birth.

Usually when a mother believes she is experiencing a letdown difficulty, the problem is actually with the baby's latch-on or sucking or with a low milk supply, (see page 97, Difficult Latch-on; page 218, Refusal to

Nurse; page 119, Tongue-tie; page 114, Sucking Problems; and page 125, Underfeeding and Weight Loss).

Milk Appearance

Whereas colostrum is usually clear, yellow, or orange, mature breast milk is white, sometimes with a bluish tint. If it resembles skim milk from the dairy, this does not mean your milk is "weak"; breast milk normally looks thin. Occasionally a mother discovers that her milk is green, blue, or pink. Such coloring is due to her intake of vegetables, fruits, food dyes, or dietary supplements and is not harmful to the baby.

Blood in the milk can usually be traced to a bleeding nipple. Occasionally, bleeding from the breast occurs during pregnancy or when breastfeeding begins. Frequently, a benign papilloma is the cause, and the bleeding generally stops within several days. Blood in the milk will not hurt the baby, though substantial amounts may make him vomit and lead to dark spots in the stool. If you are advised against nursing, pump for a few days. The problem will clear up on its own in a day or so.

Difficult Latch-on: Flat, Dimpled, or Inverted Nipples

Both mother and baby get frustrated when latching on to the breasts is difficult because of flat, dimpled, or inverted nipples. Typically, the problem is intensified if the breasts become engorged or overly full. When they do, even nipples that protruded before may suddenly flatten or dimple. Frequently, one nipple proves to be more troublesome than the other. Persistence and patience help most mothers through this problem.

Mothers with problem nipples are often more prone to soreness. This is because they tend to focus simply on getting the baby latched on rather than on getting the baby latched on well, with the nipple deep in the baby's mouth. A poor latch can lead to nipple soreness and even injury.

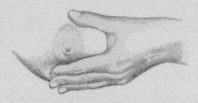 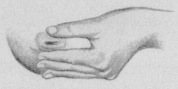

To help the baby latch on to an inverted nipple, place your thumb above the areola and your fingers below, and push your breast against your chest wall.

Don't squeeze your thumb and forefinger together, or the nipple may invert further.

Treatment Measures for Flat, Dimpled, or Inverted Nipples

1. Put the baby to the breast within the first two hours after birth. The timing of the first nursing may be critical when the nipples are flat, dimpled, or inverted. Many babies are able to latch on easily to problem nipples during this initial period, and they continue to do well.

2. To help the baby latch on to a flat nipple, make it stand out by pinching, stroking, or rolling it between your thumb and forefinger. Pinching a dimpled or inverted nipple could invert it further. To help the baby latch on to an inverted or dimpled nipple, place your thumb 1½ to 2 inches (3.8 to 5.1 cm) behind the nipple, with your fingers beneath, and pull back toward your chest. The crossover or football hold will allow you the most visibility and control.

3. Express a few drops of colostrum or milk onto your nipple or onto the baby's lips if he is reluctant to latch.

4. Stop nursing if the baby is frantic. Realize that latching when you have flat, dimpled or inverted nipples may be a work in progress.

5. If a nurse or another helper is working with you, try using the side-lying position—or, if you're large-breasted, the football hold—to allow your helper maximum visibility and control. If your nipples are dimpled or inverted, ask the helper to pull back on the breast behind the nipple rather than pinching it. Sometimes these sessions become intense and upsetting, so let your helper know when you or your baby needs a break. If you are in the hospital, let a variety of nurses or lactation professionals work with you; you can usually find one or two who are exceptionally skilled and sensitive.

6. If your baby has not latched after several attempts, hand expression and/or pumping is important to initiate milk production. Until your baby can latch, a clinical-grade rental pump is usually the best choice for collecting milk and improving the nipple shape. Before the milk comes in, you may be able to collect even more colostrum by manually expressing it. You can read about manual expression and pumping in Chapter 5, page 240. You can also learn the technique of hand expression from a lactation consultant or by viewing a helpful video made by Dr. Jane Morton of Stanford University at http://newborns.stanford.edu/Breastfeeding/HandExpression.html. Another great video from lactation consultant Maya Bolman can be seen at http://bfmed-neo.com/resources/videos.

7. Continue putting the baby to breast at most feedings.

8. Try to avoid giving the baby an artificial nipple of any kind for the first couple of days. Whether or not your baby has succeeded at latching on at first try, this may be very important. An artificial nipple can make his subsequent attempts at the breast more difficult. Options for feeding a newborn manually expressed or pumped colostrum include a dropper, a spoon, a syringe, and a soft cup.

9. Many mothers consider using a nipple shield when they have trouble getting their babies to latch on to the breast. A nipple shield is a thin, clear, soft silicone cover worn over the nipple. Holes at the tip allow milk to flow to the baby. When you use a shield, your baby may latch on and suck, but the sinuses behind the areola may not be adequately compressed unless the shield is the right size for both your nipple and the baby's mouth and the baby is well latched on to the breast and not just the shaft of the shield.

If you want to try using a nipple shield to make your nipples stand out, wait until a day or so after the birth, to give the baby a chance to learn to latch on without the shield and for your milk to come in. When using a shield, take it off after the baby has sucked for one to two minutes, and try to get him to latch on without it. Pumping just before nursing may work just as well as a nipple shield in making the nipples stand out. Use a nipple shield throughout feedings only if your milk is in and either (1) a lactation professional determines the correct shield size and makes sure that the baby is taking enough milk while you're wearing the shield, or (2) you use a clinical-grade rental pump after each nursing to guarantee that your breasts are being well emptied. Also have the baby weighed every couple of days to make sure he is gaining at least an ounce a day after the fifth day of life.

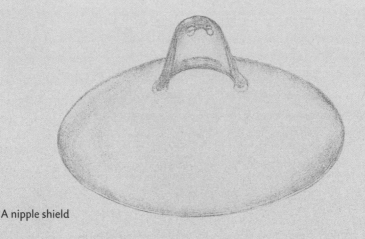

A nipple shield

10. If you and your baby are discharged from the hospital before nursing has occurred, locate a clinical-grade rental pump (see Appendix A, page 386) and use it at least eight times a day. Most hospital lactation staff members can tell you where you can get one. (See Chapter 5, page 242, for guidelines on pumping, and refer to Appendix B, page 396, for the approximate amount of milk your baby needs at each feeding.) Keep trying to nurse; at least three or four short practice sessions per day, on a soft breast when the baby is not frantic, should eventually pay off.

11. If you become engorged when your milk comes in, soften the areola by pressing on it, as described on page 78. You can also try wearing breast shells in your bra for at least a half hour before nursing; this is often essential for dimpled or inverted nipples. Many hospital maternity units have breast shells. If yours doesn't, send your partner or a friend to a maternity shop or lactation clinic to purchase a pair. Also consider purchasing Supple cups for inverted nipples. See Appendix A for purchasing information. Lastly, you can briefly pump your breasts just before nursing to pull the nipples out enough for the baby to encourage latch.

If your baby continues to be unable to latch, there may come a time when it is best to begin feeding your milk by bottle. This may be when milk production begins and if it becomes too time-consuming to feed using other methods. In this situation, you may need a great deal of support and encouragement. Finding this support will make all the difference. Seeing a lactation professional may be very helpful. Remember that most insurance companies are required to cover lactation visits under the Affordable Care Act.

It is very common for a baby to suddenly latch on one day, (usually by four to six weeks) rewarding his mother's persistence.

Fatigue and Depression

During this first week, make your life as simple as possible. Your partner or helper is essential to your recovery and adjustment. He or she can be most helpful in assuring your rest by taking over family and household duties and limiting phone calls and visitors.

Rest is necessary to your ability to cope during the postpartum period. Make a commitment to take at least one nap a day, to make up for sleep lost in labor and afterward. You may find that you are able to sleep better during naps and at night if you tuck the baby in with you. Babies often sleep better this way, too.

Turn off your cell phone or mute it. Encourage friends and relatives to leave messages or texts.

Eat a good breakfast; perhaps your partner can prepare it for you. If you lack an appetite at mealtimes, frequent snacking throughout the day on high-protein foods will assist your recovery and help maintain your energy level. Drink fluids to thirst.

If you have had tearing or an episiotomy, or if you have hemorrhoids, take a couple of baths each day or use a portable sitz bath. You can purchase a sitz bath that fits over any toilet rim, inexpensively from a large pharmacy or medical equipment company for about $12. Warm water is soothing and relaxing, and it will speed the healing of your perineum.

Don't expect to adjust to new parenthood on your own. Reach out for help or reassurance whenever you need it. Friends or relatives might welcome the opportunity to come and help out for a while, and you should feel free to call the hospital staff, a public health nurse, your childbirth instructor, or a breastfeeding counselor whenever you need assistance, reassurance, or support.

If you feel tired and overwhelmed, try not to keep it to yourself. Let your partner know; a good cry on someone's shoulder may leave you feeling much better. Avoid making your partner the target of your fears and anger. Instead of criticizing, let them know exactly what you need. One mother put it very well: "I just need him to give me hugs and let me know I'm doing okay." Your partner, after all, may be feeling as much stress as you are.

If you are alone with your baby during this first week, make a special effort to limit your activities. Perhaps you can have a friend come by to fix you lunch. Let the dishes soak all day, and tidy up the house for only ten minutes at a time, if you must.

Feeling depressed over a birth experience is not uncommon. You may be able to resolve some of your feelings by talking to your childbirth instructor or birth attendant. In a week or two, you might try to locate a postpartum or cesarean support group.

CONCERNS ABOUT THE BABY

Sleepy Baby

Many babies are sleepy during the first several days after birth. They may be so sleepy that they refuse to wake for nursing or fall asleep after just a few minutes of sucking. Sleepiness during the first few days may be related in part to recovery following labor and delivery. Pain medications and general anesthetics given to the mother during the birth process also lessen the baby's wakefulness and interest in nursing. When newborns are wrapped snugly, too, they usually sleep for long periods of time (that's why nurses bundle them tightly).

Although it may seem unkind, after the first twenty-four hours the sleepy baby should be wakened and fed at least every two and a half hours (measured from the start of one nursing to the start of the next) during the day and evening, and every three to four hours in the night. The sleepy baby needs a "mother-led" rather than a "baby-led" schedule until she begins waking on her own. This is necessary not only for her nutritional well-being but also to ensure milk production and supply. Frequent feedings will also help minimize jaundice.

Treatment Measures for the Sleepy Baby

1. While in the hospital, take advantage of the baby's normal sleeping and waking cycles by keeping her with you as much as possible.

2. Avoid supplements and pacifiers, which may decrease the baby's vigor at the breast.

3. Before attempting to nurse, wake the baby. Unwrap and undress her down to the diaper. Dim any bright lights, and sit the baby up on your lap by holding her under her chin. While talking to the baby, gently rub or pat her back (you may get a burp). Or place her against your bare chest and wait for her to begin rooting.

4. If the baby falls back asleep soon after latching on, massage or compress your breast to encourage more milk flow (see page 61). Babies are more vigorous at the breast when they are receiving milk.

5. Try the side-lying position; babies tend to nurse for longer periods in this position (get assistance, if needed, to help the baby latch on). The football hold can also be helpful in keeping a baby awake, although it may not be as effective as side-lying with a helper.

6. Burp the baby after nursing at one breast to encourage her to take the other. Sitting the baby up in your lap and bending her slightly forward usually works best. If you don't get a burp after a couple of minutes, there is probably none to be had. Change her diaper if needed.

7. If all else fails, try again in an hour.

8. Alert your physician if your baby is very lethargic and cannot be roused by the preceding techniques.

Bowel Movements

Your baby's first few stools are called meconium. Meconium is black, greenish-black, or dark brown, and it is tarry or sticky. By the second or third day, after several good colostrum feedings, the baby will have passed most of the meconium. He may have a few greenish-brown or brownish-yellow transitional stools.

Once milk production is established and the baby is nursing well, stools take on their characteristic yellow or mustard color. This usually occurs by the fifth day, unless the baby is jaundiced and receiving phototherapy, which makes the stools dark, or is not getting enough milk. Yellow stools by the fifth day are usually a sign that the baby is getting sufficient milk.

During the early days most babies have at least two bowel movements daily. The stools of a breastfed baby are generally the consistency of yogurt. They are soft or even runny, and they may appear curdled or seedy. This is not diarrhea. These stools have a sweet or cheesy odor.

Your baby may pass his stools easily, or he may fuss, grunt, and turn red in the face while having a bowel movement. This is not constipation. Constipation is not likely as long as your baby is totally breastfed.

If your baby doesn't have bowel movements every day, or if by the fifth day his stools are still dark, he may not be getting enough milk. See page 125, Underfeeding and Weight Loss, for more information on determining if your baby is getting enough.

Jaundice

A yellowing of the skin and eyes, jaundice is caused by bilirubin, a yellow pigment that is present to some degree in all blood. The skin becomes yellowish when the amount of bilirubin is higher than normal.

Bilirubin comes from the breakdown of red blood cells. These cells live only a short time; as they are destroyed, bilirubin is made. Bilirubin is then processed through the liver and finally eliminated in the stool. During pregnancy, the mother's liver processes bilirubin for the baby. After birth, the baby's liver has to begin doing the job. This usually takes a few days. Until the baby's liver is able to process bilirubin, it may increase in the baby's blood. This normal rise is referred to as physiologic jaundice. This is the most common form of jaundice, and about 40 percent of all babies develop it. It is usually noticed on the second or third day of life, and it generally disappears by one week of age.

Mild to moderate jaundice of this type will not hurt a baby, although many parents worry about it. However, the baby who nurses poorly or not at all during the first few days may become jaundiced from the lack of colostrum, which is important for the elimination of meconium. When meconium is retained in the bowel longer than usual, bilirubin cannot be eliminated as needed. The best way to treat this jaundice is to make sure the baby gets plenty of colostrum and breast milk (see page 125, Underfeeding and Weight Loss).

Some babies develop jaundice for other reasons. One type of jaundice, ABO incompatibility, occurs when the mother's blood type is O and the baby's blood type is A, B, or AB. During pregnancy, maternal antibodies cross the placenta, break down red blood cells, and cause more bilirubin to be produced in the baby after birth. On the first or second day after delivery, the bilirubin level may rise rapidly. Other, less common blood incompatibilities also produce elevated bilirubin levels. Babies of Asian descent typically experience higher bilirubin levels.

Babies with any bruises resulting from the birth process commonly develop jaundice. Jaundice is also more prevalent with vacuum and forceps deliveries. Also more prone to jaundice are babies who are sick right after birth or born prematurely, at low birth weight, or to diabetic mothers. Twins, too, are especially susceptible. Some drugs that are used during labor, including Pitocin (see page 23), can also cause jaundice.

Another type of jaundice, common only to breastfed newborns, is known as breast-milk jaundice. It occurs in approximately one-third of all nursing babies, generally on the fifth day after birth. Breast-milk jaundice usually lasts four to six weeks but can continue for as long as eight to ten weeks. When a baby's skin stays yellow beyond the first week, breast-milk jaundice is diagnosed by laboratory tests to rule out other forms of jaundice. Breastfeeding need not be interrupted to make this diagnosis. The exact cause of this jaundice is still unknown, but it has never been known to cause any problem for a baby.

If your baby looks jaundiced, the doctor may order tests to measure the level of bilirubin in the blood and determine whether treatment is necessary. If the baby was born at term and is otherwise healthy, many doctors will not order treatment unless the bilirubin level is over 20 milligrams per deciliter. Frequent breastfeeding may be all that is necessary.

Some jaundiced babies are treated with phototherapy. The "bili-lights," along with frequent nursing, help to destroy excess bilirubin. The baby usually lies under these lights from two to four days, her eyes covered with a protective mask.

Often the bilirubin level will stay constant for twenty-four hours but drop by forty-eight hours. The treatment is discontinued as soon as the bilirubin level has dropped to a normal level. Usually a baby is hospitalized for phototherapy, but in some communities home phototherapy services are available.

Rarely, usually in cases of blood incompatibility, the bilirubin climbs rapidly to high levels. On these occasions, an exchange transfusion may be done to reduce the bilirubin. Over an hour or two, small amounts of the baby's blood are taken out and replaced with donated blood.

Some doctors ask the mother to stop breastfeeding temporarily whenever a baby becomes jaundiced. However, breastfeeding is usually one of the most effective ways of eliminating jaundice.

Mothers are also commonly told that their nursing babies need water supplements to help get rid of jaundice. But water supplements do not lower the level of bilirubin in the blood. Some studies suggest, in fact, that water supplements are associated with higher bilirubin levels. In addition, babies who are routinely given water tend to be nursed less frequently, and they have a higher rate of early weaning.

Since 1994, the AAP has recommended a different approach: Healthy, full-term babies over seventy-two hours old with bilirubin levels below 20 milligrams per deciliter (or 340 micromoles per liter) should be nursed frequently, at least eight times every twenty-four hours, and should receive no water supplements.

Treatment Measures for Jaundice

1. Let the baby's physician know you prefer to continue nursing throughout the period of jaundice.

2. Nurse frequently, ideally every two to two and a half hours, and encourage the baby to suck for at least fifteen to twenty minutes at each breast. If your baby needs phototherapy, taking her from under the bili-light for these feedings will not delay the

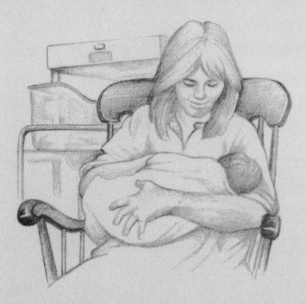

Nurse often during phototherapy; taking the baby from under the bili-light for feedings will not slow her recovery from jaundice.

effectiveness of treatment. Intermittent phototherapy is thought to be as effective as continuous exposure.

3. If your baby is sleepy, as jaundiced babies sometimes are, see page 103, Sleepy Baby, for effective measures to wake her for feedings.

4. Avoid water supplements, as these do not reduce bilirubin levels and may discourage the baby from nursing frequently.

5. To be sure your baby is getting enough milk, keep track of her bowel movements. She should have at least two each day, and preferably three or more. She should have lost less than 10 percent of her birth weight, and she should gain an ounce a day after the fifth day. If she isn't gaining this much, refer to page 125, Underfeeding and Weight Loss.

6. If you are still hospitalized or you are welcome to stay in a hospital room while your baby is being treated, ask the nurses if you can have the baby's crib and light set up next to your bed so you can care for the baby and nurse frequently.

7. If you cannot stay twenty-four hours a day with your baby, express your milk every three hours using a clinical-grade rental pump (see Chapter 5, page 242, for advice on pumping). Take your milk to the hospital for the feedings you will miss.

8. If your doctor is firm in his or her desire for you to temporarily stop nursing, again, express your milk every three hours to keep up your supply. Freeze your milk, and save it for later.

9. If you are struggling to get your baby to latch on, you may find that she becomes upset even when you bring her near your breast. In this situation, you may begin to think that your baby does not want to nurse. Nothing could be further from the truth. If your baby cries at the breast and seems unwilling to try to latch on, know that she is simply frustrated. She is crying because she wants to latch on and suck but isn't getting the signal she needs. She cannot feel your nipple far enough back in her mouth.

Difficult Latch-on: Refusal to Nurse

Latch-on problems can originate either with the baby or with the mother. Some babies fail to latch on well because they are sleepy (see page 103, Sleepy Baby). Many babies struggle to latch on when the breast becomes overly full or engorged (see page 77, Engorged Breasts), when the mother and baby are not positioned well for latch-on, or when the mother has flat, dimpled, or inverted nipples (see page 97, Difficult Latch-on: Flat, Dimpled, or Inverted Nipples). Problems other than these are as follows.

The baby who has nursed earlier. During the first week, a baby who has already nursed may suddenly refuse one or both sides. He may simply act uninterested although he is awake, or he may become upset when put to one or both breasts. This may be because he has been given a bottle or pacifier during the first week and has developed a preference for an artificial nipple. Such a baby will likely start nursing again after a few hours uncoaxed or after one or more of the following measures are taken.

Treatment Measures for the Baby Who Stops Nursing

1. If you are overly full or engorged, soften the areola by pressing it (see page 78) or by manually expressing or pumping a little milk (see Chapter 5, page 242) just before putting the baby to breast.

2. If the baby is frantic, calm him. A few drops of colostrum or hand expressed milk given by dropper on their lips or over the nipple may alert and encourage them. Occasionally, a very upset baby may need to be tightly swaddled in a thin blanket.

3. Pay attention to proper positioning (see page 52, Positioning at the Breast). When the baby turns his face from side to side with his mouth wide open, pull him in closer so the nipple is aimed toward the roof of his mouth.

4. Try letting the baby suck on your finger for a few seconds just before putting him to breast.

5. Persist. The baby who is hiccuping, having a bowel movement, or staring at his mother or something else interesting will usually be reluctant to latch on. Try again in an hour or so.

6. Coax the baby who is suddenly refusing one breast by using the football hold on that side.

7. If you can't get the baby latched on, express your milk until you can, using a clinical-grade rental pump. This may be crucial to bringing in your milk supply and to maintaining high production. Refer to Chapter 5, page 242, for information on pumping milk, and Appendix B, page 396, for the approximate amounts of milk a baby needs at each feeding.

8. Get a lot of support and encouragement until the issues are resolved. See a lactation professional.

The baby who refuses one side. Some babies latch easily to one side but refuse the other. This may happen when one nipple is more difficult for her because of the nipple size or shape (see page 97, Difficult Latch-on: Flat, Dimpled, or Inverted Nipples). Some babies may feel uncomfortable lying on one side. This can happen when a baby has a fairly common condition known as torticollis. Torticollis can be present at birth or take up to three months to develop, and most doctors believe it could be related to abnormal positioning of the fetus inside the uterus. Because the position of the jaw in utero, jaw asymmetry is often associated with this condition, making latch difficult. This condition puts pressure on a baby's sternocleidomastoid muscle, the large muscle that runs on both sides of the neck from the back of the ears to the collarbone. Extra pressure on one side of this muscle can cause it to tighten, making it difficult for a baby to turn his neck. Babies with torticollis will act like most other babies except when it comes to activities that involve turning. A baby with torticollis keeps his head in one direction when lying down and tilts the head in just one direction, and has difficulty nursing on one side. If you think your baby might have torticollis, ask your doctor to examine your baby, which involves seeing how far your baby can turn his head. If a diagnosis is made, the doctor will probably teach you neck stretching exercises to practice with your baby at home. These exercises help loosen the tight muscle and strengthen the weaker one on the opposite side. This will help to straighten out your baby's neck. In certain cases, the doctor may suggest taking your baby to a physical therapist for more intensive treatment. In the meantime, you may need to position your baby differently—for instance, using the football hold—for him to be able to latch on to the breast.

The baby who has not yet nursed. If a day or more has passed since the baby's birth and she still has not managed to latch on and suck, she may have one of the specific problems described as follows.

Recessed jaw. Some babies are born with a very recessed lower jaw. This can best be seen by looking at the baby's face in profile. A recessed jaw is problematic because a baby can latch on only if her chin reaches the breast before her upper lip; otherwise she can't take enough breast tissue into her mouth.

When you try to get a baby like this to latch on, make sure your breast isn't overly full. Extend the baby's head slightly backward as you bring her onto the breast so that her chin touches the breast first. A baby with a recessed jaw will probably begin latching on and sucking between four and six weeks of age. In the meantime, you may need to pump your milk and feed it to your baby by bottle. As a last resort, you may find a silicone nipple shield helpful to sustain the latch. (See Appendix for locating silicone nipple shield.)

Tongue-tied. Some infants who can't latch on to the breast are tongue-tied. This means that the frenulum, or string-like tissue that attaches to the underside of the tongue, is so short or connected so close to the tip of the tongue that the baby may not be able to extend, elevate, or lateralize his tongue to remove milk from the breast. Although he may be able to suck on a finger or rubber nipple that extends well into his mouth, he may be unable to grasp the underside of his mother's nipple. Not only does he fail to get milk, but nursing may be very painful for his mother even when the baby is correctly positioned. Sometimes a clicking sound can be heard as the baby sucks. Occasionally a tongue-tied baby can manage to latch on to one breast but not the other (see page 119, Tongue-tie in Sucking Problems).

Protruding tongue. A few babies have tongues that protrude. The tongue may look longer than normal; it may be visible between the lips much of the time. Some mothers have described the protruding tongue as forming a hump in the mouth that the nipple is not able to get past.

You may be able to teach the baby to nurse by encouraging her to open wide with her tongue down and pulling back behind the areola just before latch-on. The football hold is recommended for the best visibility and control.

If you manage to get the baby onto the breast, be sure she is sucking adequately. This means she does not come off the breast easily; she is taking long, drawing sucks; and she is audibly swallowing.

Tongue sucking. Other infants who have difficulty latching on to the breast are those who suck their own tongues. These babies usually slide off the nipple after one or two sucks, and their cheeks dimple with each suck. They may also make clicking noises. When the baby opens her mouth to root or to cry, you may notice that her tongue is far back in her mouth or is curled toward the roof of her mouth.

Attempt to get the baby to latch on only when she opens wide with her tongue down. Stimulating the lower lip or slightly depressing the chin may help the tongue to drop. Pull the baby in close. The crossover or football hold is best when you are alone, and side-lying will give more control and visibility when someone is assisting you.

When refusal persists. If you have followed the preceding suggestions and your baby still has not latched on, try the following measures.

Treatment Measures for Refusal to Latch

1. Work with the baby in short, frequent sessions. If someone is assisting you, the side-lying position may give the greatest control and visibility. These sessions may become intense and upsetting for both you and the baby, so let your helper know if you need a break. If you are in the hospital, ask for help from various nurses or lactation professionals. You may find one or two who are exceptionally skilled and sensitive.

2. Encourage your baby by expressing a few drops of milk onto your nipple or onto his lips.

3. If, twenty-four hours after birth, your baby still has not latched on, begin manually expressing or pumping (see Chapter 5, page 240) and feeding the baby your expressed colostrum. But don't feed it by bottle at first; an artificial nipple of any kind could make his attempts at the breast more difficult. Express your colostrum and feed it to the baby at least eight times in each twenty-four hours. Refer to Appendix B, page 396, for the approximate amount the baby needs at each feeding. You can feed the colostrum by a soft cup, tube, medicine dropper, or syringe as your hospital lactation staff suggests.

4. Continue pumping and feeding at least eight times in each twenty-four hours.

5. If your baby "shuts down" or gets upset at the breast, let him suck on a finger, nail side down. After a minute or two, quickly offer the breast, compressing it tightly so that it extends as far as possible into the baby's mouth.

6. Pump for a few minutes just before nursing to make your nipples stand out more. Some babies latch better on a soft or half-empty breast.

7. If you use a nipple shield to help the baby latch on (see page 100), take it off after the baby has sucked for one to two minutes, and try to get him to latch on without it. Use a nipple shield throughout feedings only if your milk is in and either (1) a lactation professional has determined the correct shield size and made sure that the baby is taking enough milk while you're wearing the shield, or (2) you use a clinical-grade rental pump after each nursing to guarantee that your breasts are being well emptied, and you have the baby weighed every few days to make sure he is gaining at least an ounce a day.

8. If your baby seems to latch on but sucks only once or twice, he is probably not well attached. Take him off the breast and try again.

9. Continue short practice nursing sessions several times a day. Try to be patient but persistent; don't give up on your baby.

10. If your baby continues to refuse to nurse, there may come a time when it is best to begin feeding your pumped milk by bottle. This may be when milk production begins, if it becomes too time-consuming to feed using other methods.

11. Get a lot of support and encouragement. Ideally, see a lactation professional. Your insurance should cover this.

Many babies with latch-on problems overcome them during the first ten days, but a significant number first latch on at about one month of age. With this in mind, know that the most important thing to do until the baby finally latches is to keep your milk production as high as possible. See Chapter 5 for advice on how to do this.

Sucking Problems

Some babies seem to latch on to the breast well but suck poorly. With some, the suction is so poor that they easily slide off the breast or can be taken off effortlessly. A baby's cheeks may dimple with each suck, and frequent clicking noises may be audible. Such a baby isn't really sucking on the nipple but on her tongue, which may perhaps be a habit developed in the uterus. Other babies with poor suction may have one of the physical problems described on page 111, The Baby Who Has Not Yet Nursed. Babies with poor suction receive only the milk that drips into their mouths.

Although most babies with sucking problems have them from birth, others may develop them if they lose much weight, usually close to a pound, by the end of the first week. If this happens, and the baby cannot correct her suck after several good attempts at latching on, express your milk and feed it to her for twenty-four to seventy-two hours, supplementing breast milk with formula as necessary. After the baby is rehydrated and has regained a few ounces, she may correct her suck on her own.

A baby may have difficulty sucking at one or both breasts because he is tongue-tied. In this situation, the tongue is tethered by the short piece of tissue beneath. No matter how hard the baby tries, he may not be able to reach his tongue forward and then up far enough to strip the milk from the breast. Not only may he fail to get milk, but nursing a tongue-tied baby may be very painful for the mother, even when the baby is correctly positioned. Sometimes a clicking sound can be heard as the baby sucks. (Read more about "tongue-tie" on page 119.)

Another group of babies who have difficulty sucking and getting enough milk are those with very high palates. When the roof of the mouth is very high, the baby has trouble compressing the breast against the palate to express the milk into her mouth. Many babies with high, arched palates do little swallowing at the breast and fail to gain weight well. Few health professionals, including pediatricians, yet recognize high palates as a potential problem for nursing babies. If it is difficult to see the very top of a baby's palate without placing your head close to the baby's chest, or if the shape of the roof looks much deeper than the curve of a teaspoon, the palate may be too high. If you can get the baby to suck on your little finger (nail side down), and you feel a frequent loss of suction between your finger and his tongue, or your finger isn't in firm contact with the roof of his mouth, the palate may be too high. Another sign of a high palate may be clicking sounds while the baby is sucking.

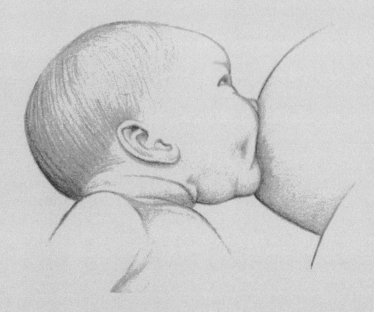

Dimpling of the baby's cheeks during nursing may signify an inadequate suck.

In the case of a high palate, the mother should use an electric pump right after each nursing to bolster her milk supply. After a few days the baby will usually start to swallow more at the breast and gain weight better, but as soon as the pumping stops, the baby may begin to take less milk and will again fail to gain sufficient weight. Usually supplemental pumping is necessary for several weeks, until the baby has grown enough to suck more efficiently. Using the football hold, or positioning the baby straddling your thigh, may help the baby suck better. Time is often the remedy for babies with sucking problems.

Lastly, babies whose mothers have large nipples—as large as or larger than a quarter—may be unable to suck effectively. Instead of latching on to the areola, behind the nipple, the baby compresses only the nipple itself, and so gets very little milk. In this case the mother needs to express her milk, using a clinical-grade rental pump, to build and maintain high production until the baby has grown enough to latch on to and compress the breast, not just the nipple. The mother will also need to obtain a large flange for effective pumping (see page 256).

Treatment Measures for the Baby with Poor Sucking

1. Remove the baby from the breast as soon as the faulty suck is evident.

2. Using the crossover or football hold, compress the breast behind the nipple, and pull the baby in as close as possible for latch-on.

3. Work with the baby in short, frequent sessions. If someone is assisting you, the side-lying position may give the greatest control and visibility. These sessions may become intense and upsetting for both you and the baby, so let your helper know if you need a break.

4. If twenty-four hours after birth or even sooner your baby still is not sucking well, begin manually expressing or pumping (see Chapter 5, page 240) and feeding the baby your expressed colostrum. You can feed the colostrum to the baby using a soft cup, syringe, or dropper and refrigerate any of the pumped milk for later use during the first few days of life. Refer to Appendix B, page 396, for the approximate amount the baby needs at each feeding.

5. Pump every two to three hours for fifteen to twenty minutes with a double collection kit, ideally eight times each twenty-four hours. If you don't have a double collection kit, pump each side twice or more, for a total pumping time of twenty to thirty minutes. In addition, use manual expression for a short period after pumping, to empty the breast thoroughly (see Chapter 5, page 242). This should insure that you'll have an abundant milk supply sooner even if your baby's sucking is ineffective. Refrigerate any of the pumped milk for later use during the first few days of life.

6. If you use a nipple shield to help the baby latch on (see page 100), take it off after the baby has sucked for one to two minutes, and try to get him to latch on without it. Use a nipple shield throughout feedings only if your milk is in and either (1) a lactation professional has determined the correct shield size and made sure that the baby is taking enough milk while you're wearing the shield, or (2) you use a clinical-grade rental pump after each nursing to guarantee that your breasts are being well emptied,

and you have the baby weighed every few days to make sure he is gaining at least an ounce a day.

7. When your milk comes in, try manual expressing or pumping a small amount of milk just before attempting to nurse. Some babies may do better on a soft or half-empty breast.

8. If you use a nipple shield to help the baby latch on (see page 100), take it off after the baby has sucked for one to two minutes, and try to get him to latch on without it. Use a nipple shield throughout feedings only if your milk is in and either (1) a lactation professional has determined the correct shield size and made sure that the baby is taking enough milk while you're wearing the shield, or (2) you use a clinical-grade rental pump after each nursing to guarantee that your breasts are being well emptied, and you have the baby weighed every few days to make sure he is gaining at least an ounce a day.

9. Continue short practice nursing sessions a few times a day. Try to be patient but persistent; don't give up on your baby.

10. If your baby continues to have sucking problems, there may come a time when it is best to begin feeding your pumped milk by bottle. This may be when milk production begins, if it becomes too time-consuming to feed using other methods.

11. If you are discharged from the hospital and the baby still isn't nursing well, find a clinical-grade rental pump (see page 245) for collecting your milk. The hospital staff will probably know where to get a rental pump. Continue pumping your milk and feeding it to the baby at least eight times in each twenty-four hours.

12. Get a lot of support and encouragement. Make an appointment to see a lactation professional. Your insurance carrier should cover visits with a lactation consultant for you and your baby.

Like babies with latch-on problems, those with sucking problems often overcome them during the first ten days, but many improve later at about four to six weeks of age. With this in mind, know that the most important thing to do until the baby finally overcomes the problem is to keep your milk production as high as possible. See Chapter 5 for advice on how to do this.

Tongue-tie

Tongue-tie, also known as ankyloglossia, is the condition in which the tongue is bound to the floor of the mouth by the frenulum or string-like tissue that attaches to the underside of the tongue. This restricts the ability of the tongue to move both forward and upwards toward the roof of the mouth, an action important in latching, sucking, and other functions.

It is believed that as many as up to 12 percent of newborns are born with some degree of tongue-tie. Boys are affected much more often than girls, and it is believed to be a congenital condition. An upper lip-tie may often be present, as well.

Some babies with severe tongue-ties may have speech problems later on. Certain letters are difficult to make if the tongue can't move to all areas of the mouth like "d," "l," "n," "r," "s," "t," and "z" sounds. Tongue-tie may also make it hard for him to stick out his tongue, lick an ice cream, play an instrument, or French kiss. While these may not seem like important skills to you as a new mother, someday they could be very important to your child. Dental development may also be affected. Lip-tie can sometimes cause a gap between the front teeth.

But, more importantly, a tongue-tie may impact the baby's ability to latch and feed effectively. Although the tongue-tied baby may be able to suck on a finger, an artificial nipple, or a nipple shield that extends well into his mouth, some tongue-tied babies may be unable to grasp the underside of his mother's nipple to latch. Occasionally, a tongue-tied baby can manage to latch on to one breast but not the other.

Often, tongue-ties go unrecognized even by a baby's doctor. And feeding difficulties due to tongue-tie can lead to the end of breastfeeding for all too many mothers.

In order to effectively get milk from the breast, the baby needs to move his tongue forward to cup the nipple and areola, drawing it back in his mouth and pressing the tissue against the roof of his mouth. Some tongue-tied babies may be able to latch on to the breast but may be unable to raise his tongue high enough to effectively express milk. The baby may get too little milk while feeding and fails to gain weight as expected. The ineffective nursing can in turn lead to developing a low milk supply.

Several feeding issues suggest the possibility of tongue-tie. Besides having difficulty latching on to the breast, some babies may end up depending on a nipple shield in order to nurse. If the newborn is able to latch, often nursing is very painful. Mothers may have nipples that become sore, cracked, and even bleeding—all due to a shallow latch. And nipple trauma may lead to mastitis. When the baby unlatches, sometimes the nipples will appear blanched and even misshaped.

Parents may be able to see the "string" of tissue leading to the tip or the underside of the tongue. The tongue may appear to be notched in the middle or to be "heart-shaped." These are known as "anterior" tongue ties. There are many photographs that can be found online that show examples of what anterior tongue-ties may look like.

Other ways to tell if your baby may have a tongue-tie is to watch his tongue to see if he can extend it beyond his lower lip. Do this while he is awake and is interested in feeding. If he cannot or you are unsure, have your baby evaluated by an experienced provider. Tongue-tied newborns may also have a tongue that appears "humped" in the back and lower in the front. Some newborns may also develop a visible white "milk tongue" in the back of the tongue. Babies who are tongue-tied may not be able to hold a pacifier in their mouth and a few may "pop" on and off the breast. Some newborns that are tongue-tied may also appear to have blistered lips from trying to compensate for their inability to form a good seal while they are on the breast.

Some tongue-tied babies may make "clicking" sounds while feeding, suggesting that the baby may be momentarily unlatching. Some mothers may even notice the baby drooling milk while he nurses.

Since these symptoms can also be caused by other reasons, it is a good idea to have the newborn evaluated by a knowledgeable healthcare provider, an IBCLC (board certified lactation consultant), if possible, to rule out causes other than tongue-tie. If breastfeeding doesn't improve, even after other measures, such as adjustments in positioning have been tried, tongue-tie should definitely be considered a possibility.

Sometimes there is no obvious tongue-tie abnormality. Even when there is no visible string of tissue below the tongue, it is possible that a baby has a "posterior" tongue-tie. This type of tie may be hidden under the mucous membrane under the tongue and is just as troublesome as, if not more than, a more visible anterior tongue-tie.

Posterior ties can be trickier to diagnose. They aren't as obvious as anterior ties, and are often missed during a visual exam. You can't see a posterior tie, but if you run your finger underneath the tongue from side to side, you may be able to feel a band of tissue under the front of the tongue.

The solution to fix a tongue-tie is simple: the frenulum should be clipped to release the tongue. Some physicians are reluctant or unwilling to perform this procedure, called a frenotomy, but more doctors and dentists are realizing the need. If your doctor does not perform the procedure, an ENT (ear, nose, and throat surgeon) or pediatric dentist often will, and it takes just a minute or two.

You can also see Dr. Jane Morton's photographs of a baby both before and after a frenotomy by following the link at http://newborns.stanford.edu/Frenotomy.html.

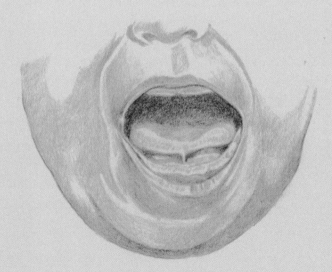

The tongue-tied baby may not be able to extend his tongue far enough or high enough to latch on to his mother's nipple.

It is thought by some experts in the field that in most cases, babies who have an anterior tie will also have a posterior tie. Clipping the more obvious anterior tie may not be enough to correct the feeding issues.

The degrees of tongue-tie range from mild to severe. An examination of the tongue by an experienced lactation professional; pediatrician; ear, nose, and throat doctor; or pediatric dentist who is experienced with this condition is usually necessary to make the diagnosis. While parents may know some of the signs suggesting a possible tongue-tie, sometimes getting a second opinion may be necessary.

Frenotomy (tongue-tie revisions) to release both anterior and/or posterior ties, are done by clipping with scissors or by laser and usually take less than a minute or two. Some pediatricians perform simple anterior tongue-tie revisions. Some pediatric dentists and ear, nose, and throat doctors perform revisions using laser treatment. Anesthesia or sutures are not necessary, although some dentists may use local pain relief. After the procedure, the baby can be soothed and nursed for comfort. Before leaving the office, the dentist or doctor may offer pain relief suggestions and any post-op care instructions, including exercises.

My own son, John, born some thirty years ago, was born severely tongue-tied. He had difficulty latching and drinking. After a couple of days, nursing was very painful, despite a good latch, and he rarely swallowed while feeding. After nursing, I then pumped and bottle-fed him. At two weeks old, I took him to see our pediatric dentist. The dentist had me sit in the dental chair holding John facing outward. It seemed to be over as soon as it began. Once snipped, I put him on the breast to comfort him, and I immediately became concerned because I could not feel him sucking at all. But soon I heard him swallowing milk.

Dr. Ghaheri of Portland, Oregon, is perhaps one of the leading experts on the diagnosis and treatment of lip and tongue-tie in the U.S. He can be found at DrGhaheri.com, which offers lots of information about tongue- and lip-tie, including photos and general information.

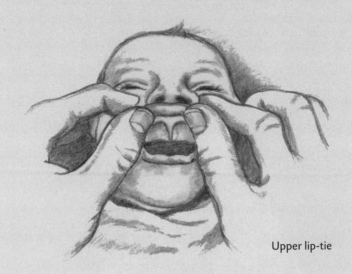

Upper lip-tie

Upper lip-tie. Some newborns are born with their upper lip "tied" to their upper gum. Usually, this poses no problems with nursings. If severe, however, it can cause the baby's upper lip to turn inward instead of outward. This may be irritating to the nipple. Few pediatricians recognize this problem, but some pediatric dentists believe that an upper lip-tie may lead to a gap between the teeth later on, can cause a problem with dental decay, and, in severe cases, can lead to trapping of food. If it seems to be causing nursing pain, an evaluation with a pediatric dentist may be in order.

Fussiness and Excessive Night Waking

It can come as a surprise when your baby suddenly becomes fussy after spending most of his first few days sleeping. It is difficult to listen to your baby's cry; it may feel like an alarm going off in your body. Sometimes parents are told it is healthy for babies to cry or that babies will become spoiled if tended to every time they fuss. But comforting your infant and responding to her needs is very important to her well-being and her development of trust. Babies are really unspoilable.

Newborns cry for a variety of reasons. Often, they are fussy during the first night home from the hospital. They may be hungry as often as every hour, especially when your milk is just starting to come in, or when feedings have been limited because of their sleepiness or for other reasons. Some babies seem to need more sucking time than others. Some seem to pass a lot of gas, which causes them discomfort. Many newborns become upset when they are not kept snugly wrapped. Perhaps they miss the close, secure feeling of the womb.

Then there are the babies who sleep most of the day and wake frequently during the night. These babies are said to have their days and nights mixed up.

Coping Measures for Fussiness

1. Nurse your baby on demand, approximately every two to three hours for at least ten to twenty minutes at each breast.

2. Massage or compress your breasts while you nurse to increase the flow of milk (see page 61).

3. Burp the baby after he finishes at each breast.

4. Wrap the baby snugly in a light blanket after each feeding.

5. Avoid water or formula supplements.

6. If the baby seems unsatisfied after a feeding, nurse him some more, or rock him or walk with him next to your body and then nurse him again in an hour or two.

7. If the baby frequently seems discontent after nursings, see page 125, Underfeeding and Weight Loss, for reassurance or steps to take.

Newborns normally wake about every three hours during the night. If your baby wakes more often than this, nurse her more often during the daytime and evening, every two to two and a half hours. If the baby has been sleeping through feeding times, wake her (see page 103, Sleepy Baby).

Your baby may be crying at night not because she is hungry but because she wants to be close to you. Try tucking her in with you for at least a few nights. You may both sleep better (see page 40, A Place to Sleep).

Underfeeding and Weight Loss

During the first week, you may wonder if your baby is getting enough to eat. You may worry about whether your milk is adequate—especially if the baby seems to be nursing all the time or is fussy after feedings. Some mothers wonder if their milk has dried up when they observe the normal softening of the breast that occurs as the initial engorgement recedes.

Seeing if the baby will take a bottle of water or formula after nursing is not a reliable method of determining if he is getting enough breast milk. Feeding water to newborn babies is never recommended. Most babies will take a couple of ounces of water or formula if it is offered, even when they have had enough milk from the breast.

A baby can lose too much weight, though, when the milk doesn't come in by the third or fourth day, when nursing is infrequent, or when he has had trouble latching on and nursing well during the period of initial engorgement. Excessive weight loss can also occur when a mother uses a nipple shield over her nipple for nursing, when a newborn has a faulty suck, and, certainly, when a baby is sick. Babies who have high palates or who are tongue-tied may fail to express milk well while nursing and thus get too little milk (see page 114, Sucking Problems). Other women who may be unable to produce enough milk are those with insufficient glandular (milk producing) tissue, or hypoplastic breasts (see page 134), and mothers who have undergone breast surgery involving an incision around the areola. This includes mothers who have undergone breast reduction surgery, some who have had breast augmentation surgery, and some with polycystic ovary syndrome (PCOS) (see page 138). Sometimes laxatives the mother has taken can cause a baby to have excessive bowel movements and to lose weight or gain too slowly.

Signs of adequate milk intake include: nursing at least eight times each twenty-four hours, nursing ten to forty-five minutes at each feeding, baby seems content after nursing, baby has several periods of swallowing during each feeding, your breasts feel softer after the baby has nursed, and the baby is stooling every day and the stools are yellow by day five. If you and your baby don't show all these signs, have him weighed as soon as possible. If you find that your baby has lost 10 percent or more of his birth weight within the first five days after birth, or if he isn't gaining an ounce per day after the fifth day, take the following measures.

Treatment Measures for Underfeeding

1. See a lactation professional. Again, your insurance provider may cover these services. Check with your individual policies.

2. To estimate the amount of milk you are producing and to increase your milk supply, obtain a clinical-grade rental breast pump (see Chapter 5, page 245). Any other pump might be inadequate for estimating milk production and rebuilding a low milk supply. This includes any pump that you may have received through your insurance company.

3. If it will be a couple of days before you are able to see a lactation consultant, you can estimate your milk production. Pump immediately after nursing the baby. If you have a double collection kit, which is ideal, pump for a total of ten to twenty minutes, or longer if the milk continues to flow. If you are pumping one breast at a time, pump each breast twice or more, for a total pumping time of twenty to thirty minutes, or longer if the milk is still flowing.

   Exactly two hours after completing this pumping, pump again instead of nursing. You may very well get less milk at this second pumping than at the first. Multiply the number of ounces collected at the second pumping by twelve. This will give you an estimate of how much milk you are producing over a twenty-four-hour period; if you collect 1½ ounces (44 ml), for example, you are producing about 18 ounces (532 ml) per day. If you determine that you have enough milk for your baby and yet she has not been gaining well, it may be that she is not taking all of the milk available at some or many of her feedings. This can happen with newborns who were born prematurely, who tend to drift off to sleep while nursing, or who have sucking difficulties. Feed your baby this pumped milk and any necessary formula. See Appendix B, page 396, to determine how much milk your baby needs per day.

4. Review the video "A Perfect Latch" recommended in Chapter 2 (see page 56) to be sure your baby is latching on well.

5. Nurse at least eight times in every twenty-four hours, even if this means waking the baby for feedings (see page 103, Sleepy Baby). Nurse for ten to fifteen minutes at each breast, or for as long as the baby is swallowing. If the baby swallows for only a few minutes, compress your breast while you are nursing (see page 61) to increase the flow. You can also switch the baby from breast to breast each time the swallowing stops.

6. If you're not producing as much milk as your baby needs, stimulate greater milk production by pumping your breasts right after each nursing. Pumping both breasts at the same time not only takes less time but is more effective in stimulating increased milk production. Use a double collection kit, if you have one, for five to ten minutes, or pump each breast separately for five minutes, and then return to each breast a second time for a few more minutes. You can also spend a few minutes hand-expressing milk from both breasts after pumping to help insure more complete emptying (see Chapter 5, page 240).

7. After pumping, feed the baby whatever breast milk you've collected, along with formula if it is necessary. If the baby needs supplemental formula (see step 3), divide the amount of supplement needed daily by the number of feedings the baby is getting each day (usually eight). A baby who needs 3½ ounces (104 ml) of formula per day, for example, should get close to ½ ounce (15 ml) after each of her eight daily nursings. The goal is to offer about the same amount of breast milk and formula at each feeding so that the baby wants to nurse at regular intervals.

8. Some mothers consider using donated breast milk from friends, relatives, or even strangers. For more information on the possible risks of using unpasteurized donated milk, see page 184.

9. Consider using herbs and/or certain foods to stimulate greater milk production (see page 84 and page 175).

10. Ignore any suggestions to drink a beer or two to help increase milk production. Drinking alcohol can in fact lessen milk production.

11. If your milk production remains low, even with the use of certain foods and herbs, consider using a pharmaceutical medication, like Domperidone, to stimulate more production (see page 87 and Appendix A, page 386).

12. As long as you must provide supplemental feedings, find a method that suits you. Many lactation professionals, fearing that bottle-feeding might interfere with the baby's ability at the breast, may suggest using a nursing supplementer (see Appendix A, page 386), a cup, a soft tube with a syringe, a finger, or an eyedropper. If one of these methods is recommended to you and it works well, good. But if you find it too frustrating or time-consuming, use a bottle. After the first few days of breastfeeding, supplementing by bottle rarely causes "nipple confusion."

13. Weigh your baby every few days to make sure that she is gaining well. After each weighing, re-estimate your baby's milk needs. Then, two hours after your most recent pumping, express your milk instead of nursing and re-estimate your milk production (see step 3). If your production has increased enough to match the baby's needs, you can decrease or even eliminate any formula supplementation. If you are seeing a lactation consultant, she will probably want to follow-up to see how the baby is doing and re-evaluate if the baby requires supplementation.

14. If you are not working with a lactation consultant, consider renting an accurate electronic baby scale (see Appendix A, page 386). Use the scale before and after feedings to determine how much milk the baby takes from the breast. One gram of weight increase is equal to one milliliter of milk intake. Thirty milliliters equals 1 ounce.

15. Once your baby is gaining well, her nursing seems more vigorous, and you are supplementing nursings only with your breast milk, you might try eliminating some of the supplement. For a few days, offer the baby only half of the milk that you are expressing, and freeze the rest. If the baby gains well over these few days, continue pumping, but don't offer her any of the expressed milk. If the baby continues to gain an ounce a day without any supplement, gradually stop pumping. Continue to have your baby weighed weekly.

If treatment fails. Although the technique just outlined will normally reverse a case of underfeeding within a few days, sometimes, when breast engorgement has been severe and little milk has been removed during this critical period, the decline in milk production can be difficult to reverse. In unusual instances, a mother fails to produce enough milk even after weeks of both stepped-up nursing and pumping. This can occur if the placenta was not completely delivered at the time of the birth (see page 80). It sometimes happens to women who have had breast surgery, particularly if the surgical incision was made around the areola (see page 138, Nursing after Breast Surgery). Other women who may be unable to produce enough milk are those with insufficient glandular (milk-producing) tissue, or hypoplastic breasts (see page 134), and some with polycystic ovary syndrome, or PCOS (see page 138).

In any of these situations, lack of support from family, friends, and health professionals can make matters worse. But even with all of the best information and support, things sometimes don't turn out as we hope. If, after giving breastfeeding your best effort, you end up having to feed formula, you have not failed as a mother. Be proud of your efforts to nurse, and concentrate on providing your baby with all of the cuddling and loving that you can. Detailed information about formula and bottle-feeding can be found in *The Nursing Mother's Guide to Weaning* (see page 423, References & Reading).

Some mothers with insufficient milk production have found that continuing to nurse with a nursing supplementer has been a rewarding experience. Others have found nursing supplementers to be cumbersome and frustrating. Another option, particularly if the baby has become frustrated at the breast, is to bottle-feed and then nurse. "Comfort nursing"—nursing just after bottle-feedings, in between bottle-feedings, or during the night—may be a pleasant experience for both mother and baby.

Many mothers struggle with breastfeeding and give up in this important first week of nursing. Sore nipples, difficulty with latch, and low milk supply are common reasons that mothers stop nursing in these early days. All too often mothers feel alone and do not have the guidance of a lactation professional or the support of family and friends. Sadly, all too many mothers suffer and/or give up on breastfeeding when seeing a board certified lactation professional might have turned things around. One study suggests that only about 65 percent of mothers who have difficulties with nursing see a lactation consultant for help.

If you or your baby are having any difficulties with feeding, make an appointment to see a board-certified lactation professional for a thorough evaluation, consultation, and a feeding plan. It can make all the difference in solving problems. A lactation consultant has accurate baby scales and can determine the baby's intake of milk and evaluate your milk supply. Her experienced eyes can identify early sucking and latch issues. Under the Affordable Care Act, lactation visits are covered benefits.

Mothers Overcoming Breastfeeding Issues, or MOBI, is an online support for mothers who want to hear the stories of other women who may not have achieved their breastfeeding goals. Most mothers who turn to MOBI (www.mobimotherhood.org) are comforted to hear the similar disappointment and grief of other mothers. MOBI also has a nice library of articles on a variety of topics.

If you do have a good milk supply, you can certainly consider pumping for a while to see if other issues can turn around. Many mothers who have struggled early on may decide to provide their babies expressed milk and decide against direct breastfeeding. Having a good milk supply, though, means you can keep your options open.

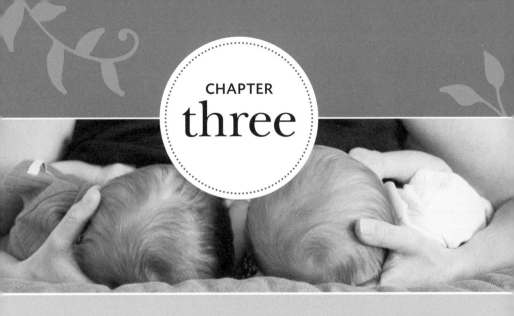

CHAPTER

three

SPECIAL SITUATIONS FOR MOTHERS AND BABIES

MOTHERS

- Infectious Conditions and Breastfeeding
- Insufficient Glandular Tissue (Breast Hypoplasia)
- Polycystic Ovary Syndrome
- Nursing after Breast Surgery
- Nursing after Gastric Bypass Surgery
- Nursing without Giving Birth
- Relactation
- Chest Feeding
- The Mother with Diabetes
- The Mother with Herpes
- The Mother with Epilepsy

- Nursing and Thyroid Conditions
- Emotional Barriers to Breastfeeding
- Maternal Substance Use and Abuse

BABIES

- Medical Reasons for Not Breastfeeding
- The Late Preterm Baby
- The Near-Term Baby
- The Very Premature or Sick Baby
- Nursing Multiples
- The Baby with Noisy Breathing (Laryngomalacia)
- The Baby with a Birth Defect
- Developmental and Neurological Problems

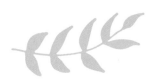

N URSING CAN BE A SPECIAL CHALLENGE in certain circumstances—situations that may result from a longstanding
condition or that may take you completely by surprise.
Either way, you may be tempted to give up the idea of
breastfeeding altogether. The specific guidelines in this chapter should
help you make a realistic appraisal of your situation and find, I hope, the
happiest solution for you and your baby.

MOTHERS

Infectious Conditions and Breastfeeding

Although most infectious conditions a mother might have pose no
harm to her nursing infant, a few are reasons to delay or even forgo
breastfeeding.

A mother with active **tuberculosis** should not breastfeed—or have
any physical contact with her baby—until treatment has been administered for one to three weeks, after which she can no longer transmit
the infection. During this period, she can express her milk to maintain
her supply, but she should discard the milk she expresses (see Chapter
5). Afterward she can safely be reunited with her infant, and she can
breastfeed.

A woman with **hepatitis** can generally breastfeed safely. If she has
viral hepatitis, also known as infectious hepatitis or hepatitis A, her baby
should be immunized with gamma globulin. If she has an active case of
hepatitis B or persistent hepatitis B surface antigen (HBsAg), her baby

should receive hepatitis B-specific immunoglobulin (HBIG) immediately after delivery. She can begin breastfeeding as soon as the shot is given, but her baby should also receive the first in a series of hepatitis B vaccines within twenty-four hours of birth. For women with hepatitis C, the Centers for Disease Control and Prevention, the AAP, and the National Institutes of Health all support breastfeeding. Although it is theoretically possible to transmit hepatitis C to a baby through breastfeeding, several research studies have shown that breastfeeding does not increase the risk of transmission. A nursing mother may be more likely to infect her baby, though, if her nipples bleed. In this situation, a mother can pump her milk (see Chapter 5) and discard it until the nipples are healed, and then breastfeeding can be resumed.

Mothers with **HIV (human immunodeficiency virus)** are discouraged from breastfeeding until more is known about the transmission of the virus.

Breastfeeding is not contraindicated for full-term infants whose mothers are seropositive for **cytomegalovirus (CMV)** as the risk for transmission through breast milk is relatively rare. There may be an association of infection for low birth weight infants, those weighing less than 1,500 grams. The AAP states that the value of feeding breast milk to low birth weight infants far outweighs the risk of illness. There has never been a reported case of long-term neurodevelopmental abnormalities in infants infected with CMV.

Freezing of milk reduces but does not eliminate CMV. Heating, either as Holder pasteurization (heating at 62.5°C (144°F) for thirty minutes) or high-temperature short pasteurization (72°C (162°F) for five to ten seconds) eliminates the viral load from the milk but also affects bioactive factors and nutrients. Thus, fresh milk from the mother is preferable for routinely feeding all preterm infants.

A mother with **herpes simplex**, in the form of either cold sores on or near the mouth or genital lesions, can nurse her baby. It is important, however, that anyone with a herpes sore take certain precautions in handling a baby to avoid transmitting the infection (see page 147, The Mother with Herpes).

Breastfeeding is also safe when a woman is infected with **toxoplasmosis**.

A mother infected with **Lyme disease** should be immediately treated, and so should her baby. The mother can breastfeed if she has begun antibiotic treatment and her baby is healthy.

Because **human T-cell lymphotropic virus type 1 and 2 (HTLV-1 and HTLV-2)** can be transmitted through breast milk, a woman infected with this virus should forgo breastfeeding. HTLV-1 is rare in North America, but it is increasingly common in other parts of the world. It is associated with the development of leukemia and lymphoma.

A woman who develops **chicken pox (varicella)** within six days before delivery should be isolated from her baby, although someone else can feed the baby the mother's expressed milk. The mother and baby can be reunited after the mother becomes noninfectious, typically after seven days.

Insufficient Glandular Tissue (Breast Hypoplasia)

Although the overwhelming majority of women are able to produce a full supply of milk for their infants, even after a setback due to infrequent nursing or inadequate sucking (see page 114), a few mothers are unable to produce enough milk for their babies. One condition that causes this is **insufficient glandular tissue (IGT)**, also known as breast hypoplasia. Perhaps because of a congenital abnormality, hypoplastic breasts contain insufficient milk-making tissue and so are typically unable to produce enough milk.

Women with IGT typically have elongated shaped breasts with a larger areola, the pigmented skin around the nipple. Some mothers have one breast that is more affected than the other. Usually the mother finds that her breasts did not enlarge during pregnancy and did not undergo any changes (such as becoming heavier or fuller or leaking milk) during the first week after delivery. Most often she has tubular breasts, with 1.5 inches (3.8 cm) or more between them—in fact, it seems to be that the greater the space, the more severe the condition. The majority of mothers with hypoplasia have one breast that is significantly smaller than the other, and most also have stretch marks on their breasts despite their lack of growth.

Many times, a mother does not realize she has insufficient glandular tissue and assumes that nursing is going well until her newborn experiences a weight loss of more than 10 percent, or he fails to gain an ounce a day after the fifth day and fails to regain his birth weight by ten to fourteen days of age. Unfortunately, many healthcare providers may not recognize this condition either.

In 2000, my colleagues and I published the results of a research study in a lactation journal for health professionals (see Appendix, References & Reading, page 423).

We worked with thirty-four women whom we suspected of having breast hypoplasia. For six weeks, we had each mother pump after every nursing and take three fenugreek capsules three times a day to try to stimulate more milk production. Many of the mothers who had mild cases of hypoplasia achieved normal milk production by six weeks postpartum, but none of the mothers with the most severe form of hypoplasia achieved adequate production.

As time went on, we added other therapies to help these mothers produce more milk. Specifically, we suggested Motherlove Herbal Company's More Milk Special Blend (a combination of fenugreek, blessed thistle, nettle leaf, fennel seed, and goat's rue) as well as Domperidone, both of which boosted the women's overall milk production in many cases.

Domperidone is not manufactured in the United States, but it can be ordered by mail (without a prescription and less expensively) from pharmacies outside of the U.S. (see Appendix A, page 386). More Milk Special Blend, an herbal blend, is available from local distributors or directly from the manufacturer (see Appendix A, page 386).

Through our research, we also discovered that some mothers who had had breast augmentation surgery to enhance the size and shape of their breasts in fact had breast hypoplasia. Breast augmentation surgery does not improve the milk-making tissue of the breast, so whenever a mother tells us that she has breast implants and that her infant is failing to gain weight well, we ask about the appearance of her breasts prior to having the surgery.

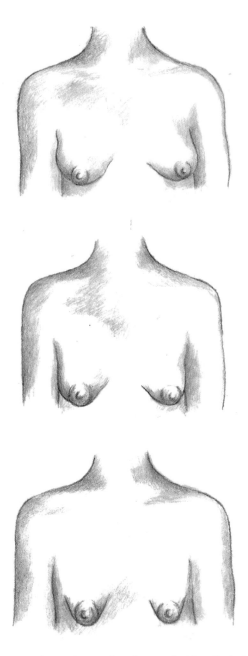

Hypoplastic breasts vary in appearance, but they can be identified with certainty when they fail to grow during pregnancy, are widely spaced, and do not swell in the first week after birth.

With the help of a lactation professional, if possible, monitor your milk production and your baby's weight (see page 125). If you can't build an adequate milk supply, you can still continue breastfeeding, but you'll need to provide supplemental formula while you nurse. Some mothers supplement their babies after nursing, by bottle (see page 125, Underfeeding and Weight Loss), while others choose to use a nursing supplementer system (see Appendix A, page 386). A supplementer, with its thin, soft tubing attached to a bottle-like container of formula or expressed milk, allows the baby to be fed supplemental milk while nursing at the breast. This may be the best way to supplement if the baby fusses at the breast or simply drifts off to sleep.

We saw some women with breast hypoplasia again, years later, with a new baby. Surprisingly, we found that these mothers produced more milk with their subsequent babies than with their firstborn.

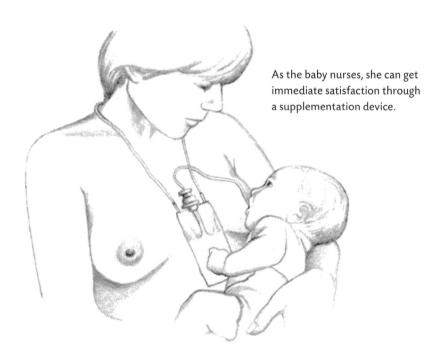

As the baby nurses, she can get immediate satisfaction through a supplementation device.

Polycystic Ovary Syndrome

Another condition that can sometimes cause a low milk supply is **polycystic ovary syndrome (PCOS)**. Occurring in up to 8 percent of women, PCOS is a complex syndrome of ovarian and other metabolic and hormonal abnormalities that develop during adolescence. Women with PCOS can have an array of problems, including ovarian cysts, menstrual irregularities, infertility, obesity and large waist size, excessive hair growth in a male distribution pattern, acne, insulin resistance and adult-onset diabetes, and depression. Not all mothers with PCOS have low milk production; some actually have overabundant milk. But it's a good idea for all mothers with PCOS to ensure good milk production by working with a lactation professional and pumping after feedings if milk is slow in coming in or is lower than what the baby needs. Some women with PCOS have succeeded in increasing their production by taking the medication metformin, which reduces insulin and testosterone levels, and some have reported improvement using herbs like fenugreek and goat's rue, both of which are components of More Milk Special Blend capsules and extract (see page 84).

Nursing after Breast Surgery

When performed prior to a woman's giving birth, minor breast surgery such as a biopsy or removal of a lump seldom affects the woman's ability to nurse unless the incision was made around the nipple or areola. A woman who has undergone a mastectomy can nurse on the remaining breast, and by nursing frequently she may be able to provide most or all of the milk that her baby needs. A breast that has been subject to radiation therapy produces little or no milk, but, again, the other breast should produce milk normally.

When a surgical implantation has been performed to alter the size and shape of the breasts, milk production is usually not affected unless the milk ducts have been severed (this may be the case if the incision was made along the edge of the areola). In the case of a breast reduction, milk production depends on the extensiveness of the surgery. When the nipples have been relocated on the breasts, some or all of the ducts have usually been severed, and so the milk supply is often threatened.

When a mother's milk ducts may have been severed, her baby should be observed closely for signs of low milk intake. I recommend a weight check by three to four days of age and every couple of days thereafter. A weight loss of 10 percent or more, or failure to gain an ounce a day after five days of age, indicates that a baby needs supplemental feedings.

If you have had breast surgery involving an incision around the areola, you may benefit from securing a breast pump and using it starting on the third day after birth or earlier. Pump for five minutes or so on each breast right after each daytime and evening nursing; if possible, pump both breasts at once. This can help bring in a more plentiful milk supply. For further guidance, see Chapter 5, as well as page 125, Underfeeding and Weight Loss.

I have worked with many women who have brought in a full supply of milk after breast reduction surgery. For many of these women, using a breast pump after each nursing helped a great deal in building an initially low supply. Herbal preparations such as fenugreek and blessed thistle capsules or Motherlove Herbal's "More Milk Special Blend" tincture have also helped boost production (see page 84). Taking the medication Domperidone (see page 87 in Survival Guide for the First Week) may also help in increasing milk flow following breast reduction surgery. Some mothers have also experienced that using a nursing supplementation device (see Appendix A, page 386) helped to increase production as well. In all cases, however, two to eight weeks' effort was required before milk production entirely met the baby's milk needs. When the milk supply is clearly insufficient and shows no signs of increasing, a mother can still continue breastfeeding indefinitely, if she wishes. A nursing supplementation device may help keep the baby from preferring the bottle.

Nursing after Gastric Bypass Surgery

Mothers who have undergone gastric bypass surgery to lose weight need nutritional guidance for both pregnancy and breastfeeding. This surgery reduces the body's intake of calories both by making the stomach smaller and by bypassing part of the small intestine, where nutrients are absorbed. Iron, folate, zinc, vitamin B_{12}, and calcium are the nutrients most often lost. Everyone who has undergone bypass surgery needs daily vitamin and mineral supplements, and pregnancy and breastfeeding increase nutritional demands even more. Particularly important are iron and vitamin B_{12}; a deficiency of either of these nutrients can lead to anemia in the mother during pregnancy and lactation, and even in the infant (signs of B_{12} deficiency in breastfed infants include diarrhea, vomiting, constipation, and poor weight gain). Ordinary prenatal vitamins may not be adequately absorbed after gastric bypass surgery, and the mother's impaired ability to absorb fat can make her milk too low in fat and calories. For these reasons, a doctor must carefully monitor both mother and baby from the start of pregnancy through weaning.

Mothers who have undergone a gastric lap-band procedure do not need to worry about lost nutrients, as this procedure does not affect the small intestine.

Nursing without Giving Birth

More and more mothers who are planning to adopt babies or are having a baby through surrogacy are considering breastfeeding them. An infant's suck can stimulate some milk production whether or not the mother has ever had or nursed a baby before, and even if she has reached menopause.

Women who have breastfed their adopted children often say that it has been one of the most memorable and rewarding experiences of their lives. You may especially enjoy nursing your adopted baby when she is older and you needn't concern yourself so much about milk production. Moments spent soothing a tired, hurt, or frustrated baby or toddler at the breast are priceless for any nursing mother.

Most adoptive mothers, however, need to supplement their breast milk, some for the entire time they are nursing. Probably the safest and most convenient way to supplement breastfeeding is with a nursing supplementation device specifically designed for this situation (see Appendix A, page 386).

Some women's enthusiastic claims of producing abundant milk for their adopted babies may set up other adoptive mothers for disappointment. It is impossible to predict whether an adoptive mother will be able to produce milk, or how much she will produce, even if she is currently nursing or has recently nursed another baby. Nursing without giving birth will be most successful if you focus on the relationship between you and your baby, rather than on your milk production. Measure your success by whether the experience truly helps make the baby yours.

Before the baby arrives, it is wise to learn as much as possible about breastfeeding and adoptive or surrogacy nursing. Be sure that the pediatrician you're choosing for your baby will be supportive of your efforts. A lactation professional may be experienced in helping you find other mothers who have nursed their adopted babies.

Nursing a baby doesn't necessarily require any advance preparation; you can simply put the baby to the breast and see what happens. In this case, though, you may or may not eventually produce significant amounts of breast milk. But if you know at least several weeks in advance that your baby is coming, you may be able to increase your chance of producing ample milk by following one of the treatment plans developed by Jack Newman, a physician, and Lenore Goldfarb, a lactation professional (see below).

When your baby arrives, he may be easily persuaded to begin nursing, or he may require a great deal of patience and persistence. In general, the younger the baby is, the easier the transition from the bottle to the breast will be. See page 110 for assistance in getting the baby to nurse.

Most mothers need to supplement their milk with formula. Some women try to increase their milk production by using formula in only minimal amounts or by overdiluting it. But these practices often result in stress and underfeeding for the baby.

If you've decided to use a supplementation device, you may be hoping for donations of breast milk to use in it, and perhaps you've already received offers of donated milk. But don't expect others to continue donating indefinitely. It can be a real effort for a nursing mother to collect extra milk. There is also the remote possibility that infectious diseases could be transmitted through donated milk.

The Newman-Goldfarb Protocols

These regimens have helped thousands of adoptive mothers, relactating mothers, and "intended" mothers, (those who have used surrogates to carry a baby to term) to bring in substantial milk supplies. Each protocol involves pumping, preferably with a clinical-grade rental pump and a double collection kit (see Chapter 5), and taking both an oral contraceptive, to hormonally mimic pregnancy, and a galactagogue, a medication that stimulates milk production. There are three protocols: a regular one, an accelerated one, and a third just for postmenopausal women. As a rule, the longer you follow your protocol, the more milk you will produce.

The protocols are designed to mimic what happens before, during, and after pregnancy. During pregnancy a woman's body produces increasing amounts of progesterone, estrogen, and lactogen, via the placenta, and prolactin, via the pituitary gland. These hormones ready the breasts for breastfeeding. Once pregnancy is completed, progesterone and estrogen levels drop and prolactin levels increase, resulting in lactation.

These protocols can be found at asklenore.info. Click on "Breastfeeding" and then on "Induced Lactation and Adoptive Breastfeeding." It is important to discuss the induced lactation protocols with your primary care provider especially if you have a history of depression or any cardiac issues, including hypertension.

If you will be present at the baby's birth, ask if a lactation consultant is available at the hospital or birthing center for assistance on getting the baby to the breast as soon after birth as possible.

Deciding Whether to Use a Protocol

The decision whether or not to follow the Newman-Goldfarb protocol may depend on how much time you have. The regular protocol might increase your milk supply more than other measures would, but only if you can follow the regimen for six months or more. This may be easy if you're using a surrogate mother, in which case you'll know about the pregnancy from the beginning. If you're adopting you may learn about your baby several months before you bring the baby home.

But sometimes a baby's homecoming is postponed, for as long as two months or more. A baby four months old or older who has been regularly bottle-fed is likely to refuse the breast. Unless you're willing to go to great lengths to persuade him to nurse, you may not want to take on the protocol.

Many adoptive parents don't know until weeks or just days in advance that they can bring their baby home. Sadly, the earlier in the pregnancy that an adoptive family is told they have been matched with a baby, the more likely it is that the birth mother will change her plans. Many women start the protocol in anticipation of adopting and then end up with no baby to nurse, or they continue pumping month after month with no news of the baby. Even those who are able to pump an impressive amount of milk find they cannot bear to keep up the pumping indefinitely.

For every mother who follows the regular protocol, brings in a good milk supply, and whose baby nurses within a reasonable amount of time, several others run into problems. Side effects can be difficult. Some women following the protocols experience weight gain, depression and tearfulness, exhaustion, swollen legs, and extremely sore and swollen breasts. Some fail to get a full milk supply even after four months or longer on the protocol. After such an investment of time and energy, this is a great disappointment.

The accelerated protocol often works well for women who have two to six months to prepare, but some lactation consultants feel that mothers who have less than sixty days to prepare will get a milk supply established faster by pumping and taking Domperidone without birth control pills, which suppress milk production as long as they are taken and for several weeks afterward. In fact, some adoptive mothers bring in a full milk supply without Domperidone, using only breast stimulation and herbs that promote milk production. An herbal preparation that is especially effective for adopting mothers is the More Milk Special Blend tincture (see page 84).

A potential risk for women who use the protocols is coming to view a nursing supplementer as evidence of failure, rather than as the important tool it is for both nurturing a baby and stimulating milk production. When a mother with a low milk supply nurses as much as possible, using a supplementer as needed, her supply often increases. More important, she establishes a long-term nursing relationship with her baby, which is beneficial in so many ways.

A more recent resource is the book *Breastfeeding Without Birthing*, written by Alyssa Schnell, a board-certified lactation consultant who nursed her third child by adoption. Her companion website can be found at www.BreastfeedingWithoutBirthing.com. This site offers mothers alternative approaches to bringing in a milk supply outside of the protocols by Goldfarb and Newmann.

Relactation

For a variety of reasons, a mother may want to begin nursing after initially starting her baby on the bottle, or to resume nursing after weaning her baby. A woman who has previously nursed her own baby may be interested in nursing another baby following adoption or surrogacy.

In general, the less time that has elapsed since weaning, the easier bringing back a full milk supply will be. A mother with a five-day-old baby who has never nursed, or with a six-week-old who has been weaned for just a few days, should be able to bring in a full milk supply within several days. After longer periods without nursing or expressing milk, the ability to re-establish full milk production will vary from woman to woman.

Always critical to milk production is frequent and regular stimulation and emptying of the breasts. This means that either a vigorously nursing baby or a clinical-grade rental breast pump should drain both breasts at least every two to two-and-a-half hours during the day and evening and twice at night. Even when a baby is willing to nurse, using a rental pump with a double-pump kit for five to ten minutes right after nursing can be very helpful in stimulating further milk production. See Chapter 5 for guidance on expressing your milk.

Herbal preparations such as fenugreek and blessed thistle capsules and More Milk Plus capsules or tincture can be very helpful in rebuilding a milk supply (see page 84 for more information).

If you find that herbs do little to increase your milk production, consider using Domperidone to stimulate more milk production (see page 87 and Appendix A, page 386).

Regardless of the time that has elapsed between weaning and attempting relactation, a baby will need supplemental feedings until full milk production has been established. You can continue bottle-feeding, but offer the bottle only after nursing and give slightly less formula than before. Or you can use a nursing supplementation device (see Appendix A, page 386), which allows you to feed your baby supplemental milk or formula while he sucks at the breast. This option may be most helpful if your baby acts frustrated while nursing.

Knowing how much supplemental milk and formula to give a baby can be a bit of a guessing game. If you are renting a clinical-grade pump, you can use the method described in Underfeeding and Weight Loss, page 125, to estimate your milk production and your baby's supplemental milk needs. Without this type of pump, you will need to rely solely on weight checks, and your breasts may not be stimulated as much as they will be with a clinical (rental) grade pump.

Whether or not you're using a rental pump, have your baby weighed every day or two during the first week or so after you start trying to relactate. Until your baby is three months old, he should gain about an ounce a day. Gaining less than this amount indicates that he needs more supplemental breast milk or formula; gaining more may mean that the supplement can be cut back a little. Always weigh your baby naked, on the same scale, at about the same time of day, and just before a feeding.

Very accurate electronic baby scales for home use are available for rent. Such a scale can also be used before and after feedings to determine how much milk the baby takes from the breast. See Appendix A, page 386, for information on renting or purchasing a scale.

Chest Feeding

Transgender individuals and non-binary birth parents may be interested in breastfeeding and will likely need a good deal of guidance as to how they can bring in as much milk as possible. Recently, the term "chest feeding" has been used by some transgender people and non-binary birth parents who want to nurse their babies. The terms "nursing" and "feeding" may also be used interchangeably by this community.

In part, however, a big problem for transgender and non-binary parents who are looking to nurse is that too few healthcare providers, including lactation consultants, have experience working with trans families. Not unlike adoptive mothers, trans people will likely need ongoing guidance as to how they can bring in as much milk as possible with the assistance from an experienced lactation professional. Even those who have had chest masculinization surgery to remove the female breasts often still have some mammary tissue and may have milk production begin after giving birth.

In one study of twenty-two transgender individuals who had experienced pregnancy, sixteen "chest fed" their infants. Two of the participants stopped due to upsetting feelings that they experienced while nursing. Other issues that came up were a lack of knowledge and support from health care providers.

The Mother with Diabetes

Many diabetic mothers enjoy the advantages of nursing. For them, breastfeeding often stimulates a remission-like response, resulting in a decreased need for insulin and an increased need for calories. Babies of diabetic mothers are less likely to develop the disease themselves later in life if they are breastfed rather than formula-fed.

If you are diabetic, your requirements for insulin and calories will need to be closely monitored—especially during the early hours after delivery, when your insulin needs will drop dramatically. Also, diabetic mothers are at a higher risk for the late onset of milk production.

For the first day or two, your newborn's blood sugar must be closely watched as her body adjusts to receiving less glucose than it did during pregnancy. She may need frequent nursing, and possibly supplemental glucose by nipple or IV, until her glucose levels stabilize. Because the infant of the diabetic mother is commonly delivered a few weeks early, she may also have respiratory problems, and she is more prone to becoming jaundiced. If your baby is born three or more weeks early, refer to page 153, The Late Preterm Baby and the Near-Term Baby.

A trial in Australia of over 600 diabetic mothers and their babies showed that newborns receiving colostrum, collected prenatally, stabilized their blood glucose better those fed formula. Included mothers were those with gestational diabetes as well as those with pre-existing diabetes. Mothers began expressing colostrum between 34- and 36-weeks gestation. The study did not include pregnancies of multiples or those babies suspected of low birth weight. Mothers were given syringes (without needles) and shown how to manually express colostrum twice a day for no more than ten minutes. The milk, usually small in amount, was dated and frozen and brought to the hospital on admission and used as needed to manage neonatal low blood sugar in place of the use of formula supplementation.

Throughout the months of breastfeeding, careful monitoring of your glucose level, insulin dose, and caloric requirements must continue. As the baby stimulates increased milk production, you and your doctor will need to adjust your insulin dosage and caloric intake to prevent insulin reactions.

You should take particular care to avoid sore nipples and breast infections. This means giving careful attention to correct positioning of the baby, watching for signs of thrush (yeast) in the baby's mouth and on the nipples (see page 195), and getting plenty of rest. Yeast infections are very common in the diabetic mother and her infant. Plugged ducts and other early signs of breast infection should be treated promptly (see page 201).

When weaning begins and milk production declines, you'll need to readjust your insulin dosage and diet again. This will be easier if you wean the baby slowly.

The Mother with Herpes

If you have an active genital herpes lesion or a positive culture near your due date, it is important to report this to your doctor. He may want to prescribe suppression medication so that the baby will be protected during birth. Many mothers receive anti-viral medications prior to and after birth, particularly if they have frequent outbreaks. If you have an active outbreak near your due date, you will probably deliver by cesarean section.

Herpes type I lesions are generally those that develop above the waist, usually on the mouth. Frequently, they appear as cold sores or fever blisters. If you develop such a lesion, it is important to wash your hands thoroughly before touching the baby and to avoid placing her in contact with the sore. Anyone else with a herpes lesion should do the same.

So long as the lesion is well-covered and you wash your hands thoroughly before all feedings, you can nurse the baby safely without gloves. There is no reason that you cannot share a room with the baby as long as you maintain these basic precautions. Should you have a herpes outbreak at home, the same principles apply.

Occasionally a mother will develop a herpes lesion on her breast, nipple, or areola. In such a case, express your milk (see Chapter 5) until the lesion is gone.

The Mother with Epilepsy

Most medications to control the occurrence of epileptic seizures are considered safe for nursing; however, it is best to check out any drug with your pediatrician. Major anticonvulsant medications are listed in Appendix D, where their safety is discussed (see page 402).

Dorothy Brewster (1979), a nursing mother with epilepsy, offers these suggestions for others:

- Have cribs or playpens available in various areas of the house; place gates across stairways and doorways.
- Nurse in a large upholstered chair or pad the arms of a rocking chair.
- When alone on outings with the baby, tag the stroller or carrier with the name of the baby and the name of a person to contact in the event that you have a seizure.

Nursing and Thyroid Conditions

Hypothyroidism

Symptoms of an underactive thyroid gland may include extreme fatigue, poor appetite, and sometimes a low milk supply. Thyroid replacement quickly reverses these symptoms. The mother who is taking medication for hypothyroidism can breastfeed, as these drugs do not affect the baby.

Hyperthyroidism

Occasionally a doctor will discover that a nursing mother has an enlarged thyroid gland. Signs of hyperthyroidism include weight loss, increased appetite, nervousness, rapid heart rate, and palpitations. Nursing must be discontinued for at least forty-eight hours when radioactive iodine is used for diagnostic testing; however, other tests are available that do not require this interruption. If radioactive iodine is used, express or pump your milk (see Chapter 5) and dispose of it (see page 422, Radioactive Agents).

If you are taking medication for an overactive thyroid gland, you can breastfeed as long as the specific medication is considered safe for the nursing baby. PTU (propylthiouracil) is the drug of choice, since it has the least effect on a baby's thyroid gland. The baby's thyroid level should be monitored by a pediatrician.

Emotional Barriers to Breastfeeding

> WARNING: The content in this section discusses sexual abuse, including during childhood.

It has been estimated that an astounding 25 to 40 percent of women of childbearing age were sexually abused during childhood. Some of these women have emotional difficulty with the experiences of childbirth and breastfeeding, which can revive old feelings of shame, guilt, or both. Such feelings keep some women from even trying to nurse; they feel certain even before the baby is born that they will not be able to handle breastfeeding. Others discover uncomfortable feelings only once they begin nursing their newborns. Sometimes memories of abuse surface for the first time with the initiation of breastfeeding. Thankfully, many women who were sexually abused find childbirth and breastfeeding an empowering and healing experience. This is most likely for women who have undergone therapy to resolve their feelings about themselves and their bodies.

How a mother who has been sexually abused responds to the idea of breastfeeding depends on whether her breasts played a part in the abuse and how far along she is in her recovery. If you were sexually abused and are now beginning to breastfeed, the feeling of suckling may disturb you. You may feel as though you do not want to share your body, and you may dread feedings. You may feel helpless or out of control if your baby's frequent requests to be fed remind you of your abuser's inescapable demands. You may be tempted to postpone feedings or limit the baby's time at the breast, but you should try to find ways to meet your baby's needs while protecting yourself from being reminded of your abuse.

Should you find yourself having very mixed feelings about breast-feeding, during pregnancy or just after the birth, you might consider giving nursing a short trial. Even a few days of nursing is a boon to a baby's health.

If the feeling of your baby's sucking disturbs you, you might try using a nipple shield (see page 100) to lessen the sensations. Selecting the right size is important to ensure comfort for you and sufficient milk for your baby, so have a lactation professional assist you.

If your baby does too much "comfort sucking" for your comfort, you can safely use a pacifier after your milk supply is well established and your baby is gaining weight well. Offer the pacifier after a good feeding, not when the baby seems hungry.

Night wakings may be particularly disturbing for women who were wakened during childhood with sexual demands. In this case, it may be preferable to put the baby to sleep in a cradle or crib rather than in your own bed, and to have your partner bring you the baby when he cries or even set an alarm and go to the baby before he is likely to begin crying.

While many mothers feel uncomfortable nursing in front of others, you may have a heightened sense of modesty if you were sexually abused. You may feel more comfortable if you wear a specially made nursing top to expose less skin, cover up with a shawl or a light blanket (or a "nursing cover" specially made for this purpose), or bottle-feed breast milk when other people are around.

If your feelings about past sexual abuse continue to make breastfeeding difficult, consulting a psychotherapist may help. Or you might try www.solaceformothers.org, an online support group monitored by a psychotherapist that helps mothers who are dealing with trauma, including past sexual abuse.

New mothers who have experienced sexual abuse are more likely than other women to suffer postpartum anxiety or depression (see page 210). If this happens to you, your regular physician or a psychiatrist can prescribe medications that are safe to use while breastfeeding.

If your feelings about past sexual abuse continue to make breastfeeding difficult despite expert help, a good solution may be to pump your milk and feed it to the baby by bottle (see Chapter 5). Some women do this for many months, even though it is more time-consuming than breastfeeding.

If you find even pumping stressful, feeding formula may be best for you and the baby.

No matter how you choose to feed your baby, a postpartum support group may be helpful to you.

Maternal Substance Use and Abuse

When a mother is narcotic dependent, breastfeeding is encouraged, but only if she is regularly receiving supervised treatment in a methadone maintenance program. Mothers who are breastfeeding and using "street" drugs, such as PCP (phencyclidine), cocaine, amphetamines and methamphetamines, and cannabis are of concern. These drugs can be detected in human milk. Breastfeeding is contraindicated because of long-term neurobehavioral development.

Alcohol (including beer) does not stimulate milk production. In fact, alcohol may decrease the milk making hormone response to sucking and have a negative effect on an infants' motor development. Alcohol easily passes into breast milk. Large amounts of alcohol can affect the baby's development and coordination. For these reasons, alcoholic beverages should be limited to the occasional intake of no more than one standard drink. There is some evidence that non-alcoholic beer may increase prolactin, the milk-making hormone.

Maternal smoking is strongly discouraged. Smoking is associated with an increased incidence in infant respiratory issues and SIDS. Smoking should not occur in the presence of the infant so as to minimize the negative effect of secondary passive smoke inhalation. Smoking is also a risk factor for low milk supply and poor weight gain.

With the legalization of marijuana (cannabis) in various parts of the United States, mothers may consider the use of it during pregnancy and breastfeeding. See Appendix D about cannabis and CBD use during breastfeeding.

BABIES

Medical Reasons for Not Breastfeeding

There are a limited number of medical conditions in which breastfeeding is contraindicated. Infants born with **galactosemia**, a rare inherited disorder, lack the enzyme necessary to break down the sugar found in all milk, including milk-based formulas, other dairy products, and breast milk. These babies must be fed a special lactose-free formula. Newborn screening tests done at discharge from the hospital or birth center detect most cases of galactosemia.

Infants with **phenylketonuria (PKU)**, another rare metabolic disorder, require a diet with little phenylalanine, an amino acid. Because breast milk is low in phenylalanine, a baby with PKU may be breast-fed part-time provided she is also fed phenylalanine-free formula. Her blood level of phenylalanine must be monitored to be sure that it remains between 5 and 10 milligrams per deciliter. A pediatric dietitian can help set up a regimen that includes limited breastfeeding.

The Late Preterm Baby

The "late preterm" baby is born early, between 34 to 36 weeks and six days before his due date. These newborns may have health complications, including short-term respiratory problems, temperature instability, jaundice, neurodevelopmental consequences, and feeding difficulties. They make up the majority of all premature babies. Some "late preterm" infants are the same size and weight as infants born at term.

The late preterm infant may fail to give obvious hunger cues and may not be vigorous at the breast. Infrequent and sluggish feedings may cause the baby to lose too much weight and delay discharge from the hospital or even lead to re-admission to the hospital.

The Near-Term Baby

Near-term infants are born between 35- to 37-weeks of gestation or three to five weeks before their due date. They are usually treated like any other newborns by physicians and nurses, and parents are encouraged to do the same.

Like full-term infants, near-term infants tend to breathe more regularly, maintain a higher blood sugar level, and cry much less if allowed to rest unswaddled against the mother's bare chest immediately after birth. If your baby is healthy at birth, you will probably be permitted to hold him skin-to-skin right after he is dried. Your baby may crawl to your breast and latch on to it unaided within the first hour or two of life. Bathing, weighing, and eye treatment can be postponed for an hour or so or until you and your baby are able to complete the first feeding.

It is important to understand, however, that a baby born a few weeks early doesn't behave exactly like a baby born at term. You may find that your baby tends to be extra sleepy and to nurse inconsistently. He may be vigorous at some feedings and inefficient at others. He may fall asleep at the breast before he has taken in sufficient milk. Unless you wake him every two and a half to three hours, he may sleep too long between feedings. He may fail to gain weight; he may even lose weight.

Breastfeeding Management for the Late Preterm and the Near-Term Newborn

For both newborns, a few days of sluggish nursing and limited milk removal can have a devastating effect on your milk production. To ensure a plentiful supply for both the late preterm and the near-term baby, I recommend compressing your breast while the baby is sucking. Starting on the third day after birth or earlier, using a clinical-grade rental pump with a double collection kit pump for ten to fifteen minutes right after each daytime and evening nursing (freeze the milk you collect for later use). This will help you build an abundant milk supply, which in turn will help the baby get sufficient milk even when he is sleepy at a feeding. See Chapter 5 for more information on pumping milk.

Watch your baby closely for the signs of adequate milk intake— vigorous sucking and swallowing and frequent stools. Weigh the baby at four to five days of age, and at any time you are concerned about his milk intake, to be sure that he has not lost an excessive amount of weight. Refer to Appendix B, page 396.

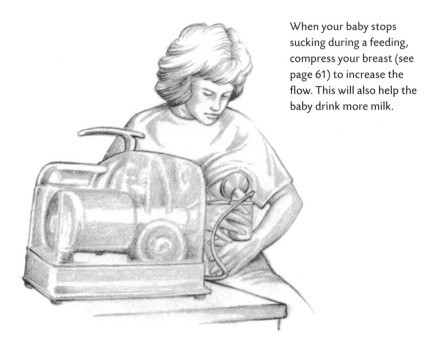

When your baby stops sucking during a feeding, compress your breast (see page 61) to increase the flow. This will also help the baby drink more milk.

If the baby is gaining about an ounce a day and has regained his birth weight at ten to twelve days, without any supplemental feedings, you can gradually stop pumping over a few days. Weigh the baby once again before returning the pump to the rental station to be sure he has continued to gain an ounce a day.

If the baby's weight loss nears 10 percent or if he is not gaining at least an ounce a day, offer him the milk you're pumping plus any necessary formula. To determine how much supplement the baby needs, see Appendix B, page 396.

A baby born three to five weeks early who is sick may be unable to nurse at first. If this is the case with your baby, you can express your milk for him until he is well enough to begin nursing. In this way he will still benefit from your milk, and you will have established your supply by the time he is ready to begin breastfeeding. For more information, see Chapter 5 and the section that follows.

The Very Premature or Sick Baby

When a baby is born sick or very immature—that is, more than five weeks early—the first days after the birth can be overwhelming. In such a case you may have doubts about many things, including your ability to nurse the baby. If your baby is too immature or weak to breastfeed, know that expressing your milk for your baby is very important to his well-being.

Your milk is easier for your baby to digest than formula, and it is particularly suited for a preemie's special growth needs. The fatty acids in human milk promote eye and brain development, which is measurably superior in preterm infants fed mother's milk than in those fed formula. Mother's milk may also reduce a premature baby's risk of developing cerebral palsy (Lucas, 1992).

Premature infants are at greater risk than full-term infants for developing infections, and preemies are less able to cope with infections when they arise. As you already know, breast milk helps protect a baby against infections. Most protective is the earliest milk, colostrum, which as a preterm mother you'll be making longer than a full-term mother. Doctors think of colostrum as a medicine for preterm babies.

Kangaroo Care

Just as a kangaroo baby, born very undeveloped, is carried and fed in its mother's pouch, a premature human baby benefits from being held next to his parent's body. More and more intensive-care nurseries are allowing and even encouraging parents to practice "kangaroo care": The preemie, dressed only in a diaper and hat, is placed upright between a parent's breasts, inside the parent's shirt or under a blanket. The baby's head is turned to one side, with his ear above the level of the parent's heart. Premature babies held this way for two hours or more once or twice a day have one-quarter the rate of apnea, or temporary cessation of breathing, of other premature infants. Even a premature baby on a ventilator can be safely moved to the mother without an increase in oxygen. Preemies held kangaroo-style experience no lowering of the heart rate, or bradycardia; in fact, their heart rates are much more stable while they are being held. Their temperatures are stabilized, too, by the warmth of the parent's body. The babies gain weight more rapidly than those kept full-time on a warming bed or in an incubator, perhaps because babies cared for kangaroo-style sleep more deeply, conserving their energy. Faster weight gain means shorter hospital stays; the length of hospitalization for a kangaroo-care baby is reduced by as much as 50 percent. Finally, the skin-to-skin contact not only contributes to parent-baby bonding but also tends to increase the mother's milk production.

As a medicine, colostrum has multiple benefits: It contains a high concentration of antibodies; it creates an environment in the intestinal tract that impairs the growth of harmful bacteria; and it has components that directly attack dangerous germs.

The first drops of colostrum contain the highest concentrations of antibodies, the second drops the next highest, and so on. For this reason, you should number each batch you collect and feed the batches in the sequence in which you have collected them. A nurse or lactation professional can show you how and where to store your colostrum.

Babies who are not yet ready for feedings but are receiving intravenous fluids instead may benefit from having just 0.1 milliliter of colostrum placed in each cheek every three to four hours. This tiny amount will not be swallowed but instead will be absorbed into the baby's lymphatic system to help protect her respiratory and intestinal tracts. If your baby is getting intravenous fluids in place of feedings, be sure to ask if she can have a small amount of colostrum swabbed inside her mouth.

Let the hospital staff know about any medications you take, including any over-the-counter medicines or herbal preparations. Although most medications are safe to take while nursing, a few could harm a sick or premature infant.

If you develop a breast infection (see page 203), you will need to discard any milk you collect, because preterm infants are more susceptible than other babies to bacteria in breast milk.

Refer to Chapter 5 for information on expressing milk in general and for a premature or sick baby in particular, on feeding hindmilk (see page 158), and on pumping for longer than a few weeks (see page 261).

Maintaining and Increasing Your Milk Supply

Bringing in and keeping your milk supply high is a problem for some mothers with sick or premature babies in the NICU. When the number of pumpings falls below eight times in a 24-hour period, milk production often drops. Mothers who are pumping eight times a day typically pump using a double collection kit every three hours around the clock or pump every two to two and a half hours during the day and evening and once in the night. Skipping or delaying night time pumpings generally leads to a drop in overall production.

If you are struggling with your milk supply, talk to the lactation staff at the hospital about the safety of using herbs and medications, such as Domperidone to increase production (see page 87). Some mothers use the timer on their phones to ring when it is time to pump.

Supplementing Breast Milk

Although breast milk alone is the perfect food for a full-term infant, a preemie, because of her small size and immaturity, may have somewhat different nutritional needs. Many premature infants need supplemental

Collecting Hindmilk for a Premature or Sick Baby

Very small premature babies and babies with heart or lung problems may be able to take only small amounts of milk at their feedings. To compensate for smaller feedings, these babies may require higher-calorie milk to grow well. When milk lets down, it starts out as low-calorie *foremilk* and gradually becomes more and more fatty. The milk expressed or fed last contains the most fat. This milk is referred to as *hindmilk*. Feeding hindmilk can be very helpful in achieving good weight gain in a preemie or a baby who has heart or lung problems.

To collect hindmilk separately from foremilk, pump for about two minutes after the milk lets down, and then stop pumping and switch collection bottles. Pump again until the breast is completely drained. Label the first bottles as foremilk, the second as hindmilk. Provide the hindmilk for the baby's immediate needs, and freeze the foremilk for the future (for use during separations or for supplementation).

Some NICU'S use a creamatocrit breastmilk fat analyzer to help estimate the lipid concentration and calories in mother's breastmilk.

nutrients, especially calcium, phosphorus, and protein. The nurses may mix commercially prepared fortifiers with your milk to provide for these special needs. Usually, the fortifiers are discontinued about the time the baby should have been born. But a preemie needs supplemental iron and vitamins even after discharge from the hospital.

Many premature babies also need a more concentrated source of calories than breast milk. In this situation, a baby may be fed a special preemie formula along with breast milk. A possible option is to feed hindmilk—the fattier milk produced after the first few minutes of pumping (see above). Feeding hindmilk exclusively will speed the weight gain of premature infants.

When Breastfeeding Begins

The preterm or sick newborn is ready to begin feedings at the breast when his overall condition is stable. It's impossible to know just when a baby will reach this point. If he has poor muscle tone, if he still requires a ventilator, or if he is not yet able to coordinate sucking, swallowing, and breathing, he may not be ready for breastfeeding.

When a baby is ready for oral feeding, breastfeeding is far better for him than bottle-feeding. Studies show that preemies at the breast have better respiratory rates, heart rates, and blood oxygen levels than preemies fed from a bottle. If there is doubt about the safety of your breastfeeding your preemie, the baby's heart rate and respiration can be observed on the electronic monitor during feedings.

When you begin nursing, try to keep your expectations modest. Preemies' abilities at the breast vary greatly, but most are unable to complete an entire feeding at first.

Have a nurse or lactation consultant help you during the first few sessions. Your goal is to position the baby well for nursing and to encourage her to latch on to the breast. These early practice sessions go best when the baby is awake and alert and the breast is not overly full. Keeping the baby snugly wrapped in a blanket could discourage her interest; it's better to hold her undressed against your skin, with a blanket draped over both of you. The nurse can check the baby's skin temperature after five to ten minutes.

The crossover hold and the football hold (see pages 54 to 56) are the positions of choice for nursing a premature baby as both of these positions support the baby's head. Place your hand around the baby's head with your fingers behind and below her ears. Support her neck and shoulders with the palm of your hand and your wrist. With your thumb at the point where the baby's nose will touch the breast, compress the breast with your fingers. Lightly stroke the baby's upper lip with your nipple to signal her to open her mouth wide. As soon as she does, pull her head and shoulders toward you so that the nipple is on top of her tongue and far back in her mouth.

While you are nursing your baby, you should eventually be able to hear her swallowing. This means she is sucking effectively and getting

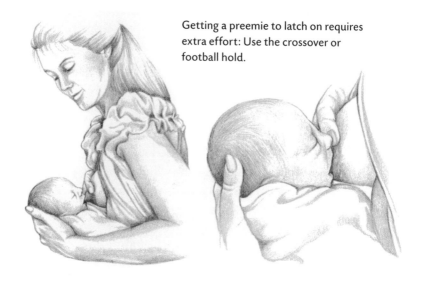

Getting a preemie to latch on requires extra effort: Use the crossover or football hold.

your milk. If you do not hear swallowing, make sure the baby is actually latched on to the breast. Her suction should be so strong that it is hard to pull her off. You should not see dimples in her cheeks or hear clicking noises as she sucks. These signs would indicate she was sucking on her tongue and not on your breast. Gently squeeze the breast while the baby is latched to increase the amount of milk the baby receives.

Once latched on to the breast and sucking, a preemie may fall asleep after just a few minutes. Again, preemies' abilities at the breast vary greatly, so be patient. As long as you have positioned your baby correctly and are encouraging her to open her mouth, you have been successful.

If the baby sucks well at the first breast and seems ready for more, you can simply transfer her to the other side without turning her, or you can reposition her in the opposite arm using the football hold.

Until she is sucking vigorously at the breast, the baby may need a supplement after nursing. Most hospitals give nursing preemies supplements by bottle; others give them by passing a soft tube through the nose or mouth into the stomach, to avoid "nipple preference." Be sure to pump after feeding sessions and collect your milk so it can be fed to your baby as a supplement. Until your baby is nursing without any supplemental feedings, you will need to continue expressing milk after each nursing to maintain your milk supply.

Difficult latch-on. Many premature infants have difficulty latching on, due to their immaturity as well as having received rubber nipples as pacifiers or for feedings. Some babies have trouble learning to lower their tongue to latch on, whereas others seem unable to identify their mothers' nipples in their mouths.

Premature infants who are having trouble latching on or drawing milk from the breast may do better with a small-size nipple shield (see page 100). Nipple shields seem to help immature babies recognize that there is something in their mouths, and this recognition stimulates them to begin sucking. You will want the help of a lactation professional in determining exactly which size shield works best for your nipples and the baby's mouth.

If your baby is unable to latch on to the breast even with a nipple shield, see page 109, Difficult Latch-on: Refusal to Nurse. In my experience, a premature infant typically learns to nurse after a period of daily practice approaching the mother's due date.

The Transition to Full-Time Nursing

While you and the baby are establishing nursing, you may wonder how much milk the baby is taking. Although mothers and health professionals often try to gauge the baby's milk intake by how long he nurses, how much swallowing can be heard, or whether the baby will take supplemental milk, none of these methods are accurate. The best way to determine the baby's milk intake is to weigh him before and after nursing, in the same diaper and clothing, on an electronic gram scale. Each gram of weight gain equals 1 milliliter of milk intake.

How much breast milk a baby should take at each feeding can be calculated by multiplying the baby's weight in kilograms by 22.5 (a pounds-to-kilogram conversion chart is in Appendix B, page 396). This will give you in milliliters the amount of milk the baby needs at each of eight daily feedings. For example, if a baby weighs 2.2 kilograms, he will need 49.5, or approximately 50, milliliters of milk each time he nurses, for a total of eight times per day. If the baby takes 30 milliliters during the nursing session, he will need an additional 20 milliliters after nursing to gain an adequate amount of weight.

While you are in the hospital, have your baby weighed on the nursery's scale before and after nursings. If you do this at each nursing, you should begin to develop a sense of how much milk the baby is taking at any feeding. Once at home, you may need weight checks only every two days or so to help you judge how much supplement the baby needs. If you want to continue pre- and post-feeding weight checks at home, rent a highly accurate electronic scale (see Appendix A, page 386).

Nursing Multiples

Needless to say, caring for two or more babies takes a tremendous amount of time and energy. Breastfeeding multiples is not only more healthful and economical than giving them formula, but in many ways it is more convenient. Mothers of twins often say that nursing is easier and less time-consuming than preparing and feeding bottles, particularly when a woman has mastered the skill of nursing two babies at the same time.

Although many mothers worry about being able to produce enough milk for more than one baby, most women are capable of producing plenty of milk for two and even three babies.

As soon as you become aware of the twins during pregnancy, you should begin some special preparations. You will want to arrange for as much help as possible for the first several weeks after the birth. It's also a good idea to get to know other mothers who have successfully nursed their twins. Many communities have organizations for mothers of twins. You might also contact your local breastfeeding support group; such a group usually provides literature on caring for and nursing twins.

Approximately half of all twins are born prematurely. During pregnancy you can do much to lessen the risk of premature delivery and other complications by maintaining a diet high in calories—at least 2,900 a day—and protein—at least 110 grams a day. Talk with your healthcare provider about monitoring yourself for signs of preterm labor. Identifying regular contractions, even if they are mild, is important to prevent premature birth.

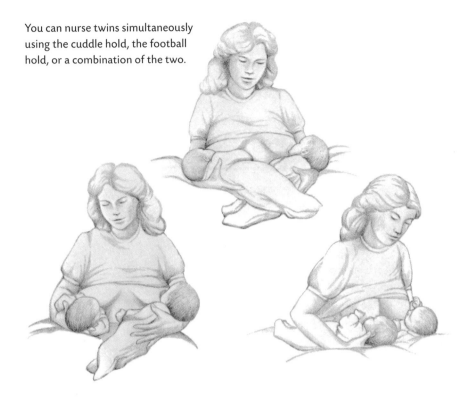

You can nurse twins simultaneously using the cuddle hold, the football hold, or a combination of the two.

Establishing an Abundant Milk Supply

Making enough milk for two or more babies depends on the frequent and complete drainage of the breasts. Multiples who are born early or of low birth weight may not consistently nurse effectively enough to stimulate abundant milk production. For this reason I recommend using a clinical-grade rental pump, with a double collection kit, whenever multiples are born three or more weeks before the due date or weigh less than 6 pounds each. See Chapter 5 for guidelines on expressing milk for near-term and very preterm infants. Even if your babies are healthy and latching on to the breast frequently, pump for five to ten minutes after each nursing to ensure complete drainage of the breasts and to stimulate abundant milk production. See page 153, The Late Preterm Baby and The Near-Term Baby, for more information on nursing premature babies and Chapter 5 for guidelines on expressing milk.

If the babies are in a special-care nursery and are unable to nurse, use the clinical-grade pump at least eight times every twenty-four hours. See page 155, The Very Premature or Sick Baby and see Chapter 5 for information on expressing milk. You should aim to produce 20 to 24 ounces (591 to 710 ml) of milk per day for each of your babies.

Breastfeeding Two or More

You should nurse each of your babies at least eight times in every twenty-four hours. This may mean waking smaller babies every three hours during the day and evening for feedings, and every four to five hours in the night, until they are gaining weight well without any supplementation.

Some mothers prefer nursing their babies together as much as possible, whereas others choose to nurse them separately. Nursing two at once certainly saves time, and it may be necessary when both of the babies are hungry. If you want to nurse the babies together, there are three basic positions you can try:

- both babies in the cuddle hold with their legs side by side or crossed over each other,
- one baby in the cuddle hold and the other in the football hold, or
- both babies in the football hold.

During the early weeks, you may need assistance getting the babies on the breast at the same time. You will also probably need a few pillows for positioning. (Special pillows are available for nursing twins. See Appendix A, page 386, for ordering information.) It may be easier to position the baby who nurses first and then put the vigorous nurser to the breast. Nursing the twins simultaneously should get easier as they get older and need less head support and assistance latching on.

Nursing the babies separately, each baby on one breast only, may be easier to manage and will allow you more time with each individually. You may decide to feed each baby whenever she seems hungry, or you may prefer to encourage the babies to eat and sleep on approximately the same schedule. To maintain a similar routine for both babies, simply offer the breast to the second baby, waking her if necessary, after nursing the first. Although most twins eventually develop a preference for one breast over the other, it is wise to alternate the babies at each feeding during the early weeks so the breasts will be evenly stimulated; this is particularly important when one baby is more active than the other. Keeping a simple written record may be helpful at first.

Mothers of triplets generally nurse two babies simultaneously and then the third baby from both breasts, or else another caregiver gives the third baby a bottle. Again, alternate the babies from one feeding to the next.

During the early weeks, if the babies are gaining weight adequately, substituting bottle-feedings for nursings is best avoided. You want to be sure your breasts are stimulated by the babies' sucking so that milk production remains adequate. Forgoing the bottle also helps minimize the occurrence of plugged ducts and breast infections.

Caring for Yourself

For the mother who is nursing two or more babies, getting plenty of rest, food, and drink is essential. Most nursing mothers are naturally hungrier and thirstier than usual. If you take on too much and become fatigued, though, you may lose your appetite and too much weight. Nutritionists recommend that a mother nursing twins consume at least 3,000 calories daily. Your diet should include high-protein foods and a quart or more of milk a day, the equivalent in other dairy products, or a calcium supplement. Vitamin C and B-complex supplements or brewer's yeast may also be beneficial.

The Baby with Noisy Breathing (Laryngomalacia)

A baby born with this abnormality has "squeaky" breathing. The larynx, or voice box, is malformed, causing the tissues to flop over and partially block the airway opening. The cause of this condition is thought to be congenital, but relaxation of the upper airway or low muscle tone may also be factors. When the baby breathes in, the larynx is partially obstructed, and you hear a high-pitched, squeaky sound known as stridor. This is the most common cause of noisy breathing in infants.

Typically, this noise begins during the first two months of life, often in the very first days. Sometimes the sound is confused with nasal congestion, but no nasal discharge is present, and the sound persists. For most infants, laryngomalacia is not serious. Despite having noisy breathing, they are able to eat and grow. The stridor is often more pronounced when the baby is lying on his back or crying, and sometimes during and after feedings. Some infants with laryngomalacia also have problems with reflux (causing spitting up and vomiting), because they have more stomach acid than other babies. The stridor commonly seems to get worse between four and eight months of age, and most babies outgrow it by eighteen to twenty months, when the laryngeal structures develop more.

Babies with mild stridor may do better with short, frequent feedings in a more upright or forward-leaning position—that is, with the mother reclined and the baby lying on top.

A small percentage of babies with laryngomalacia do struggle with breathing, eating, and gaining weight. Symptoms that require prompt attention include not breathing for more than ten seconds, turning blue around the lips, or the baby's chest pulling down, also known as retracting, without relief after being wakened or repositioned. Some babies may choke while feeding or inhale milk into their lungs. Infants with reflux may be given medications that may worsen the laryngomalacia symptoms. If the symptoms are severe, other tests are often done to evaluate the condition. A few infants may require tube feeding or even surgery.

A website devoted to helping parents whose infants have laryngomalacia can be found at www.copingwithlm.org. Although less common, tracheomalacia is when a baby's windpipe partially collapses as he breathes out. This may be aggravated when the baby coughs, cries, or feeds. Keeping the baby's head extended while feeding and allowing the baby to set the pace of the feeding can be helpful. Squeaking and noisy breathing should be reported to your baby's doctor.

The Baby with a Birth Defect

A baby with a birth defect may need breast milk, and the comfort and security of the breast, even more than other infants. Nursing such a baby is usually possible, but the mother must be supported in her efforts. Although some mothers of babies with birth defects have been discouraged from even attempting breastfeeding, many have gone on to nurse their babies successfully.

Depending on your baby's problem, you may be able to begin nursing right after birth, or you may need to express milk for a while (see Chapter 5). Whatever the circumstances, it may be helpful to seek guidance from a lactation professional.

Heart Defect

Infants with minor heart defects generally have little trouble breastfeeding. The baby with a severe defect may become easily fatigued or stressed during feedings; he may start breathing rapidly, his heart will beat faster, and his overall color may change. His growth may be greatly affected by his heart abnormality. He may also be more prone to infections and therefore in greater need of breast milk than other babies.

A baby who is getting a normal amount of breast milk but is gaining insufficient weight may grow better if he receives extra high-calorie hindmilk. Provided your milk supply is abundant, pump for two minutes or so to remove the lower-calorie foremilk, and then nurse the baby. This will provide him with a feeding that is higher in calories.

If your baby becomes stressed during feedings, nurse him more frequently for shorter periods of time. He may also be more comfortable if you hold him upright for nursing, as in the football hold.

Cleft Lip and Palate

The baby born with a cleft lip, palate, or both may have difficulty latching on and sucking effectively, so feeding her may present special challenges. Breastfeeding may be possible, depending on the location and extent of the cleft, but most of these babies, particularly those with cleft palates, are unable to get enough milk from nursing alone. Yet breast milk helps reduce the number and severity of ear and respiratory infections, which are more common in these babies than in others. Many mothers of babies with clefts, therefore, pump their milk and feed it to their babies using whatever method works best for the baby.

The baby born with a cleft lip alone may have little difficulty nursing. Until the lip is repaired, usually when the baby is several weeks old, she may need to be positioned with the cleft sealed, to permit suction. You may be able to create a complete seal just by pulling the baby close against your breast so that your breast occludes the cleft. If you find that your baby has more difficulty nursing on one side than the other, try using the football hold on that side.

Whether a baby with a cleft palate can nurse usually depends on the location and extent of the cleft. When it is in the soft palate only, the baby may or may not be able to nurse without much difficulty. It's best to position her so her head is raised; milk may come out of her nose if you feed her while she is lying flat. Ask the baby's doctor or a lactation professional about devices and techniques to help with feedings.

If the baby has a cleft palate and is unable to latch or effectively create suction, use a fully automatic electric breast pump every two to three hours around the clock, to stimulate and maintain an abundant milk supply. A clinical-grade rental pump with a double collection kit is most efficient and requires the least amount of pumping time. See Chapter 5 for more information on expressing milk.

Bottle-feeding a baby with a cleft lip or palate can also be challenging. The nursing staff should have special feeders of various types that you can try while you are in the hospital. The SpecialNeeds Feeder (formerly called the Haberman Feeder) has worked well for some of my clients. Newer on the market is Dr. Brown's Specialty Feeding System, (see Appendix A, page 386, for ordering information).

A cleft palate is generally not repaired until the baby is several months old. In the meantime, nursing can be difficult or even impossible. In this case, you will probably need to express milk for some time. Pumping and feeding your milk is far cheaper than feeding formula and may be very helpful in preventing ear infections.

Whether your baby has a cleft lip, a cleft palate, or both, closely monitor her weight to make sure that she is getting enough to eat. If you are exclusively bottle-feeding, see Appendix B, page 396, to determine how much milk she needs at each feeding. If your baby is able to latch on and suck but you're unsure whether she is getting enough milk, weigh her every couple of days, and adjust the amount of supplement as needed to maintain a weight gain of about an ounce a day. Renting an electronic scale for a few weeks may be helpful; you can use the scale before and after nursings to determine how much milk the baby is getting, or simply use it daily to check her weight. See Appendix A, page 386, to locate a scale.

Developmental and Neurological Problems

Babies with Down syndrome, hydrocephalus, spina bifida, cerebral palsy, and other neurological problems benefit greatly from breastfeeding. Because nursing provides frequent physical contact, it may be especially valuable to such a baby's development.

If the baby's sucking ability is affected, teaching him to nurse will require a great deal of patience. You may need guidance from a lactation professional experienced with such problems and also from a physical therapist. In this case, start out using the pump after each nursing to bring in and maintain an abundant milk supply. Once the baby is feeding well and gaining weight at the rate of an ounce per day, you can gradually stop pumping.

If your baby is unable to suck, he may need to be fed with a feeding tube. But some babies with neurological issues may be able to nurse with a nursing supplementation device (see Appendix A, page 386) or to drink your expressed milk from a special bottle like the SpecialNeeds Feeder from Medela or Dr. Brown's Specialty Feeding System (see Appendix A, page 386).

Down Syndrome

Many infants with Down syndrome are able to nurse. Not only does nursing further their development, it also provides them with much-needed protection from illness, as they are at greater risk than most babies for developing infections.

Some babies with Down syndrome have difficulty learning how to latch on and suck effectively. The baby may have weak muscle tone; he may act sleepy and uninterested in the breast. In this case, rouse him frequently for nursing (see page 103, Sleepy Baby) and pump after nursing until he is gaining weight as expected.

Typically, the baby with Down syndrome grows slowly. If your baby's suck is weak and inefficient, you may need to pump out the milk he leaves in the breast. Regular pumping will allow you to maintain sufficient milk production and provide the baby extra milk, which you can feed as a supplement after each nursing.

Hydrocephalus and Spina Bifida

These birth defects are usually corrected surgically as soon as possible. Until the baby can begin to nurse, the mother must express milk (see Chapter 5). For many such babies, positioning at the breast requires special attention so that they are protected and comfortable.

Cerebral Palsy

Babies with cerebral palsy may also be able to nurse, depending on the severity of their condition. Breastfeeding problems that occur are usually related to either (1) poor muscle tone and a weak suck or (2) excessive muscle tone (rigidity and abnormal posture), tongue thrusting, clenching of the jaw, and difficulty swallowing. Both of these situations usually lead to slow weight gain. Some infants with cerebral palsy are able to breastfeed successfully with a nursing supplementation device (see Appendix A, page 386). A baby with cerebral palsy who struggles with bottle-feeding may do well with a SpecialNeeds Feeder or Dr. Brown's Specialty Feeding System (see Appendix A, page 386).

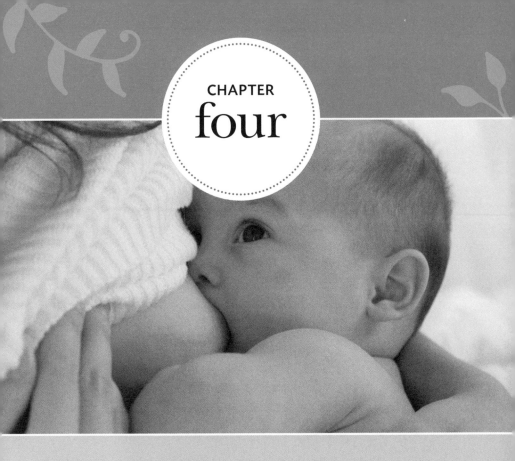

THE LEARNING PERIOD: THE FIRST TWO MONTHS

**NOW THAT YOU
ARE POSTPARTUM**

- Caring for Yourself

- Your Nutritional Needs

NURSING YOUR BABY

- Your Nursing Style

- Your Milk Supply

- Scheduled Feedings

- Infant Dietary Supplements

LIFE WITH YOUR BABY

- Illnesses: Yours and the Baby's

- The First Two Months: What's
  Normal?

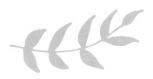

AFTER THE FIRST WEEK, you may already be feeling ener-
getic and confident in your abilities as a new mother—or
you may be exhausted, overwhelmed, and perhaps troubled by some aspect of breastfeeding. In any case, it is
important to realize that the first two months after giving birth are a
time for adjustment and learning. Mothers normally have questions and
concerns about themselves, their babies, and nursing during this period.

NOW THAT YOU
ARE POSTPARTUM

Caring for Yourself

During the six weeks after birth, all of the many changes of pregnancy
are reversed. Virtually every system in your body will go through some
readjustment. As your uterus shrinks in size and the inner lining is shed,
a new layer is formed. The vaginal flow, or lochia, decreases in amount
and progresses to pink or brown and then to white. Many women continue bleeding throughout the first month. Intermittent spotting is common. Too much activity may cause the lochia to become heavier and
turn red again—a signal that you should slow down.

If you have had a vaginal birth, your vagina, perineum, urethra, and
rectum have undergone considerable stress. Frequent warm baths, (or
sitting on a warm sitz bath, which fits on the rim of any toilet), can be
purchased inexpensively from a pharmacy, and will speed healing and
help relieve discomfort. Should you have hemorrhoids, ice packs may be

preferable. Menstrual pads soaked with witch hazel and then frozen are very soothing for hemorrhoids.

Kegel exercises will help this area return to normal by strengthening the entire pelvic floor. These exercises are simple and can be done anytime, anywhere. Several times a day, tightly squeeze the muscles around your anus, then around your vagina and urethra. Gradually work up to one hundred Kegels a day.

If you have had a cesarean birth, keep in mind you are recovering from major abdominal surgery. Most likely, you will need to take pain medication for the first week or so. Using a mild pain reliever such as acetaminophen (Tylenol) or ibuprofen (Motrin, Advil) every few hours may be enough to keep you feeling comfortable. If you are prescribed a narcotic pain reliever, use it only when over-the-counter medications are not enough. Taking a narcotic pain reliever often and for more than one week could make your baby sleepy and could possibly even cause you to have withdrawal symptoms—depression and anxiety, crying, difficulty sleeping, nausea, vomiting, diarrhea, excessive sweating, and dilated pupils—when you stop taking the medication.

You may be bothered by an uncomfortable sensation that your abdominal organs could fall out. A lightweight girdle or a wide band such as the Belly Bandit (available in maternity stores and online) might provide some welcome support.

Constipation is a common complaint in the weeks after giving birth. You can best prevent it by drinking plenty of fluids, eating foods with a lot of fiber, and getting regular exercise. Be aware that some laxatives could affect the baby through your milk, causing cramping, excessive stools, and even weight loss. For advice on safe laxatives, see Appendix D, page 402.

Night sweats are very common in the first few days after birth, and they sometimes continue for several weeks.

Starting at approximately six to twelve weeks after birth, some women experience generalized hair loss called *telogen effluvium*. Because of the hormonal changes following birth, hair follicles simultaneously move from the growing phase (which they were in during pregnancy) to the resting phase of their development. Postpartum hair loss is seldom severe, and women never go bald because of it. The period of hair loss lasts three to six months. It has no relationship to breastfeeding.

Most women experience emotional changes during the postpartum period, and some notice problems with mental function, too. Anxiety, moodiness, and irritability are common responses to the hormonal changes that occur after giving birth, as well as to the tremendous responsibility of caring for a new baby. Forgetfulness, inability to concentrate, and difficulty expressing thoughts are also common complaints. All of these problems normally pass with time, good food, plenty of rest, and social support.

Because of the rapid physical changes of the postpartum period and the tremendous amount of time and energy needed to care for and nurse a baby, rest should take high priority for all new mothers. Fatigue can slow recovery from birth and may lead to tension, inability to cope, poor appetite, and depression. Try to take at least one nap every day during these important first weeks. Do essential household chores and activities while the baby is awake so that you can nap together. Tucking the baby in with you at naptime and bedtime may help you both sleep better. Getting plenty of rest now will contribute greatly to your sense of well-being and your breastfeeding success.

After a couple of weeks, some light exercise can do much to renew your energy. A brisk twenty minute walk with the baby can be invigorating; the fresh air will do you both good. Many community centers offer exercise programs for new mothers. Often the babies are included in the exercises, and sometimes infant care is provided. Some people have claimed that exercise causes lactic acid to build up in breast milk, and that this makes babies refuse to nurse, but in fact moderate exercise has little or no effect on the composition or volume of breast milk. With whatever activity you choose, however, you will want to start out slowly.

You may feel isolated as a new mother, especially if you have left work or school—and most of your friends—to care for the baby. You need adult companionship. Check with your childbirth educator or public-health nurse about groups for new mothers. Attending La Leche League meetings, taking a mother-baby exercise class, or socializing with women from your childbirth class are excellent ways of getting out with the baby and getting to know other new mothers.

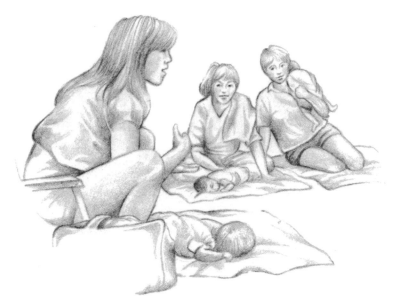

New mothers' groups provide opportunities for socializing as well as learning about infant development.

Your Nutritional Needs

Drinking Enough

Maintaining an adequate intake of fluids is usually not a problem for the nursing mother. Most women are naturally thirstier while they are breastfeeding. Contrary to popular belief, forcing fluids beyond satisfying natural thirst does not increase milk production. But when a nursing mother does not drink six to eight glasses of fluids every day, dark, concentrated urine and constipation usually result. You may need to make a conscious effort to increase your fluid intake.

Eating Well

Provided you established good eating habits during pregnancy and gained an adequate amount of weight, you probably won't need to change your diet much at all. Nursing mothers are often told to add about 500 calories, including 65 grams of protein, to their pre-pregnancy diets. Recent research, however, indicates that many mothers may

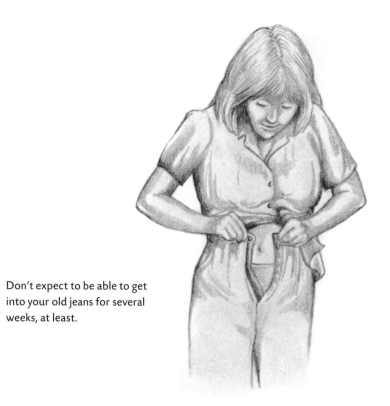

Don't expect to be able to get into your old jeans for several weeks, at least.

not need this much food, so don't feel you must eat more than you want. You can get extra nutrients in between-meal snacks, perhaps during nursings: Half a sandwich and a glass of milk or a half cup of nuts will supply about 500 calories. Some mothers experience a temporary loss of appetite during the first couple of weeks after delivery. Eating smaller, more frequent meals or snacks may be more appealing than three big meals each day.

You may feel discouraged that your body is not back to pre-pregnancy shape. The clothes in your closet may seem as if they belong to someone else. Although you lost some weight when you delivered, you are probably still pounds away from your usual weight. During the early months of breastfeeding, this extra fat is a useful energy store. If you let your appetite guide you as you continue nursing, you will probably lose the excess weight gradually and feel good while doing it. Dieting during the early weeks is not a good idea.

If you prefer to monitor your caloric intake closely, you can estimate your daily caloric needs by multiplying your current weight by fifteen. Add 500 to your total to meet the caloric needs of nursing (if you are nursing twins, add 1,000 calories).

Example:

$$
\begin{array}{rl}
135 & \text{pounds} \\
\times\ 15 & \\
\hline
2{,}025 & \text{calories} \\
+\ 500 & \text{calories} \\
\hline
2{,}525 & \text{calories}
\end{array}
$$

A moderately active woman can expect to lose a pound every two to three weeks on this caloric intake. If you are very active and have no problem controlling your weight, or if you burn calories slowly, you will need to adjust the figures somewhat: Multiply your weight by seventeen (high activity) or thirteen (low activity). The minimum safe food intake for a nursing mother of average size is about 1,800 calories per day.

Milk production is largely independent of nutritional intake during the first few months of breastfeeding. This is partly because the fat accumulated in pregnancy is available as a ready supply of calories. When a mother's diet is inadequate, however, milk production usually continues at her expense—leading to fatigue, listlessness, and rapid weight loss. Some women have trouble finding time to fix nutritious meals for themselves when they are at home alone with the baby. If you find yourself in this situation, start the day with a good breakfast, and then snack throughout the day on nutritious foods such as hard-boiled eggs, left-over chicken or beef, cheese, peanut butter, yogurt, seeds, and nuts. Don't forget the fiber: Whole-wheat bread, whole-grain crackers, and raw fruits and vegetables will provide it. Some mothers have developed their own favorite recipes for high-energy blender drinks using ingredients such as milk, yogurt, nuts, and bananas or other fruits.

Low-carbohydrate diets are not recommended while nursing. Whole grains and other high-carbohydrate foods supply nursing mothers with vitamins, minerals, and energy. Low-carbohydrate diets are dehydrating, and they often cause constipation, fatigue, and sleeping problems.

Avoid snacking on foods or drinks that are high in sugar. Refined sugar provides only "empty" calories—empty, that is, of vitamins and minerals. Soda, cookies, and candy will not provide sustaining energy and may diminish your desire for more nutritious foods.

Mothers who are vegetarians can certainly maintain a diet to support their nutritional needs. But since vitamin B_{12} is found only in foods that come from animals, deficiencies may occur with a vegan diet, which excludes eggs and milk products as well as meat. For vegans, supplementation with up to 4 milligrams of vitamin B_{12} per day is recommended.

Although most nutritionists recommend that a nursing mother drink three 8-ounce (237 ml) glasses of milk a day, there is no need to drink milk if you don't like it or can't tolerate it. A woman's bone density tends to decrease somewhat during lactation even when her calcium intake is relatively high. This causes no long-term harm. The bones grow denser again after weaning, and some studies suggest that women who breastfeed actually reduce their risk of developing osteoporosis later in life.

SERVING	MILLIGRAMS CALCIUM
yogurt (8 ounces [237 ml])	288
cheese (1 ounce [30 ml] cheddar or Swiss)	222
cottage cheese (½ cup [125 ml])	110
tofu (½ cup [125 ml])	68
corn tortillas (2)	84

Still, nutritionists recommend that breastfeeding women consume 1,000 milligrams of calcium per day. If you don't drink milk, which contains about 300 mgs per 8-ounce glass, make sure you're getting enough calcium from other sources, such as those listed in the table above.

Although dark green vegetables in general are rich in calcium (100 milligrams per half cup), the calcium they provide is poorly absorbed by the body. Broccoli is the one exception to this rule. If you do not use dairy products at all, calcium supplements may be necessary. The least expensive supplement, with the highest concentration of calcium, is calcium carbonate. Avoid bone meal, dolomite, and oyster shell, as some types have been found to be contaminated with lead.

Dietary Supplements

If you are well nourished, vitamin supplements are unnecessary while you are nursing, although you may need iron supplements if you are anemic after birth. Also, some nursing mothers develop vitamin B deficiencies, experiencing depression, irritability, impaired concentration, loss of appetite, and tingling or burning feet. A daily B-complex supplement is often prescribed to reverse these symptoms.

Sometimes nursing mothers are advised to take brewer's yeast, a natural source of B vitamins, iron, and protein. Some mothers feel it improves their milk supply or increases their overall energy level. Health-food stores carry brewer's yeast in a powdered form that can be mixed with juice or milk.

If you decide to take vitamin supplements or brewer's yeast, remember that they are no substitute for a varied diet of nutritious foods, and in large quantities they can sometimes be dangerous. There have been reports of fussiness in babies whose mothers take brewer's yeast or/and large doses of Vitamin C. Vitamin B_6 supplements in large doses have been reported to reduce milk production.

Foods and Other Substances You May Be Wondering About

Food. There are no foods that should be routinely avoided by nursing mothers, but occasionally a baby will be bothered by something the mother has eaten. Some babies fuss for up to twenty-four hours after their mothers have eaten garlic, onions, cabbage, broccoli, Brussels sprouts, cauliflower, or chiles. Citrus fruits and their juices, chocolate, and spices such as chili powder, curry powder, and cinnamon can also bother young nursing babies. If your baby has unusual symptoms such as sudden or persistent refusal to nurse, vomiting, diarrhea or green stools, gassiness, redness around the anus, fussiness at the breast, or colic symptoms, see page 103, Concerns about the Baby.

Caffeine. Caffeine in the mother's diet has been known to cause irritability and colic symptoms in some babies. Caffeine is present in coffee, tea, and many soft drinks. You may want to limit your intake of these beverages.

Alcohol. An occasional glass of wine or beer is not believed to harm a nursing infant. Because alcohol passes through the breast milk, however, moderation is essential. Alcohol does not stimulate milk production. In fact, high doses of alcohol may decrease the milk-making hormone response to sucking. Also, frequent alcohol use may have a negative effect on an infant's motor development. For these reasons, the ingestion of alcoholic beverages should be limited to the occasional intake of no more than one standard drink of alcohol per day. There is some evidence that non-alcoholic beer may increase prolactin, the milk-making hormone.

Nicotine. Mothers who smoke have lower levels of vitamin C in their milk than nonsmokers. Also, secondhand smoke increases a baby's risk of contracting bronchitis, pneumonia, and ear infections, and succumbing to sudden infant death syndrome (SIDS). If you smoke, try to limit the amount, and don't do it in your home or anywhere around the baby. Don't let others smoke around the baby, either.

Cannabis. There are few reports of the effects of cannabis in breastfed babies. Early studies on the psychoactive component, tetrahydrocannabinol (THC) in milk have been inconsistent, and there is even less information is available on cannabidiol (CBD oil), which may have some medical uses. See Appendix D for more detailed information about cannabis and breastfeeding.

NURSING YOUR BABY

Your Nursing Style

During the early weeks, each mother develops her own style of nursing. Many women feel comfortable putting their babies to breast whenever the baby signals the desire to nurse. Others expect their babies to fall into a predictable feeding schedule. They may be troubled when their babies nurse irregularly or want to nurse again soon after being fed. These mothers may worry that perhaps they have too little milk or that it is somehow inadequate. Sometimes they feel they must hold the baby off until a certain number of hours have passed since the last feeding.

But the breasts do not need to rest for any period of time to build up a supply for the next feeding; they produce milk constantly. The expectation that a baby should nurse on some type of a schedule usually leads to frustration for both mother and baby—and sometimes to breastfeeding failure.

Because breast milk is digested quickly, the newborn infant nurses often—typically between eight and twelve times in a twenty-four-hour period, or about every one to three hours. Not only must a baby nurse frequently to satisfy her hunger and thirst, she also seeks out the breast to satisfy her needs for sucking, security, and comforting. Human infants want to nurse so often that they have been described as continuous feeders.

It is a common misconception that the breast empties in a certain number of minutes, and that a baby should be taken from the breast after those minutes have elapsed. In fact, most mothers experience the release of milk several times during a feeding. The length of time required to complete a feeding varies from baby to baby. The all-business nurser, who swallows continuously with few pauses, may be done in ten minutes, whereas the dawdler may take up to 40 minutes. The length of nursing time may vary in the same baby from feeding to feeding. Before long, most mothers can tell when their babies have had enough.

Some babies nurse from only one breast at a feeding some or most of the time. This is fine, so long as the baby seems satisfied and is gaining weight adequately. You may prefer to offer only one breast per feeding, in fact, if you have an abundant milk supply. Your baby is more likely to drain the breast completely this way, and complete drainage helps prevent plugged milk ducts and breast infections. Your baby will also be sure to get the rich hindmilk, which is produced in increasing amounts as a feeding progresses.

I strongly recommend that your baby be weighed at ten to fourteen days of age. Although many infants are not scheduled for a routine well-baby exam until three to four weeks of age, a weight check at two weeks can be very beneficial. If the baby is back to her birth weight or beyond, you can be reassured early on that your nursing relationship is progressing well. On the other hand, if the baby has not yet regained her birth weight, you can usually correct this easily. When poor weight gain is not discovered until three or four weeks, it is more likely to upset everyone and may be harder to correct than it would have been at two weeks.

You may find that nursing is the most enjoyable part of your day—a time to sit back, relax, and simply enjoy being with your baby. But it may be difficult at times for you to break away from what you are doing or sit still long enough for the baby to have a leisurely nursing. It may help to make a special little nursing nook for yourself—or two or three nooks in different parts of the house. You might include a book, some magazines, or a note pad within reach. Having your phone nearby may also be handy. Some mothers routinely grab a snack or something to drink just before sitting down to nurse.

Many babies seem to get hungry whenever food is served. To avoid interruptions at dinnertime, you might offer the baby the breast just before preparing your meal. Some parents have found that taking the baby for a walk just before dinner lulls her to sleep so that they can eat without interruption.

Your Milk Supply

During these early weeks your milk production may seem somewhat erratic. At times your breasts may feel as if they are bursting with milk. At other times you may worry that there is not enough milk, especially if your breasts seem empty and your baby wants to nurse all the time. Many mothers notice this happening around two to three weeks postpartum and then again at six weeks, when a baby normally experiences appetite spurts and nurses more often to stimulate increased milk production. You can expect fluctuations in your milk supply as production becomes regulated according to the baby's requests.

By six to eight weeks after birth, many mothers notice that their breasts seem smaller or feel less full. This does not usually mean that less milk is being produced, but only that the breasts are adjusting to the large amount of milk within and to the baby's feeding pattern.

Some mothers misinterpret their babies' increased requests and their own softer breasts and begin offering supplemental bottles. Usually, this marks the beginning of the end of breastfeeding. The mother begins to assume that she cannot make enough milk for her baby, and she offers more and more formula instead of allowing the baby to increase the mother's own supply of milk. After receiving formula, the baby sleeps longer and nurses less often. He becomes increasingly frustrated at the breast as his mother's milk supply dwindles, and breastfeeding is soon over.

Some mothers try to satisfy their babies' hunger with solid foods. But introducing solids during these early weeks is inappropriate, because a young infant is both physiologically and developmentally unable to manage them. His digestive system and kidneys are not mature enough to handle cereals and other baby foods. Because his immune system is still immature, he may develop allergies to solid foods given during this period.

Fluctuations in the fullness of your breasts and in your milk supply will probably pass by the end of the second month after birth. In the meantime, you can be reassured that your milk supply is probably fine if you are nursing at least eight times in each twenty-four-hour period and letting the baby suck for as long as he wants. If you are worried about your milk supply, though, have your baby weighed. A weight gain of at least an ounce a day will tell you that your baby is getting plenty to eat. If you have additional concerns about your milk supply, see page 233, Underfeeding.

Donating to a Milk Bank

While some women are unable to produce sufficient milk, others produce more than their babies can use. Therein lies the beauty of a milk bank, which serves both those in need of milk and those who wish to donate it. If you are considering donating your milk, it is best to wait until your baby is nursing well and gaining weight as expected. Your doctor may even be required to confirm that your baby is thriving before you are permitted to donate. It is also wise to freeze an extra supply of milk for your own baby in the case of an unexpected need, and definitely if you will be returning to work or school. Or you may be a mother who decides to wean and later regrets doing so because your baby is not tolerating infant formula.

Milk banks save babies' lives. The thirty-one accredited nonprofit milk banks in the United States and Canada help protect the most medically vulnerable infants, who are usually in hospitals. Donors are not paid; rather, the cost of the milk (which is sometimes covered by insurance or by the state) goes to the screening of donors, bacteriologic testing of the milk, pasteurization of the milk, and monitoring a chain of control from the donor to the receiving infant. (There are also for-profit milk banks, like Prolacta, which solicits milk to make a human milk fortifier for premature babies.)

If you are blessed with an abundant milk supply, consider donating some of your milk to a nonprofit milk bank. Like blood banks, milk banks very often experience serious shortages of human milk. Nonprofit banks send milk most often to the sickest babies, whose need for your milk could make the difference between life and death, or serious disability. Visit the Human Milk Banking Association of North America at www.hmbana.org to locate a milk bank site near you, and see Appendix A, page 386. You can be a breast milk heroine!

Casual Milk Sharing

If you are a mother considering accepting milk from a casual milk-sharing organization (such as Eats on Feets or Human Milk 4 Human Babies), keep in mind that someone else's milk may contain toxins, including medications, illegal drugs, tobacco, or alcohol. Certain diseases can be transferred through breast milk as well. Are donor mothers always honest about their intake of tobacco, illegal drugs, and medications? Are all mothers aware of their health history or that of their partners? There is some evidence that this is not always the case. Many milk banks find that donated milk is contaminated with bacteria and must be discarded. Casual peer-to-peer sharing of breast milk could cause harm to a baby receiving milk that has not gone through the process of maternal screening, and culturing and pasteurization of the donated milk. Furthermore, casual milk sharing diverts much-needed milk away from the accredited milk banks, where it can be given to the most medically needy infants.

Scheduled Feedings

Some parenting books and classes have promoted a philosophy of scheduled breastfeeding. Called "Parent Directed Feeding," the program teaches parents to feed babies on a rigid three- to four-hour schedule and to eliminate nighttime feedings at an early age. The purpose is to relieve parental anxiety and instill a sense of order and discipline in the infant. Although most parents like the idea of predictable, widely spaced nursings and full nights of sleep from the early weeks on, these practices are often associated with low milk production, poor weight gain in the baby, and early weaning. Some babies subjected to this method have become dangerously thin and dehydrated.

Babies do best if they are nursed when they seem hungry. Parent Directed Feeding fails to take into account two important facts about breast milk and breastfeeding. First, nature has designed breast milk to be taken frequently. Low in protein, it is easily and quickly digested. Second, a mother's milk supply depends on frequent, complete drainage of the breasts. If she nurses fewer than seven times in a twenty-four-hour period, her milk production generally declines. Although some mothers can meet their babies' needs with fewer than seven daily feedings, most cannot.

The AAP, and every other organization that supports breastfeeding, recommends that babies be fed whenever they show signs of hunger.

Infant Dietary Supplements

Supplements sometimes given to nursing babies include vitamin D, iron, and fluoride.

Vitamin D

Known as the "sunshine vitamin," vitamin D is actually a hormone manufactured by the body when the skin is exposed to sunlight. Dietary sources also provide some vitamin D; fatty fish, especially salmon, herring, and tuna, provide high amounts of the vitamin if they are eaten two to three times a week. Some other foods, such as cow's milk, orange juice, and dry cereal, are "fortified" with small amounts of vitamin D.

Vitamin D is important in multiple ways. Because it promotes calcium absorption in the intestinal tract, it is essential for the health of bones. Infants and children who get too little vitamin D are at risk for developing rickets, a painful bone-softening disease that has recently been reported in some American babies. Vitamin D is also a vital part of the immune system and so may make babies less prone to infection. A deficiency of vitamin D is associated with the onset of type 1 diabetes, multiple sclerosis, rheumatoid arthritis, and cancer.

Sunlight, not food additives or supplements, is "the biologically normal and most common way for humans of all ages to develop adequate levels of the hormone 'vitamin D,'" according to Cynthia Good Mojab, a research associate at La Leche League International. The amount of sunlight exposure needed to prevent vitamin D deficiency depends on such factors as latitude, season, altitude, weather, time of day, air pollution, how much skin is exposed, whether sunscreen is applied (since sunscreen prevents vitamin D production), and skin pigmentation. In general, babies achieve adequate vitamin D levels when exposed to sunlight for thirty minutes per week while wearing only a diaper or for two hours per week while fully clothed without a hat. Infants living in northern latitudes may need more sun exposure than this; infants living closer to the equator may need less. Dark-skinned infants may need more sun exposure than light-skinned infants, although researchers have yet to ascertain this. In any case, the exposure must be direct; sunlight that has passed through window glass, Plexiglas, or almost any other plastic does not allow the body to produce vitamin D, because these materials absorb ultraviolet B radiation.

Pediatricians and dermatologists, however, warn parents to keep their babies out of the sun, particularly during the first six months of life. Because sun exposure in infancy has been associated with an increased risk of skin cancer later in life, the AAP now recommends that all children, including babies who are exclusively breastfed, consume at least 400 IU (international units) of vitamin D per day beginning as soon as possible after birth and continuing through childhood. All infant formulas, like commercially produced cow's milk, are fortified with vitamin D, and babies fed at least 500 milliliters (17.6 ounces) of formula daily get as much vitamin D as the AAP recommends.

But breast milk contains little vitamin D unless the mother takes the vitamin orally in high doses. For exclusively breastfed babies, vitamin D is available in over-the-counter liquid supplements, to be given to the baby by dropper. D-Vi-Sol, made by Enfamil, contains 400 IU of vitamin D per dose; Tri-Vi-Sol, made by the same company, contains vitamins A and C as well as 400 IU of vitamin D. Because breastfed babies don't need supplemental A and C, D-Vi-Sol is generally the better choice between these two. Although the daily dose of each of these preparations is only 1 milliliter, it must be given slowly so that the baby does not gasp, gag, and cough.

Cod liver oil, a supplement much hated by children of generations past, also contains vitamin D as well as vitamin A. The oil is no longer recommended for babies, however, because it can contain mercury and can be toxic at high doses.

There is some controversy about giving oral vitamin D to babies. According to Cynthia Good Mojab, no one has investigated the potential risks, such as aspiration of the liquid, harmful changes in the baby's gut, or increased susceptibility to infection. Since vitamin D is often given in combination with other vitamins, future studies should include the risks of supplementing with those vitamins, too.

An alternative to liquid vitamin-D supplements are the more concentrated Baby Ddrops, which are made by Carlson Laboratories and available at health food stores and through online pharmacies. One daily drop, providing 400 IU of vitamin D, is placed on the nipple for the baby to take while nursing. The drops are odorless, tasteless, and colorless. One bottle is enough for an entire year and costs about $13.00.

The AAP recommends that a breastfed baby be given supplemental vitamin D until she is weaned to infant formula or, preferably, until she is at least a year old and is drinking at least 2 cups of whole milk per day.

If you want to avoid giving your baby vitamin D supplements, you have a couple of choices. While you're pregnant, you can get plenty of sunshine and dietary vitamin D. This will ensure that your baby is born with enough vitamin D stores to last two months even if she is never exposed to the sun. Then you can postpone giving supplements at least until your baby is two months old.

After your baby is born, you can also take supplemental vitamin D yourself, in the amount of 4,000 to 6,000 IU per day. This will increase the amount of D in your milk enough to protect your baby. The recommended form of supplemental vitamin D is cholecalciferol, or vitamin D_3.

Iron

The full-term newborn has sufficient stores of iron for at least the first six months after birth. The small amounts of iron in breast milk are very well utilized by the nursing infant, so iron supplementation is unnecessary. Furthermore, iron supplements can interfere with the anti-infective properties of breast milk.

The baby born prematurely, however, is likely to use up her iron stores earlier than the full-term infant. Supplemental iron is recommended for the premature infant beginning at two months of age or earlier.

Fluoride

This mineral, taken from infancy in water or in supplemental drops, has been shown to reduce childhood dental cavities by 50 to 65 percent. Because little fluoride reaches a baby through breast milk even if the mother drinks fluoridated water, fluoride supplements have sometimes been prescribed for exclusively breastfed babies. Too much fluoride, however, can cause spotting of the developing tooth enamel, and some infants are reported to become fussy and irritable and to have gastro-intestinal upsets after being given fluoride. For these reasons, the AAP recommends delaying fluoride supplements until a baby is six months old and then using them only if the local drinking water is severely deficient in fluoride, with less than 0.3 parts fluoride per million.

The usual dose of supplemental fluoride is 0.25 milligram per day. Fluoride is available by prescription, either alone or in combination with vitamins A and C, which breastfed babies don't need.

LIFE WITH YOUR BABY

....

Illnesses: Yours and the Baby's

When you come down with a minor illness such as a cold or flu, you need not interrupt breastfeeding. Most likely your baby will have already been exposed to the virus that caused you to get sick. In fact, the antibodies you produce against the illness will reach the baby through the milk and may protect him from getting the same sickness. Even though you may not feel much like eating, try to drink extra fluids to keep from getting dehydrated. Should you need to take a medication, even an over-the-counter drug, be sure to check on its safety for the baby (see Appendix D, page 402). Some over-the-counter cold remedies contain pseudoephedrine, which can decrease milk production, sometimes permanently.

Temporary weaning is also unnecessary if you suspect you have a case of food poisoning, provided your only symptoms are vomiting, diarrhea, or both.

Your milk supply may seem low during or just after an illness, but a few days of frequent nursing will usually bring milk production back to normal.

Should you require hospitalization or surgery, you can continue breastfeeding. If you know ahead of time that you'll need a hospital stay, you can pump and save milk for any time that you may be unavailable to your baby. You may be able to arrange to have your baby stay with you, although the hospital will probably require that another adult be there to care for the baby. Ask if the hospital has a fully automatic breast pump for you to use when you cannot nurse; if not, arrange to bring one along, with a double-pump kit. The hospital may even have a lactation professional on staff who can assist with any breastfeeding problems that arise during your hospitalization.

You won't need to express and throw out milk contaminated by an anesthetic or pain medication. By the time you awaken from anesthesia, there will not be enough of the drug in your body to be a problem for your baby. Pain medications are also safe. If you take this book to the hospital with you, you can refer to Appendix D, page 402, for information on other medications.

When you are not able to nurse your baby, express your milk every two to three hours during the day and evening and as often during the night as you usually feed the baby. Wake as often as you need to pump. The nurses should be able to refrigerate your milk in clean containers that you can take home to your baby.

Should your baby become ill, nursing should certainly continue. Breast milk is the best source of fluids and nourishment for recovery and nursing the best source of comfort. But be aware that sickness often changes a baby's nursing pattern. He may nurse more than usual, or he may lose interest in nursing. Ear infections, sore throats, and fever blisters may make nursing painful for the baby. As long as he is nursing infrequently or is refusing to nurse, be sure to express your milk every couple of hours to keep up your supply.

Colds and stuffy noses can make nursing difficult for a baby. Holding your baby upright while feeding, using a humidifier in the room, or administering saline nose drops and cleaning out his nose may make nursing more comfortable for him. Try the NoseFrida, a safe, gentle nasal aspirator that captures the baby's nasal discharge and prevents it from contaminating the device, unlike a traditional bulb aspirator. The NoseFrida is available at many stores and online.

Fever is a sign of infection. During the first four months, a temperature above 99°F (37°C) if taken in the armpit, or 101°F (38°C) if taken rectally, should be reported to the baby's doctor. If, besides having an elevated temperature, the baby doesn't act like his usual self or he nurses poorly, he should be checked by the doctor. The severity of a fever does not always correspond with the seriousness of an illness; a high fever may appear with a minor infection, and a low fever may accompany a serious infection. Because a fever may lead to dehydration, frequent nursing is very important.

Diarrhea in the breastfed baby, although less common and usually less severe than in the formula-fed baby, is characterized by frequent (twelve or more per day), extremely loose or watery bowel movements. Often the stools are foul-smelling, and they may contain mucus or blood. Since babies lose a great deal of fluid with diarrhea, they can easily become dehydrated, so frequent nursing is important. With its high water content, breast milk helps replace the lost fluids. Diarrhea generally improves within three to five days. Fever, infrequent feedings, or signs of dehydration (dry mouth, few wet diapers, listlessness) are reasons to notify your doctor. In cases of severe diarrhea, doctors occasionally recommend supplements of an electrolyte solution, such as Pedialyte, in conjunction with nursing.

The First Two Months: What's Normal?

During the first two months, you can expect your baby will nurse between eight and twelve times a day, including at least once at night. If your baby sleeps four to six hours at a stretch at night or takes a three-to four-hour nap during the day, she will probably want to nurse often during the next few hours to make up for the meal she missed. The baby who is nursing fewer than eight times in a twenty-four-hour period or who is sleeping longer than six hours at a stretch at night is typically the infant who fails to gain enough weight during the early weeks of nursing.

Generally, eight or more wet diapers a day are a sign that the baby is getting enough milk. By two weeks, most nursing infants have regained their birth weight. A gain of at least an ounce a day is normal.

The breastfed baby typically has very loose and seedy-looking stools. During the first month most infants have at least one bowel movement daily. After the first month it is not uncommon for a baby to go several days without a bowel movement. As long as the baby seems comfortable, there is probably no need for concern; your baby is unlikely to be constipated or underfed. The baby who is not getting enough to eat typically has small, and usually infrequent, brown or greenish stools and is gaining less than an ounce a day.

Many mothers continue to experience dripping or spraying milk during or between nursings. But some women stop leaking altogether after the first several weeks, and most gradually notice less leakage.

At some point during the first two months you will probably start to experience the sensations of milk letdown. You may notice this tingling, pins-and-needles feeling in your breasts just before or during a feeding or at any time your baby signals you with his cry.

Occasionally babies spit up after a feeding. Some babies spit up after every nursing. This is usually due to an immature digestive system; what comes up is normally just a few teaspoons. If your baby spits up more, the cause may be certain foods or beverages in your diet (see page 216, Spitting Up and Vomiting, and page 219, Fussiness, Colic, and Reflux). In any case, spitting up passes with time; until it does, keep a diaper or small towel handy.

A baby cries for any of a number of reasons. She may be hungry or tired, or she may just want to suck and be held. Sucking at the breast is soothing and comforting for her. Babies usually have a fussy period in the evening. Although many theories have been suggested to explain why this is, most babies are comforted by extra nursing. Try not to assume your milk is somehow lacking. Many mothers who interpret their babies' cries this way begin supplementing with formula and soon find the babies weaned. See page 219, Fussiness, Colic, and Reflux, for more on why babies cry and how to cope with crying.

During the appetite spurts at about two to three weeks and six weeks of age, your baby may act more fussy than usual and want to nurse more often. After a few days of frequent nursing, your milk supply will increase to meet her needs and she will return to her usual nursing pattern.

Some babies cry hard, as if in pain, for prolonged periods every day. They are said to have colic, which is just a name for extreme irritability that continues day after day—for any of a number of reasons. Some cry at the breast or refuse nursing entirely. If your baby has colic symptoms, see page 219, Fussiness, Colic, and Reflux.

You may have heard that tending to your baby each time she cries will spoil her or will reinforce her behavior and cause her to cry more often. Nothing could be further from the truth. Babies do not cry to exercise their lungs, but because they are in need of something. If your baby's needs are met in infancy, she will develop a sense of security, and she will grow to trust in you and others as well.

During these early weeks, while you are learning about your baby, caring for her needs, and learning to breastfeed, you are apt to experience some feelings of concern, confusion, and perhaps even inadequacy regarding your mothering abilities. Motherhood and breastfeeding may not be exactly what you expected. Your baby's crying and the unpredictability of her sleeping and wakeful periods may be upsetting. The baby's nursing schedule (or lack thereof) and her many needs may make it impossible to feel organized or productive. Perhaps you are disappointed by the lack of help from your healthcare providers. Early motherhood may also bring feelings of loneliness and isolation.

It is normal to have mixed feelings about nursing. Try to keep in mind that new motherhood brings a period of uncertainty and adjustment, and that nursing, like mothering, gets easier with time.

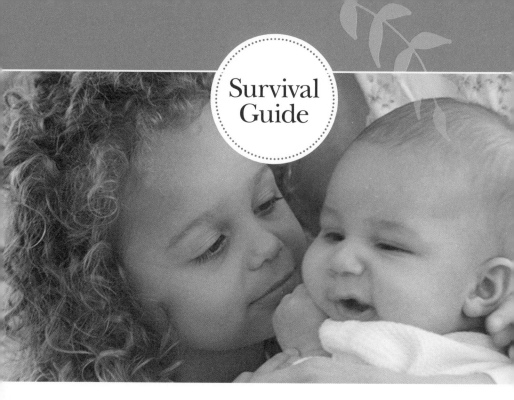

THE FIRST TWO MONTHS

CONCERNS ABOUT YOURSELF

- Sore Nipples
- Breast Pain
- Plugged Ducts
- Breast Infection (Mastitis)
- Breast Abscess
- Breast Lumps
- Leaking Milk
- Overabundant Milk
- Lopsided Breasts
- Nausea or Headache

- Depression and Anxiety
- Dysphoric Milk Ejection Reflex
  (Bad Feelings while Nursing)

CONCERNS ABOUT THE BABY

- Spitting Up and Vomiting
- Pulling Away from the Breast
- Refusal to Nurse
- Fussiness, Colic, and Reflux
- Underfeeding

CONCERNS ABOUT YOURSELF

Sore Nipples

It can certainly be discouraging when sore nipples persist beyond the first week. If this happens to you, review the information on sore nipples (see page 76, Survival Guide: The First Week). It may be helpful to have your partner or a friend observe your latch-on technique and compare it with the descriptions of latch-on (see page 52, Positioning at the Breast). Babies who are tongue-tied may also cause painful nipples (see page 119). But don't discount the possibility that your nipples are irritated due to thrush or another dermatologic condition.

Thrush nipples. If your nipples suddenly become sore after a period of comfortable nursing, thrush is the most likely cause. This problem occurs when a yeast (monilia) infection in the baby's mouth spreads to the mother's nipples. The nipples become reddened and shiny, swollen, tender, and sometimes cracked. Occasionally, peeling or a red, dotty rash can be seen on the nipples and areola. Some mothers complain of itching; others complain of burning. Thrush sometimes begins after the mother has taken a course of antibiotics or when she has had a vaginal birth and had a yeast infection (symptomatic or not) during pregnancy. Those who have given birth by cesarean section may have received antibiotics during surgery making yeast a possibility. Mothers who are diabetic or who become diabetic during pregnancy are more susceptible to yeast.

If you suspect a case of thrush, carefully inspect the baby's mouth. You may see white patches on the inside of the cheeks, lips, and possibly on the tongue. Yeast on the tongue is creamy white. If white areas are only seen on the back center area on the tongue, this may not be yeast. The fat in breast milk can linger on the back of the tongue.

Sometimes a baby will have no symptoms in the mouth but will have a diaper rash caused by yeast. A yeast rash often resembles a mild burn; it may be scaly and peeling. There may be "satellite" areas apart from the main rash, and the rash may appear scaly. It is usually well defined, very red, and a bit raised. Sometimes it looks like just a patch of red dots.

It usually appears in the genital area but may also be noticeable in the folds of the baby's diaper area. A yeast rash will not respond to typical remedies like frequent cleaning and the usual diaper rash creams. For treatment, see page 221.

Treatment Measures for Thrush Nipples

Your doctor can prescribe Nystatin cream or ointment for your nipples, which can also be used for your baby's diaper rash, if one is present. Instead of getting a prescription, you can purchase over-the-counter antifungal creams such as Lotrimin AF, Micatin, or Monistat 7, which is the same strength of the prescription cream/ointment.

1. Apply the medication to your nipples after each nursing. Some lactation professionals recommend rinsing the nipples for the first few days of treatment with water or a mild solution of vinegar (1 tablespoon [15 ml] vinegar to 1 cup [235 ml] water) before applying the medication.

2. To prevent reinfection, your baby's mouth must be treated at the same time as your nipples. Many pediatricians will prescribe Nystatin suspension (Mycostatin) for the baby, which is only available with a prescription. The typical treatment recommendation for thrush is 1 milliliter of Nystatin suspension by dropper into the baby's mouth after every other nursing (or four times daily for fourteen days). Wait a few minutes after nursing before giving this prescription medication so it won't be washed out of the baby's mouth by the milk. Half the dose should be dropped into each side of the mouth. Even if the symptoms are gone after a few days, continue the treatment for the full fourteen days.

3. Because Nystatin inhibits yeast growth for only about two hours after you swab the baby's mouth, it is often ineffective when used as prescribed. If your baby's mouth isn't clear of thrush after five to six days of treatment, ask your doctor about more frequent dosing, or try using gentian violet, as described in Step 4, instead.

4. Gentian violet, an anti-fungal liquid, can be purchased without a prescription to treat oral thrush. A 1 percent solution of gentian violet can be purchased at most, but not all, drugstores, so

call around before making the trip, or have the pharmacy order it for you. If you can find only 2 percent gentian violet solution, you can have the pharmacist dilute the solution, or you can do it yourself by placing a few drops in the cap and adding an equal amount of water. Thoroughly swab the affected areas in the baby's mouth using a cotton-tipped applicator once or twice a day for three days. The solution will stain the baby's mouth purple; take care in applying it so that nothing else turns purple. Some lactation professionals recommend painting the mother's nipples with gentian violet, too, but I don't recommend this treatment if the nipples are tender. Gentian violet costs around $5.

5. Canadian pediatrician and breastfeeding specialist Dr. Jack Newman recommends using grapefruit seed extract (available at most health food stores) as a nipple solution. Mix five to ten drops of the liquid into 1 ounce (30 ml) of water and rub some of this solution on the nipples and areolas after nursings. The concentration of the grapefruit seed extract can be increased gradually to up to twenty-five drops in 1 ounce (30 ml) of water. You can use this solution in addition to any topical antifungal cream by alternating it with the cream. If you find that your nipples begin flaking, stop using this solution.

6. If the weather allows, briefly expose your nipples to the sun two or three times daily to hasten healing.

7. Sanitize your breastfeeding supplies to prevent reinfection. If you're using nursing pads, change them at each feeding. If you are using a pump, wash all the parts thoroughly after each use. Bottle nipples, plastic breast shells, and pump parts that come in contact with the breast or the milk should be boiled in water for five minutes daily. If your baby uses a pacifier, make sure you boil it daily as well.

8. If thrush and accompanying sore nipples aren't cured by the usual treatment measures, some mothers try fluconazole (Diflucan), an oral antifungal agent. The usual dosage is 400 milligrams on the first day followed by 100 milligrams for the next thirteen days. This medication is very expensive, though, and I find that most mothers can overcome yeast infections by using

antifungal cream on the nipples and treating the baby's mouth. If you try a course of fluconazole and still suffer with nipple soreness, yeast is probably not the problem.

9. If after the treatment just described your baby shows no signs of thrush but your nipples are still irritated, see a dermatologist. In the absence of visible thrush, pink, burning nipples may indicate nipple dermatitis.

Nipple dermatitis. If you experience pink, tender nipples beyond the first week of nursing and your baby shows no signs of thrush, you may have another dermatologic condition. A dermatologist can probably both uncover the cause of the soreness and offer effective treatment. Before seeing a dermatologist, though, you might ask your regular physician to prescribe Dr. Jack Newman's all-purpose nipple ointment, or APNO. A topical medication that must be specially made up in a pharmacy, APNO includes 2 percent mupirocin ointment (15 grams), an antibacterial; 0.1 percent betamethasone ointment (15 grams), an anti-inflammatory; and 2 percent miconazole or clotrimazole powder, an antifungal. An optional fourth ingredient, ibuprofen, is helpful for pain relief. The ointment is applied sparingly after nursings or pumpings until the nipples are free of pain for a few days, and then gradually used less often.

If your nipples are still tender after treatment with APNO or an antibacterial ointment, I highly recommend seeing a dermatologist.

Painful, blanched nipples. Some women notice that their nipples become painful and pale at the end of nursing sessions. Often, this pain and blanching results from poor positioning of the baby at the breast. The compression of the nipples probably causes a vasospasm—a spasm in the blood vessels—which prevents blood from getting to the nipples. You may be able to solve this problem by correcting your latch-on technique (review page 52, Positioning at the Breast) and by applying warm compresses to the nipples right after nursing.

Sometimes vasospasm in the nipples results from Raynaud's disease or Raynaud's phenomenon (these two are different; the less common Raynaud's disease occurs on its own, whereas Raynaud's phenomenon is associated with illness such as rheumatoid arthritis or repetitive trauma or injury and affects some 22 percent of twenty-one- to fifty-one-year-old women). In both conditions, blood-vessel spasms brought on by a drop in temperature prevent blood from getting to a particular area of the body. Most commonly, Raynaud's occurs in the fingers, typically when a person goes outdoors from a warm building on a cool day. In this case, the fingers turn white and the tips hurt.

When Raynaud's affects the nipples, it causes nipple blanching just after a feeding, probably because the ambient air is cooler than the inside of the baby's mouth. When the baby comes off the breast, the nipple is its usual color, but it very quickly turns white. This blanching is accompanied by burning pain. Then the nipple turns blue; this is caused by deoxygenation of the blood. As the blood starts flowing back to the nipple, the nipple returns to its normal color, and the mother may experience a throbbing pain. The three-phase color change—from white to blue to red—suggests a diagnosis of Raynaud's phenomenon rather than poor positioning. The nipple colors and the types of pain may alternate for several minutes or as long as an hour or more.

If you have Raynaud's phenomenon, avoiding cold is important. Your entire body needs to be kept warm. Breastfeed in a warm place, wear warm clothing, and avoid exposure to cold at all times. If you experience a painful vasospasm, applying warm, moist cloths to your nipples may help. Avoid smoking and caffeine.

Dietary supplements may help alleviate vasospasms caused by Raynaud's phenomenon. Some women have used a combination of calcium (2,000 milligrams per day) and magnesium (1,000 milligrams per day). So far, however, no studies have tested the effectiveness of this remedy. Jack Newman, a pediatrician, reports that vitamin B_6 often helps with Raynaud's phenomenon and is safe to use. He suggests a dosage of 150 to 200 milligrams once a day for four days. If the symptoms don't lessen in this much time, vitamin B_6 probably won't help at all, Newman says. But if the pain resolves, he suggests taking a reduced dose of 25 milligrams once a day until you are pain-free for a few weeks. If the pain returns with the smaller dose, you can return to the higher dose (Newman and Pitman, 2006).

Various drugs have been investigated for the treatment of Raynaud's phenomenon. The most effective among them is nifedipine, which is primarily used to treat hypertension. Nifedipine is probably safe to use, since very little of the drug (less than 5 percent of the total dose) appears in the breast milk, and side effects in the mother are uncommon (the most frequent side effect is a headache). The usual dosage of nifedipine is one 30-milligram slow-release tablet per day for two weeks. If the nipple pain returns, as it does in about 10 percent of mothers, a second course can be taken. Women rarely require more than three courses.

Eczema and impetigo. Eczema can appear on the nipple and areola, making the area burn, itch, flake, ooze, or crust. Women with a history or current outbreak of eczema elsewhere on the body are most often affected. If you suspect eczema, seek treatment from a dermatologist.

Impetigo is a severe infection that causes continual sloughing off of the skin. When it occurs on the nipples, impetigo is very painful, but it can be quickly cured with an oral antibiotic or an antibiotic cream. Bactroban (mupirocin) is a prescription antibiotic cream commonly used to treat impetigo.

Breast Pain

For a variety of reasons, your breasts may begin to hurt during nursing or become perpetually tender or sore. If this happens, it is important to identify the cause so that you can take any necessary action.

Uncomfortable engorgement can occur any time the breasts become overly full—when the baby misses a feeding, for example, or when he begins to sleep longer at night (see page 77, Engorged Breasts).

Most mothers begin noticing normal letdown sensations during these early weeks. Letdown may be experienced as a mild ache at the start of nursing or a tingling, pins-and-needles sensation.

A deep pain, often described as "shooting" that occurs just after nursing is thought to be related to the sudden refilling of the breast. These pains disappear after the first few weeks of nursing. Blocked nipple pores can also cause stabbing pains (see next page).

Pain during nursing, often described as burning or stinging, is usually associated with thrush. The nipples may be pinker than usual.

Sometimes a rash may be visible. See page 195, Thrush Nipples, for additional information on causes and treatment.

If you can feel a tender area or painful lump in your breast, see the following section.

Plugged Ducts

You may experience a plugged milk duct as a small, tender spot or as a large area of the breast that feels overly full and does not soften with nursing. If you look in a mirror, the skin over the area may appear slightly reddened.

Occasionally a plug in one of the nipple openings blocks the milk flow and causes a backup of milk in the breast. If the nipple looks normal in color but you can see a white pimple (a "bleb") on the end of the nipple, particularly right after the baby comes off the breast, the problem may be a plugged nipple pore. Plugged nipple pores are often associated with stabbing breast pain, especially right after nursing.

Plugged ducts are most common during the early weeks of nursing, but they can occur at any time during breastfeeding. They occur for various reasons. In the early weeks and months, they frequently seem to be caused by incomplete drainage of the breast. Mothers with high milk production, including those nursing twins, tend to be more prone to plugged ducts. Interrupting the baby's nursing to switch to the other breast before the baby signals that he is finished may lead to a plugged duct. A plugged duct may follow a missed feeding or a long stretch at night without nursing. Overly tight bras, especially underwire types, may obstruct milk flow and lead to plugged ducts. Baby carriers with tight straps can also cause this to happen.

For unknown reasons, plugged ducts seem to be more common during the winter months. Some breastfeeding specialists feel that mothers who drink an insufficient amount of fluids, who become slightly dehydrated due to a cold or flu, or who are overly fatigued may also be more susceptible to developing plugged milk ducts.

Any breast lump that does not get significantly smaller within a week should definitely be examined by a doctor. Plugged milk ducts rarely last more than a few days, and breastfeeding mothers can develop breast cancer.

Treatment Measures for Plugged Ducts

1. Remove your bra if there is any question that it may be too tight or may be pressing into part of your breast.

2. Before nursing, apply moist heat to the breast for fifteen to twenty minutes.

3. Nurse frequently, at least every two hours. Begin each nursing on the affected breast.

4. While nursing, gently massage the breast just behind the sore area. Some lactation consultants suggest trying a vibrator, including an electric tooth brush, to dislodge the clog. If the plugged area is still there, consider using your fingers to perform manual expression to clear the duct. Watch the video by lactation consultant Maya Bolman (http://bfmedneo.com/resources/videos/). Apply moist heat for a few minutes and massage the breast well using an edible oil. Next, perform hand expression removing the milk between the plugged area and the nipple. After getting milk out below the plugged area, try nursing again.

5. If you are following the preceding recommendations but notice no change in your breast after a feeding or two, try positioning the baby with his chin close to the plugged duct, if possible, to promote better drainage. Another approach is getting into a warm shower. With your breast well-soaped, try using hand expression again.

6. Increase your fluid intake so that you urinate more frequently.

7. If the blockage seems to be in the nipple, look for dried milk secretions or a clogged nipple pore, which may resemble a whitehead. If necessary, you can gently remove a visible plug from a nipple opening with a sterilized needle. (Wash your hands well. To sterilize a needle, place the needle in a cup of rubbing alcohol or hydrogen peroxide, and leave it there for thirty seconds. Wash your hands again, and then pick up the needle by the blunt end.)

Using the needle to open the "bleb" may cause a little bleeding, but you probably won't feel any pain.

8. If nursing is too painful or if you suspect the baby isn't draining the affected breast well, begin pumping your breasts after or instead of nursing. Renting a clinical-grade pump for a couple of days may be best. If you are pumping instead of nursing, pump very often. Some mothers have found that using Pumpin' Pal Super Shields while pumping can clear up a plugged milk duct (see page 256). Occasionally a mother who pumps while having a plugged duct will get pink milk from a bit of blood coming from the plug opening up. There is no need to be alarmed, but avoid feeding that milk to your baby, as blood is a gastric irritant and can cause her to vomit.

9. Be alert for signs of a developing breast infection—fever, chills, and achiness—so you can treat it promptly (see the section that follows).

10. Should you get a second case of a plugged milk duct, see page 345, Recurrent Plugged Ducts and Breast Infections in Survival Guide: Months Two through Six.

If a plug does not resolve after a few feedings with the above measures, some lactation professionals suggest using an old-fashioned treatment for swelling: Apply castor oil to a warm, moist washcloth, lay it over the sore area, and place a heating pad over the washcloth. Keep the compress and heating pad in place for about 20 minutes before nursing or pumping. This can be repeated before each feeding.

Breast Infection (Mastitis)

Up to 20 percent of all nursing women develop mastitis, or infection of the breast. It occurs most often in the first three months after birth and, interestingly, it is more common during the winter months.

A breast infection is caused by bacteria, often the same ones normally present on the nipples and in the baby's mouth. A breast infection often follows an untreated cracked nipple or a plugged milk duct. It is more likely to occur when the baby (or a pump) is ineffective at draining the breasts. Other possible causes include poor-fitting bras, skipped feedings, infrequent changing of wet breast pads, anemia, stress, and fatigue.

Since mastitis causes flu-like symptoms, women sometimes mistake it for the flu. Headache, general achiness, and a reddened area of the breast are the early symptoms; they are usually followed by fever (typically over 101°F [38°C]), chills, and weakness. Usually only one breast is affected; it becomes quite tender in the infected area.

Women who promptly apply moist heat to the breast and work on getting it as empty as possible may recover quickly without antibiotics, usually in one or two days. In one study of women with mastitis, half used no antibiotics, and none of them suffered complications (Riordan and Nichols, 1990). I have come to believe, however, that prompt treatment with antibiotics is indicated whenever a nursing mother has flu-like symptoms and a reddened breast, and especially if she has a fever. Some women have permanently lost their milk production from the affected breast following a breast infection, although this has usually occurred when treatment has been delayed. Late treatment can also result in an abscess, which may require surgical drainage. This risk may be greater if you are anemic.

Effective treatment with an antibiotic requires the right choice of antibiotic. The bacterium involved in mastitis is usually *Staphylococcus aureus*, or "staph," which is resistant to amoxicillin, penicillins G and V, and many other antibiotics.

Usually, the most effective antibiotics against this organism are cloxacillin and dicloxacillin, and cephalosporins, such as cephalexin (Keflex). Another frequently prescribed penicillin is Augmentin, a more potent form of amoxicillin. Erythromycin, clarithromycin, azithromycin, and clindamycin are used in women who are allergic to penicillin. All of these antibiotics are safe to take while breastfeeding unless the baby is allergic to them (the allergy usually causes a rash).

Recently, some staph infections have become resistant to all penicillins, so if you are not markedly better in three or four days, contact your healthcare provider. You may need a different antibiotic, such as clindamycin, co-trimoxazole (Septra), or doxycycline. Mothers who fail to respond to antibiotics may have contracted MRSA, or methicillin-resistant *Staphylococcus aureus*. This bacteria has been cultured in the milk of some mothers who do not seem to be responding to the antibiotics normally used to treat mastitis. If you are still sick after a few days, speak with your doctor about this possibility.

In general, antibiotic treatment for mastitis should continue for ten to fourteen days. It is important to take the antibiotic until it is used up, even if you feel better, because you could develop a resistant infection if you stop too soon.

With prompt and proper treatment, the symptoms usually subside within forty-eight hours. Nurse frequently during this period; discontinuing nursing would slow healing and might lead to the development of a breast abscess. Unless you are expressing milk for a premature or sick baby who is hospitalized, you don't need to worry that the baby will get ill, since the infection involves only the breast tissue, not the milk. Try to identify the probable cause of the infection so you can prevent a recurrence in the future.

Mastitis in both breasts, though rare, can be a sign of B-streptococcal infection, which is transmitted by the infant to the breasts. When both breasts are affected, the baby's doctor should be promptly notified so that the baby can be tested and treated, if necessary.

Treatment Measures for Mastitis

1. Go to bed, if you haven't already.
2. Remove your bra if you are more comfortable without it or if there is any question that it may be pressing into part of your breast.
3. Nurse frequently, at least every two hours, and begin each nursing on the affected breast. Giving up nursing could slow healing and lead to a breast abscess. Use an edible oil to massage the breast from the painful area toward the nipple while nursing.
4. If nursing is too painful or if you suspect the baby isn't draining the affected breast well, begin pumping your breasts after or instead of nursing. Renting a clinical-grade "rental" pump for a couple of days is usually best (see Chapter 5 for advice on expressing milk).

If you are pumping instead of nursing, pump very often with a clinical grade pump.

5. Call your doctor, who will probably prescribe antibiotics. Antibiotics should be taken for the entire time they are prescribed, even though the symptoms may disappear.

6. Increase your fluid intake enough that you notice an increase in urination.

7. Apply moist heat to the breast for fifteen to twenty minutes before nursing or pumping and intermittently between feedings.

8. Monitor your temperature. A mild pain reliever, such as ibuprofen (Motrin, Advil), may help reduce your fever and discomfort more than Tylenol.

9. Consider taking vitamin C. Some women report that a dosage of 1,000 milligrams four times a day speeds healing and recovery.

10. After you have completed a course of antibiotics, watch for symptoms of yeast growth in the baby's mouth and diaper rash caused by yeast (see page 195, Thrush Nipples).

11. See page 345, Recurrent Plugged Ducts and Breast Infections, if you have a recurrence.

Breast Abscess

On very rare occasions, a breast infection develops into an abscess. A breast abscess is an accumulation of pus walled off within the breast. It may occur when a mother stops nursing during a breast infection, when treatment for mastitis is delayed, or when a mother has trouble fighting a breast infection because she is anemic.

A breast abscess should be suspected whenever mastitis symptoms last for more than a couple of days and a lump persists. The lump may be hard or soft but does not change with nursing. An abscess must usually be drained by a physician, either in an office or a hospital. After it is drained, recovery is rapid.

Some doctors are willing to avoid surgical drainage by performing a series of needle aspirations, by which a needle is inserted into the abscess and the pus is withdrawn into a syringe. This is much less invasive than opening the abscess to drain over a period of a couple of weeks.

The development and treatment of an abscess can be traumatic. You may be advised to stop nursing entirely, or you may doubt yourself whether you should continue. Although you need not abandon nursing completely, you may be advised against nursing from the affected breast for the first few days after it is drained. In the meantime, you can rent a clinical-grade electric pump to maintain your milk flow until the baby resumes nursing on both sides. The incision may leak milk for a short while, but it will heal and close over. I developed an abscess six weeks after giving birth and went on to nurse successfully without any further difficulties.

Breast Lumps

Lumps in the breast are very common during the early weeks and are usually related to lactation.

The breast may feel generally lumpy when it is overly full or engorged. A tender lump that arises suddenly is usually a sign of a plugged milk duct or, when it is accompanied by fever and flu-like symptoms, a breast infection. A lump that appears just before nursing and seems to get smaller or disappear afterward is probably a small cyst that fills with milk.

Whenever a lump shows no change in size for longer than a week, it should be examined by a doctor. It is probably a harmless cyst or benign tumor; cancer is rarely the cause. But some breastfeeding women with persistent lumps have been found to have breast cancer, so see your doctor for a thorough breast exam as soon as possible. If further diagnosis is recommended, you don't need to wean your baby, although a doctor unfamiliar with the lactating breast may recommend doing so.

Some mothers may need a mammogram, ultrasound, MRI, or breast biopsy to rule out breast cancer. Mammograms and ultrasounds can be performed while you are nursing, but they are best done on an empty breast, so drain the breast as completely as possible just prior to these procedures. When a mother needs a breast MRI, the contrast agent used is generally considered safe to allow her to resume nursing after the procedure (see Appendix D, page 402). Needle biopsies, both fine-needle and core biopsies, can also be done while a mother is nursing, but mothers are often told to wean because a biopsy can cause a milk fistula. In reality, fistulas are very rare. Any necessary incisions should be done so as to avoid the nipple and areola, especially the lower outer border, to keep from injuring the fourth intercostal nerve. A radial (horizontal) incision is also recommended. The use of local anesthesia is safe for immediate nursing or pumping, and bottle or cup feeding the baby afterward is safe. In fact, the breast should be kept well drained after the procedure by nursing or pumping. Pumping may be preferable if there is much blood coming through the milk—blood can be irritating to the baby's stomach, so he might vomit up the milk.

Consider getting a second opinion whenever drastic measures are recommended.

Leaking Milk

See page 76, Survival Guide: The First Week, for basic information on leaking, dripping, and spraying milk.

After a few weeks of nursing you may notice that leaking diminishes or stops entirely. This should not be a cause for concern so long as the baby is nursing frequently and gaining weight.

If continuing leakage becomes bothersome, you might want to try stopping it by pressing your wrist or the heel of your hand against your nipples whenever they start to drip. You might also try LilyPadz, sticky silicone pads that can be worn with or without a bra (see Appendix A, page 386).

If leaking at night continues to be troublesome, you might try nursing the baby just before you go to sleep.

Overabundant Milk

Some mothers seem to produce too much milk. Besides feeling weary of the jokes about being able to nurse twins, you may feel uncomfortably engorged much of the time. Leaking and spraying may be bothersome. Your baby may gasp and choke as the milk lets down.

Most women find this less of a problem after the first two months of breastfeeding. In the meantime, nursing your baby on just one side at each feeding should make your breasts feel more comfortable. When your baby is draining your breasts more completely, they will feel less engorged, even though each is nursed on less often. Decreasing your fluid intake is not recommended. Nor is wearing plastic breast shells or pumping after or between feedings, either of which would probably increase, not decrease, milk production.

If your baby has difficulty nursing because the milk lets down forcefully, see page 217, Pulling Away from the Breast. Refer to page 346, Overabundant Milk, if you continue to produce milk in overabundance after two months.

Lopsided Breasts

When one breast receives more stimulation than the other, milk production in that breast increases, commonly resulting in a lopsided appearance.

Providing more stimulation to the smaller breast will usually even out the size difference between the two. Start each feeding on the smaller side for a day or so. If your baby nurses there for only a few minutes, encourage her to take the smaller breast again after she has nursed at the fuller one. As soon as your breasts become closer in size, you can begin alternating the breast at which the baby begins each feeding.

Nausea or Headache

Rarely, a new mother experiences nausea when nursing her newborn. This is thought to be a gastric hormonal response to suckling. Eating something before nursing may help. Fortunately, nausea generally decreases in severity and frequency as nursing is established, and the problem usually disappears completely by six to eight weeks after birth.

Headaches in new mothers have various causes. A woman who has had spinal or epidural anesthesia may suffer from a severe headache whenever she raises her head. This occurs when spinal fluid, which cushions the brain, has escaped from the spinal canal, causing the brain to sag down into the opening at the base of the skull. Remaining in bed, increasing fluid intake, and drinking beverages containing caffeine may help. When spinal headaches continue for more than a day or two, some doctors offer a "blood patch," by which they inject the mother's own blood into the spinal canal. This often produces immediate relief.

Several case reports in medical literature have concerned "lactational headaches." These occur during feedings as the milk lets down and may be related to the hormone oxytocin. Some writers have said that pain relievers such as acetaminophen (Tylenol) and ibuprofen (Motrin, Advil) are helpful and that these headaches gradually become less severe and stop by two months after birth. But other writers have described cases in which relief came only with weaning.

Another type of headache associated with lactation occurs when one or both breasts are overfull. This type of headache may be a sign of an impending breast infection. Relief comes from draining the breasts well and heading off mastitis.

Other causes of headaches include drop-in hormones in the first week postpartum; low blood sugar; eye, dental, or sinus problems; allergies; or migraine.

Regardless of the suspected cause of your headaches, you may want to consult with your doctor or a neurologist if they are frequent or severe. Keeping a headache log can be helpful in determining a diagnosis.

Depression and Anxiety

Many new mothers experience moodiness, mild anxiety, or an occasional "blue" day during the first two weeks after delivery. These feelings are due to the sudden hormonal changes that follow birth, fatigue from labor and lost sleep, and the stress that becoming a mother entails. But when emotional symptoms are severe, when they continue beyond the first two weeks after birth, or when they start later and last for more than two weeks, they may indicate postpartum depression or anxiety.

Often, new mothers who complain that they are feeling depressed or anxious are told that their feelings are normal and to be expected. But there could be more to it. Postpartum emotional disorders are often misunderstood or unrecognized by family, friends, and health professionals. Co-parents are also believed to experience postpartum depression, including sadness, irritability, anger, low motivation, distancing away from friends and family, and sleep and appetite disturbances.

As many as one out of every nine or ten new mothers' experiences postpartum depression, postpartum anxiety, or both. Much rarer is postpartum psychosis, characterized by delusions, hallucinations, or extreme mental confusion. Postpartum emotional disorders are more common in women who have had a stressful pregnancy or difficult birth, previous psychological problems, or relationship difficulties. Occasionally, a thyroid disorder may mimic postpartum depression.

Symptoms of postpartum depression or anxiety usually include several of the following:

- Change in eating habits (poor appetite or overeating)
- Change in sleep pattern (difficulty falling or staying asleep, oversleeping)
- Tenseness, nervousness
- Panic attacks with physical symptoms such as shakiness, palpitations, shortness of breath, or lightheadedness
- Fatigue or lack of energy
- Poor concentration, forgetfulness, or confusion
- Crying every day
- Feelings of hopelessness
- Withdrawal, lack of interest in usual activities
- Excessive worry or guilt feelings
- Recurrent disturbing thoughts or compulsive behaviors that cause distress or take up a great deal of time
- Failure to keep appointments

Symptoms that call for immediate assistance from a mental-health professional include these:

- Thoughts of suicide
- Fears of harming the baby
- Sounds and voices heard when no one is around
- Thoughts that seem not your own or out of your control

- Sleeplessness lasting forty-eight hours or longer
- Inability to eat
- Inability to care for the baby

There are many helpful books available on the topic for mothers suffering from postpartum depression or anxiety. I especially like *This Isn't What I Expected: Overcoming Postpartum Depression*, by Karen Kleiman and Valerie Raskin (see page 423, References & Reading). Many women with mild cases have helped themselves without professional assistance. Try the coping measures that follow.

Coping Measures for Depression and Anxiety

1. Tell your partner, a supportive friend, or a relative how you are feeling. Although some people may not understand, you may find valuable support close by.

2. Talk to your doctor or midwife about how you are feeling. Ask about blood tests to make sure something else, such as a thyroid disorder, isn't the problem.

3. Call Postpartum Support International (800-944-4PPD) to find out whether there is a postpartum support group in your area. Or visit www.postpartum.net and click on "Get Help." Postpartum Support International is a not for profit organization that provides telephone support, including referrals to resources for help. Their phone number is 1-800-944-4PPD and you can leave a message at any time. Find more details, along with information and articles about pregnancy and postpartum mood disorders, at www.postpartum.net.

4. Make getting extra rest a priority; being tired makes depression and anxiety worse. Nap when your baby naps. Maximize your baby's sleep stretches at night by feeding him every two to two and a half hours during the day and evening.

5. Enlist the help of others to relieve you of some mothering and household duties. Eliminate or lessen your daily chores until you are feeling better. If you want to do some chores, set minimal goals for yourself.

6. Maintain a well-balanced diet. If you have little appetite, fix small, nutritious snacks for yourself throughout the day. Avoid all caffeine and sugary foods and beverages; these are associated with worsening symptoms. Increase your intake of foods made up of complex carbohydrates, such as whole-grain breads and cereals, potatoes, rice, and pasta. Eat more fruits and vegetables. Using powdered milk or yogurt, wheat germ, and fruit or juice concentrate, you can make nutritious blender drinks. If you find it difficult to prepare food for yourself throughout the day, your pharmacist can recommend a high-calorie nutritional supplement such as Ensure or Sustacal.

7. Consider increasing your intake of the long-chain omega-3 fatty acids DHA (docosahexaenoic acid) and EPA (eicosapentaenoic acid), which have been shown to help prevent and remedy post-partum depression and other mental problems in new mothers. The main dietary source of DHA and EPA is fish, but you would have to eat a great deal of fish every week to achieve the necessary levels. Kathleen Kendall-Tackett, a psychologist, suggests taking omega-3 supplements, which can be found at almost any drugstore or health-food store. To prevent depression, she recommends 200 to 400 milligrams of DHA daily. To treat depression, she recommends 1,000 to 2,000 milligrams of EPA daily. These levels are recognized as safe by the U.S. Food and Drug Administration.

8. Get some exercise every day. Many people find that exercise has an antidepressant effect. Join an exercise or dance class; many offer free childcare. Take a brisk walk every day with or without the baby.

9. Nurture yourself as much as possible. Take long bubble baths, get a massage, ask your partner to hold you, spend the afternoon watching a video or reading a light novel. Even just making a point of getting dressed and fixing your hair when you get up can be the first step in feeling better about yourself. It may not fix things on a clinical level, but a little self care can go a long way.

10. Make an effort to spend time with other adults. Invite friends over, join a postpartum group, or make friends with other mothers from your childbirth class. Your childbirth instructor may have additional suggestions. If you have just moved to the area, ask at your pediatrician's or family practitioner's office about social resources for new parents.

If your distress is severe or unrelieved by these measures, consider seeking professional help. Low-cost mental healthcare is available in most communities. Ask your doctor, midwife, or childbirth educator to refer you to a therapist, ideally one who has a special interest in postpartum mental illness.

Postpartum Support International is a not for profit organization that provides telephone support, including referrals to resources for help. Their phone number is 1-800-944-4PPD Pacific Time and you can leave a message at any time. Experts are available by phone during weekly chats on Wednesdays. Find more details at www.postpartum.net/resources.

Also, Postpartum Support has a website that has information and articles about Pregnancy and Postpartum Mood Disorders.

Depending on your symptoms, a therapist may recommend medication. Some antidepressants are safe to use during nursing; others may not be. Safe antidepressants include sertraline, which is sold under the trade name Zoloft; nortriptyline (Pamelor); and paroxetine (Paxil). All of these are also available generically. When nursing mothers take one of these drugs, it is usually undetectable in their babies' blood.

Your doctor may recommend weaning your baby before taking antidepressants; however, in Appendix D, you'll find what information is available about the safety of various antidepressants. You may want to share this information with your doctor while discussing what is best for you and your baby.

You may be tempted to try St. John's Wort, a popular herbal remedy for depression. This herb, however, has not yet been proven safe to use during breastfeeding.

A new option for mothers with severe postpartum depression is the intravenous administration of Zulresso, which is given by continuous infusion over a total of 60 hours (2.5 days or longer) in a certified health-care facility. The cost of this treatment may be covered by insurance. Side effects may include sleepiness, dizziness, and loss of consciousness. In younger mothers, under the age of 24, there is also a risk of suicidal thoughts and actions. Studies suggest that improvement in symptoms occurs quickly over the course of treatment. The cost which can be as much as $35,000 may be covered by insurance. Zulresso is safe to take while breastfeeding.

Dysphoric Milk Ejection Reflex (Bad Feelings While Nursing)

Some nursing mothers experience negative emotions beginning just before their milk lets down and continuing from several seconds to as long as a minute or two. This newly recognized syndrome, called dysphoric milk ejection reflex (D-MER), is apparently caused by a sudden drop in dopamine, a hormone and neurotransmitter.

Mothers with D-MER variously describe a sinking feeling in the stomach; a low mood; a brief feeling of hopelessness, depression, apprehension, or dread; "an urge to get away"; or simply "a yucky feeling." A few mothers experience feelings of impatience, frustration, agitation, or anger. The feelings quickly disappear after the milk releases but may recur as the milk lets down throughout the feeding.

D-MER is not postpartum depression or a psychological response to breastfeeding; it is a physiologic response. Happily, many things can help with this problem. Some women just distract themselves while nursing. Others get relief by keeping well hydrated, exercising, sleeping more, or taking small amounts of beverages with caffeine. Nutritional supplements such as omega-3 fatty acids and evening primrose oil may also relieve symptoms. The prescription antidepressant bupropion (the active ingredient in Wellbutrin) may be helpful as well. The website at www.d-mer.org is full of helpful information on managing D-MER.

Similar in some ways to D-MER is BAA (Breastfeeding Aversion and Agitation). This unexplained phenomenon includes experiencing negative feelings while the baby is latched on to the breast. Mothers typically feel agitated, irritable, itchy, and even disgusted while their baby or toddler is actively sucking. Mothers may experience a strong desire to end the feeding. After nursing, some women are left feeling shame and guilt. For some, this reaction to nursing is more common while they are menstruating. Some have theorized that this may be the body's way to encourage toddler weaning.

CONCERNS ABOUT THE BABY

Spitting Up and Vomiting

Spitting up small amounts of breast milk is common; some babies do this after almost every nursing. Recently, it has become common for doctors to diagnose these babies with gastroesophageal reflux, or GER (see page 219, Fussiness, Colic, and Reflux).

Occasionally a baby may vomit what seems like an entire feeding. Although there may be no apparent cause, this can sometimes be traced to something the mother recently ate. Vomiting can also be a sign of infection. You will want to notify your doctor if the baby has a fever or if the vomiting continues.

When a baby continues vomiting forcefully after most feedings, you should suspect that either he is sick, sensitive to something in your diet, or he has pyloric stenosis, a muscular obstruction of the bottom part of the stomach that typically develops at about two to four weeks of age. It is thought to occur in four of every 1,000 babies. Although this condition is most common in first-born males, it can occur in females, and one study found it is more common in babies with an allergy to cow's milk. Typically, the vomiting becomes progressively worse; the baby eventually stops gaining weight, or loses weight, and may become dehydrated. In the breastfed infant, the condition may go undiagnosed longer than in the bottle-fed infant, since breast milk is digested much more easily than formula. The baby's weight may not be affected until the obstruction becomes nearly complete. Frequently, waves can be seen moving across the baby's lower abdomen from the left side to the right just after a feeding and prior to vomiting. X-rays confirm the diagnosis.

The obstruction is corrected with a relatively simple surgical procedure. Breastfeeding can resume within a few hours after the obstruction is removed. At this time breast milk is especially good for the baby because of its digestibility. Some mothers notice a temporary reduction in the milk supply after the baby's surgery. Rest, frequent nursing, and switching the baby from side to side during the feeding usually reverse this situation.

Pulling Away from the Breast

Babies pull off the breast while nursing for a variety of reasons. Often it is because they have had enough to eat or they need to be burped. If your baby has a cold, she may pull away because she is having trouble breathing through her nose. Try to position her so her head is more elevated during nursing. A warm-mist humidifier can be helpful in thinning nasal secretions, as can saline nose drops. You can also use the NoseFrida (see page 190) to remove excess nasal discharge from the baby's nostrils.

Some babies pull away from the breast gasping and choking as the milk suddenly lets down. This is usually a temporary problem; the baby gradually learns to keep up with the rapid flow of milk. In the meantime, positioning the baby differently may help. Try sitting the baby up, using the football hold, or lying on your back with the baby's head over you. You can also try laying the flat of your hand against the breast and pressing inward until the flow of milk seems to subside. Some mothers manually express or pump milk until the initial spray has subsided, but this could work against you by increasing the overall production of milk, which would strengthen the letdown response.

Refusal to Nurse

If your baby pulls away from the breast crying or refuses to nurse, don't assume he is ready to wean. There are a number of possible reasons for such behavior, but when it persists, it can frequently be traced to certain foods in the mother's diet to which the baby is sensitive. Typically, this behavior starts when the baby is about two weeks old. He may also act fussy and have very frequent, sometimes greenish stools. Other symptoms may include gassiness, redness around the rectum, a mild rash anywhere on the body, or a stuffy nose. Fussiness while nursing and refusal to nurse may occur sporadically or may increase as the day goes on. Although the baby refuses the breast, he may eagerly take breast milk from a bottle. The reasons for this are unclear.

Babies with gastro-esophageal reflux also sometimes refuse to nurse. When accompanied by frequent spitting up and fussiness, refusal to nurse is most likely caused by a painful irritation of the esophagus.

A baby who has developed a yeast infection, or thrush, may also become fussy at the breast and refuse to nurse. Besides having a characteristic white coating on his tongue, the insides of lips, cheeks, or all, the baby with thrush may be gassy. There may also be a bright red, dotted or peeling rash around the baby's genitals or on your nipples. Your nipples may burn or itch.

Babies with ear infections also sometimes fuss at the breast and refuse to nurse. Although ear infections are less common in breast-fed than in formula-fed babies, especially in the first two months after birth, even in this period an ear infection may accompany or follow a runny nose.

Occasionally a baby will refuse to nurse because his mother is wearing perfume or a scented deodorant.

When a baby has been fed supplemental formula and the milk supply has lessened, he may lose interest in the breast, preferring the immediate flow from the bottle. He may fuss and cry when his mother tries to breastfeed him.

Treatment Measures When the Baby Refuses to Nurse

1. As long as your baby refuses to nurse, express your milk every two to three hours so your supply will not be affected. Use a clinical-grade rental pump or a near-clinical-grade personal pump (see Chapter 5). Feed the baby by bottle.

2. See the next section, Fussiness, Colic, and Reflux.

3. Check your baby's mouth and your nipples for signs of thrush (see page 195, Thrush Nipple).

4. If you can find no reason for your baby's irritability and refusal to nurse, have a doctor examine the baby.

Fussiness, Colic, and Reflux

You may be surprised to learn how much crying a baby can do and how uncomfortable it can make you feel. The sound of a baby's cry is intended to be distressing so adults will be alerted to his needs and answer them.

Many mothers tend to blame themselves for their babies' crying, wondering if their inexperience, nervous feelings, or milk supply is somehow responsible. Keep in mind that most babies fuss and seek out the comfort of the breast when they are tired, bored, lonely, or uncomfortable as well as when they are hungry, and that all babies have fussy periods during appetite spurts.

If you are worried that the baby is not getting enough milk, have him weighed. A weight gain of 1 ounce (28 g) a day or more in the exclusively breastfed baby means she is getting enough milk (see page 235, Underfeeding).

Some babies are extremely irritable during the early weeks, with periods of intense crying. If your baby's crying makes you feel that something is wrong, trust your instincts. By all means have your baby examined by your doctor.

Outlined below are common reasons that babies cry and suggestions for relieving their distress.

Missing the womb. Harvey Karp, a California pediatrician, theorizes that much of the fussing babies do in the early weeks results from missing the uterine environment. In *The Happiest Baby on the Block: The New Way to Calm Crying and Help Your Baby Sleep Longer*, Dr. Karp suggests that parents calm their babies through the five S's:

Swaddling. Many societies have used this technique to imitate the secure feeling of the womb during late pregnancy. A baby is wrapped tightly in a thin blanket with his arms at his sides. Securing the arms and hands keeps the baby from flailing them and makes him more receptive to the other four calming techniques.

To swaddle your baby, lay the blanket out flat, turn in a corner, and place the baby's neck on the folded edge. With the baby's right arm straightened at his side, pull the right corner of the blanket tightly over his body, and tuck it under his lower back on the left side. With his left arm straight at his side, pull the bottom corner of the blanket up over the right arm and shoulder and tuck the blanket under his right side; don't worry about scrunching the baby's legs. Now wrap the left side of the blanket snugly across his body.

Side or stomach position. Although it is now known that laying a baby to sleep on his stomach raises his risk of succumbing to sudden infant death syndrome (SIDS), laying a baby on his back tends to make him startle—to extend his arms and cry out as if he feels he is falling backward. To prevent startling—or the Moro reflex, as it is sometimes called—swaddle the baby and lay him down to sleep on his side, or let him rest on his stomach over your lap or shoulder.

Shushing. Loud white noise calms a baby because it sounds like the flow of blood from the placenta. The louder a baby cries, the louder the shushing he needs. Hair dryers and vacuum cleaners work as well as vocal shushing sounds.

Swinging. Swinging is also reminiscent of uterine life. The swinging should be in rapid, small movements back and forth with the baby face down across your lap. You can swing your baby by wearing him as you walk, by rocking him, or by using a baby swing after the baby is one month of age (see page 232, Coping Measures for Fussiness, Colic, and Reflux).

Sucking. You can calm a baby who is upset but not hungry by either nursing or offering a pacifier. If your baby seems to need a great deal of comfort sucking, a pacifier may be appropriate. You can introduce one when your baby is between two and six weeks old. Before two weeks a pacifier could interfere with the establishment of breastfeeding, and after six weeks your baby might be much less willing to accept it.

Appetite spurts. You will probably notice that your baby is fussier at around two to three weeks and again at around six weeks, when most babies experience appetite spurts. During an appetite spurt, a baby nurses more frequently for a few days, and this stimulates an increase in milk production. Fussiness in the late afternoon or evening is typical.

The baby's temperament. Every baby is born with her own distinct personality. Some babies tend to be quiet, whereas others are more active. Some babies are highly sensitive to their surroundings and overreact to any sudden stimulation. They are tense, jumpy, and often fussy. They may go almost instantly from sleepy or calm to full-blown crying. Once crying, they may be difficult to soothe. Although some of these babies need to be carried around or entertained continually, others may actually resist being held or cuddled.

Learning how to mother a highly sensitive baby takes time and patience. You will soon develop a sense of what your baby enjoys and what she does not, how much stimulation she can tolerate, and how to help her settle down. If your baby does not enjoy touching, try not to take it personally. With time and a gradual increase in physical closeness, she will eventually be able to tolerate and enjoy being held. Most babies outgrow their early fussy months and grow to be happy children.

Diaper rash. A baby may fuss a lot if she has a diaper rash. At each diaper change for an entire day, gently wash the baby's bottom and apply a zinc oxide ointment (such as Desitin). Expose the baby's bottom to the air as much as possible, and leave off disposable diapers or plastic pants. The rash should improve dramatically, unless it is caused by yeast (see the following section).

If the baby's stools are green, he may be reacting to certain foods in his mother's diet. See Colic and Reflux, below.

Yeast infection. Although common in infants, yeast infections are frequently overlooked as the cause of excessive fussiness. A baby with a yeast infection usually shows signs in his mouth—on his inner lips or cheeks, and sometimes also on the tongue. This is known as thrush. The baby is typically very gassy, as the yeast is frequently present in the intestinal tract as well. The yeast may also cause a dotty, red rash or a peeling rash that resembles a mild burn, typically in the genital area. The mother's nipples are often reddened; they may show a rash, and they may itch or burn. One nipple may be more affected than the other.

Nystatin suspension (Mycostatin) is usually the drug of choice when a baby has a yeast infection. Because Nystatin is swallowed, the yeast in the bowel is usually eliminated. Sometimes, however, a diaper rash appears only after treatment with the oral medication, and in other cases a rash gets worse during the first few days of treatment. Nystatin ointment can be used to treat both the mother's nipples and the baby's diaper rash.

The other common oral medication, gentian violet, mainly kills yeast in the mouth and therefore may not be as helpful for the baby who is fussy and gassy.

See page 196, Thrush Nipples, for a complete discussion of treatment measures for yeast infections.

Colic and reflux. Colic is a catchall term for unidentified infant discomfort characterized by periods of intense crying and apparent abdominal pain. Although the causes of colic have been much debated over the years, it is often dismissed as something parents must simply endure until the baby is three to four months old, when the symptoms are expected to lessen or disappear. In the meantime, the baby is unhappy, and her mother may wonder if breastfeeding is to blame.

Recently, many babies who might in the past have been labeled colicky have been diagnosed instead with gastroesophageal reflux, which is also called GER or simply reflux. Reflux is the backward movement of food and acid from the stomach into the esophagus and sometimes into the mouth and out onto your shirt. Nearly all babies have episodes of reflux; most parents consider it normal for their babies to "spit up" after feedings. Some babies who regurgitate frequently show no apparent discomfort. Others, however, seem to suffer painful heartburn, even if they don't spit up their milk.

The main reason babies spit up is that the lower esophageal sphincter isn't fully developed in infants. Also, babies take in a lot of milk relative to the size of their stomachs, and many also swallow a lot of air when they nurse or suck on a pacifier. When the baby burps, milk may come up with some air.

Breastfed babies generally have fewer and less severe episodes of reflux than formula-fed babies. Sucking at the breast triggers peristaltic waves along the gastrointestinal tract; these muscular contractions help move the milk down into the stomach and on to the small intestine. Also, human milk digests more completely and almost twice as fast as formula. The less time the milk spends in the stomach, the less opportunity there is for it to acidify before backing up into the esophagus. In addition, breastfed babies are generally fed in a more upright position than bottle-fed babies. Gravity may help to keep the milk and gastric acid in the stomach, where they belong.

Still, breastfed babies can suffer painful reflux. Symptoms of this problem can include sudden or inconsolable crying, arching of the back during feedings, refusing the breast or bottle, frequent burping or hiccuping, bad breath, gagging or choking, frequent throat inflammation, and poor sleep patterns. In extreme situations, some babies have slow weight gain, frequent ear infections, and, less commonly, respiratory problems—wheezing, labored breathing, asthma, bronchitis, pneumonia, and apnea.

Some babies with reflux want to nurse all the time and therefore may grow very fast, although it may seem as if they spit up all the milk they take in. On the way down, breast milk is very soothing, as is sucking itself. But if a baby overfills her stomach, her reflux symptoms can worsen. For such a baby, it may be helpful to nurse on one breast at a time; the slower flow of milk may soothe the baby's heartburn without overfilling her stomach. Some mothers have reported that pacifiers help such babies.

Other babies with reflux seem to find nursing painful. They not only cry after and in between feedings, but they fuss at the breast and sometimes refuse nursings altogether. Oddly enough, they may take the same milk from a bottle that they wouldn't take from the breast.

Many parents try to minimize reflux by keeping their babies upright or semi-upright for thirty to forty-five minutes after feedings. Recent research has found, however, that putting a baby in an infant seat (elevated to 60 degrees) actually increases reflux. Reflux is reduced, the studies have found, when the baby is laid on her left side or on her stomach. But putting babies to sleep on their stomachs has been associated with a higher rate of sudden infant death syndrome (SIDS). Perhaps the best idea is to carry the baby on her left side in a sling, both to minimize reflux and to soothe the baby with the motion of your body. You might also try laying the baby stomach-down on your forearm; parents say that the pressure on the belly seems to be soothing.

Jostling or other rough or fast movement of a baby after feeding may add to the problem of reflux. Burp the baby before switching breasts, but don't jiggle her. Just hold her over your shoulder or sit her upright, and pat her back gently. Let her suck at the breast until she falls asleep.

Some babies seem to suffer more with lower belly discomfort than with regurgitation and heartburn. Besides crying, these babies' symptoms may include gassiness; stools that are very frequent or green, mucous, or even bloody; and redness around the rectum. A baby may have a stuffy nose or a rash on her face or upper body. She may want to nurse all the time.

Something in your diet. Whether or not your baby has bloody stools, if she exhibits colic or severe reflux symptoms every day or nearly every day, you should try writing down everything you have eaten and drunk during the past three days. Include any nutritional supplements or medications. Make notes, too, of any particularly fussy periods the baby has had during the past three days. If you are producing a lot of milk, also have your baby weighed to see how fast she is gaining. A baby who is gaining much more than an ounce a day may be having symptoms of what I call hyperlactation syndrome, which is described on page 228.

Most foods that bother breastfeeding babies, as either intestinal irritants or allergens, fall into one of several major food categories. When a baby has been fussy at particular times, a suspect food can often be identified by looking back one to two meal periods or about two to six hours back from the start of the symptoms. If eating chocolate, say, seems to cause your baby's symptoms, you can try giving up chocolate and see if she does better. But because more than one food may be making your baby fussy, you might be wise to avoid all of the commonly offending foods for a while, and then reintroduce them to your diet one by one. This way, you'll know exactly what bothers your baby.

Completely eliminating all of the following foods for three days may bring speedy relief to your fussy baby. Be sure to check the ingredients in any commercially processed food before eating or drinking it.

Although streaks of blood in a baby's stool or diaper rarely indicate an emergency, for a parent they are alarming, and when they appear, it's a good idea to call the baby's doctor. In most cases, however, blood in the stool results from either an anal fissure or a food intolerance. An anal fissure—that is, a small tear in the anus—usually results from constipation and straining during a bowel movement. Since exclusively breastfed babies cannot be constipated, anal fissures are unusual for them. A sensitivity or allergy to something in your diet is the more likely cause. Some doctors may say that a baby with bloody stools should be temporarily weaned from the breast and fed hypoallergenic formula instead of breast milk; however, in most cases, the bleeding stops after the mother removes the offending food from her diet and the baby's gut has time to heal.

- *Chocolate and spices.* The major offender in chocolate is theobromine; even in small amounts, this ingredient is a potent irritant in the digestive tract of many infants. In the example given on page 227, the chocolate frozen yogurt was probably responsible for this baby's (and mother's) difficult night. Many spices and other strong flavorings, including cinnamon, chiles, garlic, and curry, can also bother young infants.

- *Citrus.* A frequently overlooked cause of digestive disturbances is citrus fruits and their juices. Oranges, lemons, limes, tangerines, and grapefruits can all bother a baby's intestines. Other strongly acidic fruits, such as pineapples, kiwis, and strawberries, affect many babies similarly. In the chart on page 227, the mother had grapefruit juice at breakfast and pineapple juice in the afternoon. Her baby may have been bothered by these.

- *Gas-producing vegetables.* Certain vegetables can also cause temporary digestive problems for young babies. These include onions, broccoli, cauliflower, Brussels sprouts, cabbage, bell peppers, and cucumbers. Prepared mustard can cause a similar reaction. Onions, an ingredient in so many dishes, can cause gastric upset for a baby even when they are cooked, ingested in small amounts, or eaten as onion powder. The stir-fry dish in the chart contained one of these offending foods.

- **Cow's milk.** Some infants are allergic to cow's milk and cow's milk products, including cheese, yogurt, sour cream, cottage cheese, and ice cream. Researchers have estimated that nearly half of all cases of severe reflux and colic are associated with an allergy to cow's milk. If a baby is truly allergic to cow's milk products, cutting back on milk will probably not eliminate the baby's symptoms. You must eliminate from your diet all dairy products, including those in commercially processed foods like creamed soups, certain types of salad dressings, and puddings; cow's milk may be identified as "casein" or "whey" on the label. You should not feed the baby any infant formula made from cow's milk. The baby in the chart may or may not be reacting to dairy products.

If possible, do without certain medications and dietary supplements while you're avoiding these four food categories. Laxatives taken by a nursing mother can disturb her baby's intestinal tract. Aspirin and the chemical phenylpropanolamine, a decongestant, can make a baby fussy; both of these drugs are in many headache and cold remedies. Certain dietary supplements taken by the mother or given directly to the baby, such as vitamin C, brewer's yeast, and fluoride, have been known to cause colic symptoms. Fluoride is very helpful in preventing cavities, but it is best delayed until the baby is six months old and need be given only if your water supply contains less than 0.3 parts per million.

During the three days of eliminating all the commonly offending foods from your diet, write down what you eat and drink along with observations of your baby. If the baby has particularly difficult times, look back one to two meal periods, or about two to six hours before the symptoms began, and try to identify any suspect foods. You may find that you ate something forbidden without realizing it, or perhaps another food seems to be at fault. Other foods that can cause reactions include tomatoes, eggs, peanuts and peanut butter, corn and corn syrup, wheat (in breads, crackers, cookies, cakes, and noodles), soy (the basis of some infant formulas and an ingredient in many processed foods), apples, and bananas. If you decide to eliminate any one of these foods, you

THURSDAY	
8:30 a.m. Grapefruit juice Prenatal vitamin Granola with milk Toast with butter	10:30 a.m.–12:00 noon Fussy, spitting up
12:15 p.m. Roast beef and cheese sandwich, with mayonnaise and lettuce Potato chips Milk	2:00 p.m.–5:00 p.m. Crying
3:00 p.m. Pineapple juice	
6:45 p.m. Chicken–green pepper stir-fry Spinach and mushroom salad, Italian dressing Rice Milk	
8:15 p.m. Chocolate frozen yogurt	11:30 p.m.–2:00 a.m. Very fussy, vomited

Sample chart of a mother's diet and her baby's reactions.

should continue to avoid the original four food categories, too. More than one food group may be affecting your baby.

If your baby is much better after the three days and having very few fussy periods or other symptoms, try adding milk products back into your diet. Have a lot of milk products early in the day and then watch the baby for twenty-four hours. If the baby reacts, avoid milk products completely for the next couple of days.

After this period, you might experiment with small amounts of milk, cheese, yogurt, or ice cream to see which of these, if any, your baby can tolerate, and in what quantity. Although some babies cannot tolerate any milk products, others do fine when their mothers have hard cheese, and some can tolerate small amounts of any milk products as long as their mothers take them only once every few days. (If you must cut dairy products from your diet completely, be sure you are taking sufficient calcium in another form; see page 178).

After you have established which dairy products are safe, and in what quantity, add another food category to your diet every few days. Eat a lot of the food in question. If the fussiness recurs, eliminate the offending food category from your diet again. Continue adding food categories until you have tested all the foods that you had eliminated. Again, more than one food may be a problem for a very sensitive baby.

Hyperlactation syndrome. Researchers have also identified a kind of colic that is characterized by gassiness, frequent stools, spitting up, and general discomfort and fussiness (Woolridge and Fisher, 1988). Although these babies may seem to be sensitive to something in their mother's diet, they show little or no improvement with the elimination of suspect foods and beverages. Typically, these babies nurse frequently from both breasts and are gaining more than an ounce per day. Their mothers often have overabundant milk supplies.

Some lactation professionals refer to these symptoms as overactive letdown syndrome. I don't think that letdown is really the problem. More likely, the underlying cause of the colic is the baby's disproportionate intake of low-fat foremilk, the milk that is available early in the feeding. When a baby consumes large amounts of foremilk and little of the fatty hindmilk, his stomach rapidly empties, dumping excess lactose into the bowel. This results in increased gas and colic symptoms.

Relief is achieved by getting the baby to empty one breast at each feeding so that he receives not only the foremilk but the fatty hindmilk, too. Allow the baby to nurse from the first breast until he spontaneously pulls away satisfied; do not interrupt the feeding at any point to switch the baby to the second breast. If this doesn't help, try limiting the baby to one side for one and a half to two hours before nursing on the other side. Some lactation professionals advise limiting the baby to the same breast for several feedings in a row until the colic subsides, but I feel that this is unnecessary. Keeping the baby at just one side per feeding should solve the problem.

Treatments and tests for colic. Because tests for colic are invasive, many doctors treat the problem without testing for it. They choose from three kinds of pharmaceutical drugs. First are antacids, which neutralize stomach acid without known side effects. Among these, Mylanta and Mylicon are best known for colic and are available over the counter. They contain simethicone, an anti-foaming agent intended to reduce bloating, discomfort, and pain caused by excess gas in the stomach or intestines. The drops are given right after feedings. Rarely do they seem to help.

Second among kinds of drugs for reflux are those that suppress acid production in the stomach. These include cimetidine (Tagamet), famotidine (Pepcid), nizatidine (Axid), ranitidine (Zantac), and the "acid blockers." Medications in the last group prevent any acid production at all. Among these, omeprazole (Prilosec) and lansoprazole (Prevacid) are approved for use in children, although others are sometimes prescribed. Since not all infants react in the same way to these drugs, you may have to try several before you find one that works well. It may take about two weeks before you can tell whether a particular drug works.

The third group of medications prescribed for reflux increase motility—that is, they improve the muscle tone of the digestive tract to keep food moving through it. These medications are more helpful in older babies who are eating solid foods; exclusively breastfed babies generally have fast digestion. Bethanechol (Urecholine), erythromycin, and metoclopramide (Reglan) are the motility drugs currently used in the United States. They can cause gastric cramping and diarrhea. Long-term use of metoclopramide in children (that is, over a period of weeks) hasn't been well studied; in fact, there are concerns about its long-term use in adults.

Some mothers turn not to pharmaceutical drugs to ease their babies' colic symptoms but to old-fashioned "gripe water," which has been marketed since the mid-nineteenth century and is today used around the world. There are many brands of gripe water, but they are similarly formulated; most contain different herbs, and some contain sodium bicarbonate. Although some mothers feel that gripe water has helped their fussy babies, a study published in the *New England Journal of Medicine* found it generally ineffective against colic symptoms.

A new approach to treating colicky babies uses "good" bacteria, or probiotics. In a study published in *Pediatrics* (Savino et al., 2007), exclusively breastfed infants with colic symptoms who were treated with *Lactobacillus reuteri* improved within seven days of the start of treatment. At the end of one month, they had reduced their average crying time by 95 percent. During the same period, colicky breastfed babies treated with simethicone reduced their crying time by only 7 percent. By changing the balance of bacteria in the intestinal tract, researchers speculate, probiotic supplementation may reduce the effects of both gastrointestinal infection and allergic disease. Other studies suggest that *L. reuteri* inhibits pain by reducing the sensitivity of nerves in the intestinal tract.

The probiotics used in the 2007 study were produced by Bio Gaia, a Swedish company. These drops have been purchased by Gerber and are now called Gerber Soothe Colic Drops.

Gerber now has additional formulations for babies: two named Soothe, both containing *L. reuteri* and one of which also includes vitamin D. Another Gerber probiotic is Gentle Everyday Probiotic and Vitamin D Drops, which contains *B. Lactis* and vitamin D and was specifically developed for babies born by c-section. The final product is Good Start Protect, which is meant to be used for occasional intestinal upset. You can find more information about ordering these drops in Appendix A, page 386. Depending on the formulation, the price is between $80 and $120.

Another newer probiotic preparation for infants suffering with colic symptoms is Evivo, a preparation that contains activated *Bifidobacterium infantis*. This bacterial strain is known to restore the infant gut microbiome after the use of antibiotics and/or c-sections have interrupted the transfer of "healthy bacteria" to the newborn infant during childbirth. Intended for infants who suffer with colic symptoms, this rather expensive product is mixed with breast milk and given orally once a day for as long as the baby is being breastfed. Evivo is kept either refrigerated or frozen before being mixed with breast milk and given to the baby.

A one-month supply of Evivo is about $80. See more about ordering Evivo at Evivo.com. You can find more information about these drops in Appendix A, page 386.

Medical tests for reflux and other digestive disorders are rarely advised unless the baby shows signs of poor growth, severe choking, or lung disease. In such a case, the best test for severe reflux is the pH probe, in which a tube is put down the baby's throat to measure the acid level at the bottom of the esophagus. Less invasive is the barium swallow, in which the baby drinks a barium mixture, an X-ray is taken, and then the X-ray is examined for any blockage or narrowing of the stomach valves that may be causing or aggravating the condition. The X-ray, however, will not identify whether a baby's stomach contents are more acidic than normal or if the esophagus has been damaged by reflux. Damage to the esophagus is determined through a more invasive procedure, endoscopy with biopsy. All of these tests should be used cautiously; they do not always provide conclusive results, and they are stressful for both the baby and her parents.

When nothing works. Whether your baby has painful reflux or other colic symptoms, the extreme stress of caring for her may make you consider another feeding method in hopes that the symptoms will lessen. Keep in mind that these conditions usually improve without any such change. Switching to formula, in fact, might well make the problem worse instead of better. Continuing to breastfeed will provide important health benefits for both you and your baby and, most important, a strong bond that can help you both get through this difficult time.

Needless to say, a baby with colic or severe reflux may sleep poorly and fuss a great deal. Your baby may need to be held upright most of the time. She may deprive you of sleep and, by refusing the breast, make you feel rejected. The risks of postpartum depression and even child abuse are higher when a baby has severe reflux or colic. Since this can be a very challenging period even for the most stable family, it is important that you get emotional support, find practical help, and limit your commitments until the problem passes.

Cereal for Colic?

Some doctors recommend thickening milk with cereal for babies who suffer with reflux or colic, on the theory that heavier food stays down better. But there is no proof that this helps; in fact, adding cereal to a baby's milk may slow the emptying of her stomach, increase episodes of reflux, and possibly cause choking. Regurgitated solids are more irritating than regurgitated human milk, and if bits of cereal are aspirated into a baby's lungs, they can cause pneumonia. Besides, cereal replaces rather than supplements breast milk in a baby's diet, and it can thus cause a decrease in the milk supply. Since many babies with severe reflux or colic have allergies, introducing cereal to them early can lead to fussing at the breast, refusal to nurse, and early weaning.

Coping Measures for Fussiness, Colic, and Reflux

1. Offer your breast—it is a source of comfort as well as nourishment for your baby.

2. Try a pacifier. Pacifiers are soothing to many babies who need a lot of extra sucking, who are fussy, or who have difficulty calming themselves. If your baby won't take a pacifier at first, try different kinds.

3. Be sure to burp your baby frequently while he nurses or sucks on a pacifier.

4. Try swaddling your baby tightly in a light blanket.

5. Soothe both yourself and the baby with a warm bath.

6. Most babies love motion. Try walking or using a baby pack, sling, or stroller. Rocking can also be comforting—borrow a rocking chair if you don't already have one. Most babies are lulled to sleep by car rides. Do not place your baby in an inclined infant sleeper. These are now associated with infant suffocation. Infants need to sleep on a flat surface, so that should they attempt to turn over or should they tuck their chin onto their chest, they will not occlude their airway or suffocate.

7. White noise may calm a crying baby. Try helping him sleep by turning on a radio or a recording of a humming car or vacuum cleaner, or by placing an aquarium near the baby's bed. Or put on a white-noise CD (see Appendix A, page 386). White noise should be quiet, as recent studies have revealed hearing loss in infants exposed to loud white noise.

8. Consider sleeping with the baby, if you aren't doing so already.

9. Consider purchasing infant probiotics, specifically Gerber's Soothe Colic Drops, and give five drops once a day or the more expensive Evivo powder intended for infants who suffer from colic symptoms after being born by c-section or who were exposed to antibiotics.

10. Take a short break from the baby each day. Your partner might play with him while you take a bath, go for a walk, or visit a friend.

11. Find another mother who has a fussy baby. There's nothing like a friend who really understands. You might also visit www.colicsupport.com, a website for parents with colicky babies.

Underfeeding

For any number of reasons, you may wonder if your baby is getting enough to eat. He may seem to be nursing all the time, or he may seem especially fussy. Most young infants want to nurse eight to twelve times in each 24-hour period. Nursing this often is normal and seldom reflects a poor milk supply. You can't tell whether your baby is getting enough breast milk by offering him a supplemental bottle of water or formula after nursing. Most babies will take 1 to 2 ounces (30 to 60 ml) if it is offered, even when they have had enough milk from the breasts.

The baby is probably getting enough milk if:

- he is nursing at least eight times in a 24-hour period,
- he is nursing for ten to forty-five minutes at each feeding and seems content after feedings,
- he has several periods of swallowing during each feeding,
- your breasts feel softer or lighter after the baby has nursed, and
- your baby is having bowel movements every day during the first month.

If any of these statements isn't true of your baby, have him weighed. Even if all are true, have your baby weighed if you need reassurance. The nurse in your pediatrician's office should be happy to do this for you.

Between the fifth day and the end of the third month after birth, a baby should gain an ounce every day. A weight gain of an ounce a day reflects an adequate milk intake. If your baby was weighed at any time after the fifth day, you can see whether he has gained enough by weighing him again now. If he hasn't been weighed since the fifth day, consider that by ten to fourteen days of age most babies have regained their birth weight. If your baby is two weeks old and weighs less than his birth weight, he definitely needs more milk. If your baby is two weeks old and weighs more than his birth weight, he is probably getting plenty of milk—that is, unless the baby is being supplemented. If you have any doubt about how much the baby is gaining, weigh him.

Inadequate weight gain usually occurs when a baby has had trouble latching on or nursing vigorously during the period of initial engorgement in the first week, or when nursing has been infrequent. Underfeeding often occurs among the group of mothers and babies described on page 65, Babies Who May Not Get Enough. This problem can also occur when a newborn has a faulty suck (see page 114, Sucking Problems), is tongue-tied, or has a high palate; when a mother has used a nipple shield over her nipple for nursing (see page 100); and, certainly, when a baby is sick. Some laxatives, when taken by the mother, can cause a baby to have excessive bowel movements and to lose weight or gain too slowly even if he is taking enough milk. A baby who gains weight slowly or not at all after gaining well at first may be suffering with painful reflux. Some babies with reflux limit their milk intake because of the discomfort of heartburn (see page 219, Fussiness, Colic, and Reflux).

Usually a baby's failure to latch on or suck well during the early weeks quickly leads to low milk production. The solution is to build the milk supply by pumping after nursing, and to feed the baby the expressed milk along with any necessary formula.

Treatment Measures for Underfeeding

1. If possible, see a lactation professional. Your insurance provider should cover all the costs.

2. To estimate the amount of milk you are producing and to increase your milk supply, rent a clinical-grade breast pump. Any other pump may not be adequate for accurately estimating milk production and may be less helpful in increasing your milk supply.

3. Estimate your milk production by pumping your breasts instead of nursing. If you are pumping one breast at a time, pump each twice, for a total pumping time of twenty to twenty-five minutes. If you have a double-pump kit, use it for a total of fifteen to twenty minutes. Feed this milk and any necessary formula to your baby. (See Chapter 5 for guidelines on expressing milk and Appendix B, page 396, to determine how much milk your baby needs at each feeding.)

   Exactly two hours after completing the first pumping, pump again. This time you may get less milk than in the first pumping. Multiply the number of ounces collected at this *second* pumping by twelve. This will give you an estimate of how much milk you are producing over a twenty-four-hour period; if you collected 1½ ounces (44 ml), for example, you are producing about 18 ounces (237 ml) per day.

   Now you can compare the baby's daily milk requirement, as listed in Appendix B, with your milk production. For example, if you estimate that your baby needs 21.4 ounces (633 ml) per day and your milk production is 18 ounces (532 ml) per day, the baby needs about 3½ ounces (104 ml) of formula per day until your milk production increases.

   If you determine that you have enough milk for your baby and yet he has not been gaining well, it may be that he is not taking all of the milk available at some or many of his feedings. This can happen with newborns who were born prematurely, who tend to drift off to sleep while nursing, who have sucking difficulties, or who suffer with painful reflux. In such a case, you'll still want to take the steps that follow, feeding your baby expressed breast milk (rather than formula) after nursing until his feeding skill improves.

4. After you have estimated your milk production, go back to nursing your baby at least eight times in every twenty-four hours. This may mean waking him for feedings. Nurse him every two to two and a half hours during the day and evening (counting from the start of one nursing to the start of the next) and every three to four hours in the night, for ten to fifteen minutes on each breast. (I suggest limiting the nursing to this amount of time so that the entire nursing-pumping-supplementing session can be completed in forty to fifty minutes.) Frequent short nursings are more effective in increasing milk production than infrequent lengthy ones. Be sure to observe the baby for swallowing. If the baby is sucking but not swallowing milk, gently compress your breast to get the baby to take more milk.

5. Pump your breasts right after each nursing to stimulate further milk production. If you're pumping one breast at a time, pump for five minutes on each side, and then pump each breast a second time for a few more minutes. Pumping both breasts at once not only takes less time but increases milk production faster. Use a double-pump kit for five to ten minutes after nursing.

6. Right after pumping, offer the baby whatever breast milk you've collected along with any necessary formula. If the baby needs supplemental formula, divide the total amount needed by the number of feedings the baby is getting each day (usually eight). For example, the baby needing 3½ ounces (104 ml) of formula could take a bit less than ½ ounce (15 ml) after each of his eight daily nursings. The goal is to offer about the same amount of milk and formula at each feeding so that he wants to nurse at regular intervals.

    Many lactation consultants, fearing the bottle would interfere with the baby's ability at the breast, suggest that a baby be fed supplements with a nursing supplementer (see Appendix A, page 386), cup, eyedropper, or soft tube taped onto the parent's finger. If one of these methods is recommended to you and it works well, then continue with it. But if you find it too frustrating or time-consuming, use a bottle. After the first several days of nursing, using a bottle for supplemental feedings rarely causes latch-on or sucking problems.

7. To stimulate even greater milk production, try fenugreek capsules, blessed thistle capsules, or More Milk Plus capsules or tincture (see page 84). Go-Lacta is another herbal remedy for low milk supply and can be used with other herbs as well. There has been only one study on this herb that showed an increase in production, but some lactation consultants who recommend it in the United States are seeing good results (Estrella et al., 2000). (See page 392 for information on ordering Go-Lacta.)

8. Some mothers are told to drink a beer or two to help increase milk production. This is an old wives' tale; in fact, drinking beer can lessen milk production.

9. Weigh your baby every few days to be sure that he is gaining well. After each weighing, re-estimate his milk needs, since as he gains weight, his milk needs will increase. Re-estimate your milk production, too. Two hours after your last pumping, use the breast pump instead of nursing, and figure your milk production as explained in step 3. Hopefully your milk production will have increased enough that you can decrease or even eliminate any formula supplementation.

10. If you find that the herbs listed in step 7 do little to increase your milk production, consider using Domperidone (see page 87).

11. Once your baby is gaining well, his nursing seems more vigorous, and he is receiving supplements only of your breast milk, try eliminating some of the supplement. For a few days, offer half of the milk that you are expressing to the baby, and freeze the rest. If the baby continues to gain well, keep pumping, but don't offer the baby any of the pumped milk. Once the baby is gaining an ounce a day without any supplement, you can gradually stop pumping. Continue to have your baby weighed weekly.

If treatment fails. Although the technique just described usually ensures a weight-gaining baby and higher milk production within several days, occasionally these measures won't work. Sometimes, when breast engorgement has been severe and little milk has been removed during the first week, the decline in milk production is difficult to reverse.

In unusual instances, a mother simply cannot produce enough milk. This sometimes happens to women who have had breast surgery, particularly when the surgical incision is around the areola (see page 138, Nursing after Breast Surgery), or who have insufficient glandular (milk-producing) tissue, or hypoplastic breasts (see page 134). Mothers with polycystic ovary syndrome, or PCOS (see page 138), and mothers with retained placental fragments (see page 80) may also struggle with low milk supply.

In any of these situations, lack of support from family, friends, and health professionals can only make matters worse. But even with all of the best information and support, things sometimes don't turn out as we hope. If you have given nursing your best but finally end up having to bottle-feed, you have not failed as a mother. Be proud of your efforts to nurse, and concentrate on providing your baby with all of the cuddling and loving that you can.

Some mothers who can't produce enough milk have found that continuing to nurse with a nursing supplementer has been a rewarding, worthwhile experience. Others have found these devices to be cumbersome and frustrating.

Another option, particularly if the baby has become frustrated at the breast, is to first bottle-feed and then nurse. "Comfort nursing"—nursing after or between bottle-feedings, or during the night—may be a pleasant experience for both mother and baby.

Detailed information about formula and bottle-feeding can be found in *The Nursing Mother's Guide to Weaning* (see References & Reading, page 423).

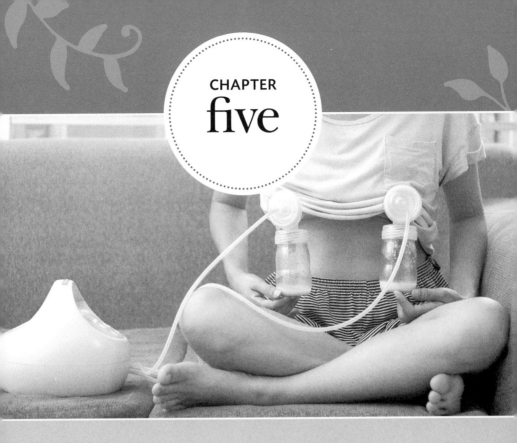

EXPRESSING, STORING, AND FEEDING BREAST MILK

- Expression Methods
- Expressing Milk for Occasional Separations
- Expressing Milk before Returning to Work
- Expressing Milk at Work
- Insurance Pumping
- Expressing Milk for a Baby Who Cannot Nurse
- Pumping Exclusively
- Increasing Your Milk Supply while Pumping
- Collecting and Storing Your Breast Milk
- Feeding Your Expressed Milk
- A Review of Breast Pump Models

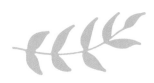

THERE ARE A VARIETY OF SITUATIONS in which mothers express milk for their babies. Some mothers, because of complications, need to express their milk full-time during the early days or weeks after birth; those who are struggling with latch-on difficulties or sore nipples, or whose babies are too premature or sick to breastfeed, may find themselves in this situation. Other mothers breastfeed full-time but need to do "insurance pumping" after nursings to maintain or increase milk production and to provide supplemental milk to their infants. Some mothers, for reasons of their own, exclusively express milk and bottle-feed it to their babies by choice. Some mothers express milk only for occasional separations. And, of course, many mothers who return to the workplace express their milk, not only to feed their babies when they are apart but also to maintain their production.

Expression Methods

Hand Expression

Although few mothers today consider regularly expressing their milk by hand, manual expression is a technique that every nursing mother should probably learn. If you need to express colostrum for a newborn, before mature milk production begins, you may well obtain more by using your hands than by using a pump, partly because the tiny amounts of colostrum produced in the hours following birth can get lost in the plastic parts of a pump. After milk production begins, hand expression can soften your breasts so the baby can latch on more easily. If you begin using a pump regularly, doing some hand expression after each pumping can be a good way to ensure complete drainage of the breast and maximize your milk production. And if pump parts get misplaced, batteries die, electricity goes out, your pump breaks, or you find yourself missing a feeding unexpectedly, hand expression may become a necessity.

When a mother is initiating lactation without a nursing baby, pumping and hand expression combined bring in higher volumes of milk than relying solely on a pump. Dr. Jane Morton of Stanford University has created a short video that shows how to use hand expression to collect more colostrum for a newborn who can't yet breastfeed. You can find this video at http://newborns.stanford.edu/Breastfeeding/HandExpression.html. Lactation consultant Maya Bolman also has a good video showing the technique. The video can be seen at http://bfmedneo.com/resources/videos/. It is worth your time to review these videos prior to implementing hand expression. It takes practice. With several practice sessions, most mothers can master manual expression. You might practice on the free side while nursing, after the baby stimulates the milk to letdown. Place a towel in front of you to catch the spray as you get started. Or practice while standing in the shower.

To start, position the pads of your thumb and index finger 1 to 1½ inches (2.5 to 3.8 cm) behind the nipple directly across from each other. Gently press your fingers straight back toward your chest and then together. Relax your fingers, and then repeat these motions several times. Avoid sliding your fingers away from their original position. Once you have the motion down, rotate your fingers around the nipple to empty other areas of the breast.

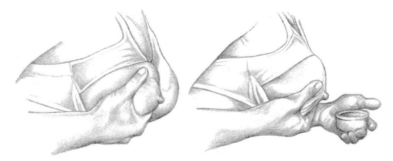

When using hand expression, catch the milk in a cup or any other clean container.

If you begin expressing milk when you're away from the baby, you will probably find that a few minutes of gentle breast massage will help the milk to letdown. You can catch the milk in any clean container. To get more milk, switch back and forth from one side to the other as soon as you notice the flow lessening. You may be able to save time by expressing milk from both breasts at once, into containers on a table in front of you. Once you have learned the technique, the whole process should take about twenty minutes.

Some mothers actually come to prefer hand expression to pumping. They feel that expressing milk by hand is quieter, more natural, and more convenient than using a pump.

Pumping

Mothers today are getting pumps in record numbers. This is mainly because so many women are returning to work or school within weeks or months of giving birth. But even many women who are planning to stay home with their babies often see a pump as a necessity, for occasional separations or to allow their partners to participate in feedings. And most mothers are now eligible to receive a pump through their insurance company under the Affordable Care Act.

The best pump for you often depends on how much time you'll be spending away from your baby. If you'll be separated from the baby only on occasion, hand expression or most any pump that has good reviews found later in this chapter will probably suffice.

If you'll be working or attending school and away from your baby on a regular basis, getting a high-quality pump is usually important in order to maintain your milk supply and provide most, if not all, of your baby's milk needs. Getting a pump that can express milk from both breasts at the same time will get the job done in half the time and help maintain your milk supply.

Some mothers may find that the pump they purchased or received through insurance is so inefficient that it may be useless. Its cycling— the speed at which the pump pulls and releases—may be too slow, its vacuum may be too low, or both. She may find that she cannot express very much milk. If she uses the pump regularly or often, her milk production may suffer.

The efficiency of a pump depends on three main factors: its cycling speed, its vacuum, and the size of the flanges. The ideal cycling speed is between 48 to 60 times per minute. The vacuum of breast pumps is measured by the movement of mercury in a hydrostatic gauge. The vacuum should reach at least 240 millimeters of mercury.

Lastly, the pump flanges are also important. Flanges that are too small or too large for a mother's nipple will not only be uncomfortable but may not drain the breast well, which could lead to low milk production. Many mothers require a flange size of 27 mms. If a pump comes with only a size 24 or 25 mms, but the mother needs a size 27 mms or larger, she may experience uncomfortable pumping and may find that her breasts do not drain completely. Poor milk emptying can lead to low milk supply if the pump is used with much regularity. Ideally, pump kits usually come with two or more flange sizes. Some mothers may have nipples that are larger and require a flange size of 30 to 31 mms that are carried by some, but not all, pump manufacturers.

A mother who buys an inefficient pump may not notice the problem at first. Some mothers may letdown milk easily with nearly any pump in the early days, weeks, or even months, but often after a time a pump seems to lose efficiency. Usually, the efficiency of the pump hasn't changed, but the mother has come to need higher speed and vacuum.

Sometimes a mother assumes that if she can't pump much milk, she must not be producing much. She worries that she is underfeeding her baby and she may work at increasing production, when in fact her baby is taking plenty of milk at the breast.

If a mother figures out, sooner or later, that her pump is inefficient, she finds that she has to purchase another one, and so she ends up spending more than she would have if she had bought a good pump in the first place. While you should purchase the best-quality pump that you can afford, keep in mind that a high-quality pump is much cheaper than a couple of months' worth of baby formula.

A high price tag, however, is no guarantee that a pump is high-performing. As you will learn later in this chapter, the quality of pumps varies greatly within a particular price range. If you are sure you want to purchase a pump, start by determining the category of pump you need, and then identify a high-quality model within that category. This chapter will help you do just that. If you need extra help, a lactation professional may also guide you to the best pump for your situation.

When's the right time to get a pump? Many women do so during pregnancy, but keep in mind that in most cases, you probably won't be using your pump until after the baby is nursing well. (If you need a pump in the early days because of breastfeeding problems, I strongly recommend renting a clinical-grade pump instead of a using a less effective personal use pump.)

You can begin pumping after the first ten to fourteen days postpartum to collect a backup supply of milk for future needs.

Pumping often and on a regular basis prior to this time may lead to an oversupply. Having too much milk can lead to other problems like plugged milk ducts or colic symptoms if the baby is drinking from both breasts and ends up taking in more of the low-fat foremilk than the fatty hindmilk.

Most mothers naturally have more milk during the night and in the morning, so one of the best times to express extra milk is during the morning hours, right after nursing. Pumping in between nursings can be taking some of your baby's next feeding. When you pump in the morning after feeding the baby at the breast, you will most likely get just an ounce or two. But by doing this every day, or nearly every day, your freezer will fill up quickly.

Most young babies will need about 3 ounces (90 ml) per feeding in your absence. So, when you pump, place the milk in the back of the refrigerator; when you get 3 ounces (90 ml), combine the cold milk and then store it in the freezer. Older babies usually need 3 or 4 ounces (90 or 118 ml) per feeding. See page 165 for information on milk storage.

Just before the baby is a month old, you'll want to start giving bottle-feedings, of an ounce or so every few days, so that your baby will continue to accept the bottle.

I divide pumps into five categories:

- clinical-grade (rental) pumps
- personal-use pumps
- cord/tubing free, wearable breast pumps
- single electric or battery-operated pumps
- hand-operated pumps (including "Drip Milk" collectors)

Clinical-grade pumps. These piston-driven pumps, built for rental use, cycle automatically about forty-eight to sixty times per minute and have certain minimum vacuum of approximately 240 millimeters of mercury. Clinical-grade pumps closely approximate the sucking action of an infant, and most drain the breasts gently as well as effectively. These pumps are available for rent at rental stations throughout the country.

Medical professionals and pump companies often refer to these pumps as hospital-grade, but usually all they mean is that a pump meets certain electrical and other standards that ensure a pump is safe for hospital use. Know that the designation hospital-grade has nothing to do with how well a pump works. I use the term clinical-grade or multi-user to designate pumps of the highest quality.

Clinical-grade or multi-user pumps are recommended for the following mothers and babies:

- Babies who fail to begin latching on to the breast and sustaining sucking within twenty-four hours after birth
- Mothers who have no signs of milk production seventy-two hours following birth
- Mothers who are pumping exclusively or nearly exclusively
- Premature or sick hospitalized newborns
- Babies with poor muscle tone, neurological problems, or birth defects such as cardiac, respiratory, or craniofacial abnormalities
- Mothers who are experiencing breastfeeding problems, such as severe sore nipples, that necessitate temporarily stopping breastfeeding
- Mothers planning for adoptive nursing or relactation
- Mothers estimating their milk supply
- Babies who are refusing the breast, because of colic or a nursing strike
- Mothers who are doing "insurance pumping" after nursings (see page 254)

Probably the finest breast pumps ever manufactured are the large, heavy, internal-piston pumps. To most lactation professionals, they are

Getting a Pump through Your Insurance Carrier

You may know that the Affordable Care Act (ACA) mandates that mothers covered by insurance are entitled to breastfeeding support and breastfeeding supplies, including breast pumps. This was signed into law in 2010, and most insurance plans began implementing this coverage on or after August 2012.

Getting a pump from your insurance company can be a bit complicated, but here is some information that should help you. Unfortunately, there is a great deal of variation in what sorts of pumps are covered, and how they are covered. Because the law's recommendations aren't very specific, coverage varies from insurance company to insurance company. Most plans require women to obtain the pumps from their designated vendors, or a DME (Durable Medical Equipment) provider, which may or may not offer the pump that a woman hopes for. This means a mother usually can't simply buy a pump at retail and submit a receipt for reimbursement. Some plans have relationships with DMEs that cover only the purchase of cheap manual, battery operated, or electric pumps that may not be effective enough, especially for mothers returning to the workplace. Also, know that there is no co-pay for your breast pump as long as you deal with an in-network provider. On the other hand, depending on what pump you want, there may be some high-end models available to you with a co-pay. Your insurance company will either list these preferred contracted providers on their website, or you can call them for the list. Going out-of-network will usually result in out-of-pocket expenses and less recourse if you are unsatisfied.

Ask your insurance provider for the name and contact information for every eligible durable medical equipment provider, then call each DME to see what pumps they offer mothers. If you are unsure about some of the models, take some time to read reviews.

When speaking with your insurance company, talk to them about what you want and need. Be sure to ask your provider what your "ordering window" is—that is, when you are eligible to place your order and when the coverage ends. Mothers may only be eligible for a pump every three years, or after each baby.

Some insurance carriers refuse to cover clinical-grade rental pumps, which may be needed soon after birth to help mothers establish adequate milk flow because of a sick or premature baby or a breastfeeding complication, like low milk supply. If your insurance carrier does cover one, a written prescription from your baby's doctor and preauthorization is usually necessary. For mothers who need a hospital-grade pump, some insurance companies will cover a standard rental up to the value of the purchase price. In some of these cases, depending on how long the pump is needed, the insurance carrier could actually purchase the breast pump for the mother. The breast pumps must be purchased through a medical equipment company that the insurance company contracts with.

While you are pregnant, try to educate yourself about the many pumps on the market. Later in this chapter, I have included a thorough review of most of the pumps on the market, indicating which ones are commonly offered by insurance carriers, and which get good, mixed, or poor reviews by both mothers and lactation consultants (including myself). It is not too early to contact the DME companies to see which pumps are offered to nursing mothers before your baby comes. In this way, you will know which are higher-quality pumps.

One recent review of insurance companies revealed that few of them allow mothers to upgrade to a better pump, even if the mother is willing to pay the difference. Some insurance companies without a contracted DME may be flexible if the pump you want isn't available, letting you choose another pump or, rarely, reimbursing your purchase from a retail store. Again, you need to ask for what you want! Because pump benefits vary from company to company, you will need to contact your insurance provider, using the number on the back of your insurance card. The National Women's Law Center can help you if your plan is denying you benefits, unless they are "grandfathered" out. They can be reached by phone at (866) 745-5487 or by email at prevention@nwlc.org.

Unfortunately, coverage for lactation services and breast pumps does not cover all women who receive Medicaid or WIC benefits. You can see if your state's WIC program complies with the ACA at www.advisory.com/daily-briefing/resources/primers/medicaidmap.

the gold standard for breast pumps. Unfortunately, most of these pumps are no longer being manufactured.

At this time lightweight pumps, including the Medela Symphony, the Medela Lactina, and the Ameda Platinum are popular choices for rental pumps. All of these pumps should only be used with a new double collection kit.

Double collection kits, which are purchased at the time of the rental, allow mothers to express milk from either one or both breasts at the same time. Double pumping can significantly cut the amount of time needed to empty both breasts and may stimulate greater milk production than pumping just one breast at a time.

You may be able to find local pump rental stations by calling the toll-free numbers provided by the pump manufacturers (see Appendix A, page 386). Rental rates can vary tremendously, so shopping around can pay off. Rates for long-term, prepaid rental are usually lowest, but in general the cost of a pump rental is far less than the cost of formula-feeding. If your doctor prescribes the use of a clinical-grade pump, your insurance company may cover the cost of the rental depending on your situation.

Some larger pump rental stations may offer "grant pumps" to a certain number of mothers who can't afford to rent them. If you do not qualify for WIC services and yet don't have enough money to rent a clinical-grade pump, discussing your situation with local rental stations may be worth your while.

Using a clinical-grade pump is usually very simple. Place the flange carefully over the nipple so that the nipple is centered in the middle of the tunnel opening. (If the nipple is off center, it will rub uncomfortably against one side of the tunnel as you pump.) When pumping in the

The Special Supplemental Nutrition Program for Women, Infants, and Children, or WIC, lends external-piston clinical-grade pumps to some of its participants. A mother who qualifies for the program and who needs a pump because she has breastfeeding complications or a premature or sick baby, or because she is working or attending school, may be eligible for the loan of a portable electric pump. See Appendix A, page 386, for more information on WIC.

early weeks, many mothers find that a thin coat of modified lanolin, olive oil, or coconut oil applied around the base of the nipples decreases the friction between the nipples and the hard plastic of the flange.

Adjust the suction until it feels strong but not painful. Pumping that is hurting is not better and may inhibit your letdown response. Most mothers start out pumping with low suction and gradually turn up the suction until it feels strong but comfortable.

Personal-use electric pumps. These pumps cycle automatically. The best pumps in this category reach vacuums of 240 millimeters of mercury and cycling speeds of at least 50 per minute. Many, but not all, personal-use pumps have separate controls for adjusting suction strength and speed, which many mothers prefer. These pumps are recommended for mothers who have normal milk supplies but are separated from their infants on a weekly basis, mothers who are wanting to collect extra milk for occasional separations, and mothers who experience a minor temporary breastfeeding issue.

Personal-use pumps are generally not designed for exclusive pumping, particularly in the early weeks. Women who are depending on a pump alone for milk removal usually get off to a better start with a more effective clinical-grade pump.

Many women borrow or are given personal-use pumps from friends or relatives or buy these pumps secondhand. As of this writing, only a few of the pumps in this category are certified by the U.S. Food and Drug Administration (FDA) as "multiple-user pumps," which can be safely passed on if the new user buys a new collection kit. Other models in this category are designated as "single-user" pumps, which means they are not to be shared or resold. These pumps cannot be sterilized, so the risk of contamination from viruses transmitted through milk, such as HIV and cytomegalovirus (CMV), cannot be eliminated, even with the purchase of a new collection kit. Airborne viruses can get into the motors of these pumps and cause contamination for the next user. The used pumps that I check out for mothers often harbor mold.

It is important to understand, too, that most personal-use pumps have a limited life, so a used pump may not function as well as it did when it was new. Some manufacturers warn that after a year their pumps may not generate as much speed and vacuum as formerly. If you pump every day with a secondhand pump, you may find your milk supply faltering as the efficiency of the pump declines. And if a borrowed pump wears out after the end of the warranty period, you may feel obligated to purchase a new pump for the woman who lent you hers. So borrowing or purchasing a used pump may not be the bargain that it seems. If you own a pump that you used with a previous baby, you will want to check all of the pieces of the kit to be sure the pump will work well for you. Some lactation consultants offer pump "checkups."

Prices vary greatly within this category, as do warranty periods. Purchasing one of the better-quality pumps in this category may save money in the long run, especially if you are going back to work, you will have other children in the future, or both.

Many of today's pumps have "Two Phase Technology." This describes the initial pumping pattern of rapid and shallow sucking when the pump is turned on. It is thought to be similar to the initial nursing pattern of a baby in the first minute or so of nursing. At around two minutes, the sucking pattern automatically changes to a slower, deeper pattern that occurs when milk letdown happens. If a mother wants to switch over to the "expression phase" sooner, she only needs to press the letdown button to change to the slower, deeper pattern.

Start with minimal suction strength, and slowly increase the suction until it feels strong but comfortable.

Cord/tubing free wearable breast pumps. New to today's market are pumps that can be worn "hands free" inside of any bra and do not have an electric cord or any suction tubing. The pump is made up of two separate flanges that fit over each breast which are held in place within the bra cups. These pumps allow for discrete pumping and are perfect for multi-tasking.

If you are using a breast pump at high altitudes—2,000 feet above sea level or higher—know that the pump will not generate as much suction as the manufacturer states. Pumps that normally have low pressures will be very ineffective at high altitudes.

Hand-operated pumps (including "drip" milk collectors). The final group of pumps comprises those that are hand operated.

These pumps are portable and relatively inexpensive; the h
comfortable and easy to use. Hand-operated pumps are re
for mothers with adequate milk supplies who need to pun
sionally, no more than a few times a week.

As with other types of pumps, you'll need to carefully center your nipple in the flange. You may also have to repeatedly squeeze and release a handle or squeeze and release a bottle to create suction and control the cycling speed. Familiarize yourself with the manufacturer's directions, and practice to see which techniques work best for you.

A pump or a collection flanges, such as the Haakaa pump or "Milkies On-the-Go Milk Savers," (www.mymilies.com) can be positioned on one breast while the other side is being nursed at the same time. These devices work somewhat like a siphon. The milk collected in the Haakaa pump or the "Milkies On-the-Go" usually contains less fat and is often called "drip milk." It is usually lower in calories but is fine to use for feeding the baby.

Expressing Milk for Occasional Separations

If you anticipate that you and your baby will be separated from time to time, you will want to begin expressing milk, by hand or with a pump, once breastfeeding is well established. For most mothers this means sometime after the first two weeks when your baby is latching well at the breast. If you are planning to buy a pump, see my reviews in the categories of "Personal-Use Double Electric Pumps," "Personal Use Single Electric Pumps," "Wearable Breast Pumps," and "Manual Pumps," starting on page 275.

Babies will usually happily accept a bottle if it is introduced before they are a month old. They will usually continue to do so thereafter as long as the bottle is offered every two to three days.

If you are offering a bottle just to keep the baby familiar with the artificial nipple, you will need to feed only an ounce or so of milk at a time. Most mothers find they can pump this much after a morning nursing, when production is a bit higher than at other times.

Expressing Milk before Returning to Work

If you are facing a return to work or school and so will be missing feedings, you will want to practice hand expression, select a very good pump, or both. If you will be getting a pump, you will probably want to purchase a personal-use double electric pump that is designed either for personal use or for multiple users. See my review of these pumps starting on page 283.

Most mothers find comfort in having a backup supply of milk in the freezer when they return to work. This extra milk may come in handy whenever you cannot pump as much in one day as you would like or the baby takes more milk than usual. You may feel reassured that you have a backup supply in the freezer should the need for more milk arise.

If your only freezer is a compartment of your refrigerator, collecting just a couple of ounces daily will quickly fill the space. Depending on how much milk you're saving, you may want to search out available space in someone else's deep freezer, or even buy your own. Breast milk will keep for three months in the freezer compartment of a refrigerator (with a separate door) and six to twelve months in a deep freezer. See page 265 for more information on storing breast milk.

Offer a little of the milk you express to your baby. Offering a bottle frequently and regularly will keep your baby willing to take it if you return to work before he is able to drink well from a cup. Use the oldest milk in the freezer for these practice sessions so that none of your milk becomes outdated. Whenever you offer thawed breast milk to your baby, you can express some milk to replace what you've taken from your supply.

You will probably discover that you produce the most milk in the night and in the morning. This means that the morning will be a good time to collect extra milk for your baby. Expressing milk right after one, two, or even three of the first nursings of the day typically yields the most milk—for most mothers, 1 to 2 ounces (30 to 60 ml). This milk will have a very high fat content, which will be a bonus for the baby when you are apart.

Mothers whose babies begin a long sleep stretch early in the evening sometimes express milk right before they retire for the night. If the baby doesn't always sleep for a long stretch, however, pumping between nursings may not be a good idea, as you might be taking half of the baby's next feeding.

Expressing Milk at Work

If you will be missing one or more feedings while you are away at work or school, you should plan to express your milk. This will help to prevent engorgement and, more important, to maintain your milk supply. The milk you express can be used later to feed your baby while you are away. If you leave your baby for longer than four to five hours three or more times a week and do not express your milk, particularly if your baby is less than eight to ten months old, your milk supply will probably diminish.

How often you should express milk depends on the age of your baby, how long you are apart, and how often the baby nurses while you are together. Babies under four months should nurse at least eight times in twenty-four hours; emptying the breast this often is necessary to maintain adequate milk production. If your baby is less than four months old, then, plan on expressing milk every two and a half to three hours while away.

Four- to seven-month-old babies typically nurse at least seven times a day. If your baby is this age, express milk often enough so that, with pumping and nursing, your breasts are emptied seven times in each twenty-four hours. If your five-month-old nurses frequently during the day and twice at night, you may not need to express milk while you work four hours a day, unless you prefer that your baby receive only breast milk when you are apart.

A baby who is eight months old or older may be nursing often or just a few times a day. The decision to express milk at this point depends not only on how much time you spend away from your baby, but also on whether he is eating a wide variety of solid foods and on how you feel about providing formula instead of breast milk.

It is important to also understand this: Extended periods of time without complete breast drainage lessen overall milk production. For most women, if the breasts aren't thoroughly drained seven times in a twenty-four-hour period, milk production declines.

This decline in milk supply involves several factors. A lessening in breast stimulation, experts think, leads to lower prolactin levels, the hormone responsible for milk production. Additionally, full breasts that go undrained for long periods of time probably release substances that cause the milk-producing cells to slow or even cease production.

Some people mistakenly theorize that when a woman regularly goes for lengthy periods without nursing or expressing milk, the breasts become "trained" to produce sufficient amounts of milk when she does put the baby to breast. Unfortunately, this is not the case. Neglecting to express milk when apart from the baby leads to an overall lessening of the milk supply. A low milk supply generally leads to a delayed milk letdown, frustration at the breast for the baby, and in many instances premature weaning.

If you decide against expressing milk, your baby will need a commercially prepared formula for missed nursings during the first year.

Insurance Pumping

There are several situations in which it may be important to express milk after nursing a baby. This is called "insurance pumping." Mothers and babies in this category include:

- babies making the transition to full-time breastfeeding (see page 161),
- babies born at 37 weeks' gestation or earlier or weighing less than 6 pounds (2.7 kg) (see page 153),
- babies who have unusual conformations in their mouths, such as a short frenulum, a high palate, or a cleft lip or palate or both (see pages 119 and 167),
- babies who are being fed with the help of a nipple shield (see page 100),

- mothers who by seventy-two hours following birth have had no signs of milk production (see page 79),
- mothers with low milk production (see page 125),
- mothers whose breasts remain engorged because the baby isn't thoroughly draining them (see page 77),
- mothers with nipples as large in diameter as a quarter, or larger (see page 116),
- mothers who have had previous breast surgery involving an incision around the nipple or areola (see page 138),
- mothers diagnosed with polycystic ovary syndrome (PCOS) (see page 138), and
- mothers with hypoplastic breasts (long, thin, widely spaced breasts that didn't get larger in pregnancy and that may differ markedly from each other in size, see page 134).

Mothers in the categories just listed are at risk for low milk production, and their babies are at risk for poor weight gain. In many of these cases, the babies may not be vigorous enough to stimulate and drain the breasts well and to bring in a full milk supply. This is often true with near-term babies and babies making the transition to full-time nursing. A mother may bring in a full milk supply, but if the baby nurses poorly, the supply may plummet. In other situations, the baby may suck well, but the breasts may need more stimulation and emptying than the baby can provide. Examples are mothers with large nipples and mothers who have had breast surgery. In these cases, pumping right after nursings is necessary to bring in an abundant supply, as well as to insure that the baby receives plenty of milk.

Generally, double-pumping for five to fifteen minutes with a clinical-grade pump right after nursing will drain the colostrum or mature milk remaining in the breasts. When a mother pumps after each nursing, not only does her milk supply usually increase, but her baby begins receiving more milk. One pediatrician put it this way: "Insurance pumping makes the breast perform more like a fire hydrant and less like a garden hose."

Newborns in the insurance-pumping categories need to be carefully monitored for signs of adequate milk intake. If your newborn loses 10 percent of her birth weight (see Appendix B, page 396), or if she fails to

How Does Your Flange Fit?

The early weeks at home provide an opportunity to see how well your pump works for you. One question that may arise is whether the flange—the part that fits over the nipple—is the right size for you. While some flanges are made of hard plastic, others are made of more pliable silicone. This piece should be centered over the nipple and form a complete seal around the areola. The vacuum from the pump gently draws the nipple in and out of the tunnel for milk removal. If it doesn't fit well, pumping may be uncomfortable and you may not be able to express milk effectively.

Flanges, also known as breast "shields," that come with a pump vary in size depending on the manufacturer. If your nipples are as wide as or wider than a nickel, the smaller 24/25 mm flanges may be too small. Even if your nipples are narrower than a nickel, they may swell in the tunnel of a flange until the fit is clearly too snug. While you're pumping, your nipples shouldn't rub against the side of the tunnel, and the areola, the dark portion around the nipple, should move a bit with each pull. Pumping should be comfortable; experiencing nipple pain is another sign that the flange may be too small. Aside from being uncomfortable, an undersized flange may not allow for complete drainage of milk. Using the wrong size shield can lead to sore nipples, clogged milk ducts, and/or lower milk supply. A video showing how flanges should fit can be seen at www.youtube.com/watch?v=TpAnNNpRwx8.

Sometimes when a mother telephones me to ask whether she may need a different flange size, I suggest pumping again twenty minutes after a regular pumping. Collecting more than ½ ounce (15 ml) of milk in the second pumping may indicate that the flange fits poorly.

Most pump manufacturers offer information about the sizing of their flanges. Usually mothers can go to the websites of the pumps they are interested in or call the company to see if they offer a tool that helps to determine the best flange size. You can probably order large (size 27 mms) or extra-large flanges (size 30 mms) from the manufacturer (see Appendix A, page 386).

Another option for getting a comfortable flange size is by contacting Pumpin' Pal who can help you find and order the perfect silicone flange size (see Pumpin' Pal on page 386).

The angled, elliptical Pumpin' Pal Super Shields can be used with various pump brands for more comfortable pumping. The shields can be used in place of the removable flanges of other brands and can be used with adapters for other pumps. The flanges come in three sizes, determined by the mother's size, shape, and elasticity. For either small or large sets of the inserts for use with Spectra, Motif Luna, or Ameda models, the price is $49.95. For either size for the Medela or Lansinoh, the cost is $39.99. A sizing quiz at www. pumpinpal.com will guide you to the correct purchase. Visit the website or call to place an order, speak with a helpful salesperson, or find a local retailer.

A new product designed for more comfortable pumping is BeauGen breast pump cushions, designed for mothers with uncomfortable pumping despite having the correct size flanges. The majority of mothers who rated the product highly say it helps with having very elastic nipples and inadequate milk flow. One set sells for $21 and purchasing two sets costs $40. Some mothers will want to subscribe to getting a pair on a regular basis and saving money over the one-time purchase price (see BeauGen on page 388 for more). There are two helpful videos online—one which shows how BeauGen cushions can help (www.beaugen.com/pages/how-it-works) and another that shows how to insert the cushions (www.youtube.com/watch?v=IC14JWlascA).

An additional product called Liquid Shields is a soft fluid silicone flange system designed for more comfortable pumping sessions with Pumpable brand flanges. The liquid inserts mold to the breast tissue, providing a soft environment for the nipple to be drawn down. When the breast pump applies suction, the liquid insert will collapse around the nipple, which compresses and massages the nipples.

The Liquid Shield insert two-pack costs $12 and the full system kit costs $24.95, which includes one single hard flange with a Liquid Shield insert. Sizes offered are 17, 21, 25, and 29 millimeters. The Pumpables brand SuperGenie breast pump includes the Liquid Shields. For more information, visit Pumpables.co.

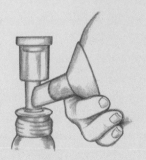

Tight fit

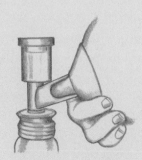

Good fit

gain an ounce a day after five days of age, you'll need to feed her some or all of the milk that you collect by pumping. If you can't collect enough milk, she may also need supplemental formula. In these cases, working with a lactation professional can be very helpful.

When your baby is gaining weight normally without supplemental breast milk, you can slowly wean yourself off the pump. After doing so, continue to monitor the baby's weight for a short while.

Expressing Milk for a Baby Who Cannot Nurse

Some mothers must bring in a milk supply without a nursing baby. If your baby is unable to nurse because of a latch-on problem, prematurity, or illness, you will want to start pumping as soon as possible, ideally within hours of delivery, so your baby receives plenty of colostrum. Colostrum is especially beneficial because it has such a high concentration of protective antibodies.

The nursing staff should provide you with a suitable pump and instructions for collecting and storing your milk. Most maternity units have a clinical-grade breast pump available; this is the type of pump you want when you must pump around the clock. (If the hospital uses the Medela Symphony breast pump, see page 276 for information on using this pump to bring in a full milk supply.) If your baby is being transferred to another hospital for care, ask the transport team about their procedures for storing and transporting your milk. If you will be following the baby to a special-care nursery in another city, try to get a pump to take along with you. See page 276 for information on renting a clinical-grade breast pump.

It is very important that you have the right size flanges for pumping. Some standard pump flanges are too small for many mothers. If your nipples are swelling in the tunnels, and especially if pumping is painful, the flanges may be too small. If they are, your breasts won't drain completely. For advice on choosing the correct flange size, see page 256.

Initially, you may be more comfortable if you apply a thin coat of lanolin around the base of the nipples before starting to pump (for sources of modified, hypoallergenic lanolin, see Appendix A, page 386). If pumping is painful even with lanolin, again, you may need larger flanges.

You may receive differing bits of advice on how often and how long to pump your breasts. Some hospital nurses suggest that women pump every three to four hours during the day and sleep all night. With such limited stimulation, most mothers would find either that they wouldn't bring in an abundant supply or that after a while it would dwindle. Keep in mind that your milk supply depends on the frequent stimulation of your breasts. You should plan on expressing milk as often as your baby would nurse, or at least eight times in twenty-four hours. Some mothers prefer to express their milk every three hours around the clock, whereas others would rather pump a little more often during the day so they can sleep for longer periods at night. Determine a reasonable schedule for yourself, but do not go more than five hours without pumping.

Studies now suggest that the effectiveness as well as the frequency of colostrum removal in the first three days is highly predictive of how much milk will be produced in the days to follow. Surprisingly, dependence on a pump alone during the first several days may be associated with lower milk production. Dr. Jane Morton and others at Stanford University have found that pumping alone may remove only a fraction of the available colostrum and milk. In this study, mothers who both hand-expressed colostrum and pumped with the Medela Symphony pump collected 80 percent more milk than women who used only the pump. For instructions on hand expression, see page 240. You can see Dr. Morton's technique in the video at http://newborns.stanford.edu/ Breastfeeding/HandExpression.html.

If you are hand-expressing for a healthy full-term or near-term baby who is unable to latch on to the breast, you can collect the colostrum in a plastic spoon or syringe, which you can then use to feed the baby. If your baby is sick or very premature, ask the hospital staff about what small container to collect and store colostrum for later use.

Once your milk is in, how much you produce will depend on how much you manage to express. Ideally, you should pump more milk than your baby requires. Building and maintaining a volume of at least 24 ounces (720 ml) per day, or for twins, 40 to 48 ounces (1,200 to 1,440 ml) per day, will allow you to have extra milk on reserve should you experience a temporary decline in production—due to stress or illness, for example—during your baby's hospitalization. Having an abundant supply will also help your baby get milk more easily once he is able to latch on to the breast and suck.

You can maximize the amount you collect by massaging or pressing firm areas of the breast while you pump. To see Dr. Morton demonstrate the hands-on pumping technique, go to http://newborns.stanford.edu/Breastfeeding/MaxProduction.html.

It may be easier to massage and compress your breasts if you pump one side at a time. Alternatively, you can wear a hands-free bra, also known as a pumping bustier, which will hold the pump flanges in place (see page 388). A tight sports bra with the centers cut out can also allow you to massage and pump both breasts at once.

After pumping, you can collect even more milk by hand-expressing for a few minutes, alternating breasts several times.

With practice and experimentation, you will develop your own method for collecting the most milk possible. Most mothers find that once they are able to pump 3 to 4 ounces (90 to 120 ml) at a time, they can gradually eliminate the other measures to increase milk production.

Whenever possible, provide freshly expressed or refrigerated milk for your premature or sick baby. Freezing breast milk preserves many but not all of its protective substances. You can keep your milk for twenty-four to forty-eight hours in the refrigerator (ask the intensive-care nurses for a more precise limit) or for up to three months in the freezer.

Depending on your baby's maturity or general progress, you may find yourself expressing milk for several weeks. It is important that you eat well, get plenty to drink, and rest enough to maintain your own energy as well as your milk supply.

If you notice that your milk production is declining for a few days in a row, you will need to assess the situation and make whatever adjustments are necessary. The most common causes of decreasing milk production are infrequent expression—fewer than eight times in twenty-four hours— and an inefficient pump. Although a few mothers can maintain a good milk supply while expressing less often than this or while using a non-clinical-grade pump, most can't do so for longer than a few weeks.

If you have been using a hand pump or an inexpensive battery-operated or plug-in pump, or even a personal-use pump, rent a clinical-grade pump. Most mothers find that a clinical-grade pump requires less effort to operate and works more efficiently. Using Dr. Morton's methods to increase milk production, as described in this section, may also help improve your overall production.

Occasionally you may notice that your milk production drops when you and your baby have a difficult day. Stress can temporarily decrease a mother's milk supply; this is normal and usually temporary. The following suggestions have proven helpful when this occurs:

- Pump regularly, every two to three hours.
- Take a short nap or a warm bath just before expressing.
- Apply moist heat to your breasts before expressing.
- Massage each breast as you pump, and perform hand expression right after each pumping.
- Ask someone to rub your back between the shoulder blades while you are pumping.
- If possible, hold the baby while you are pumping at the hospital, or keep a photo of your baby with your pump.
- Hold the baby skin-to-skin as much as possible.

Pumping Exclusively

For any of a variety of reasons, a woman may find herself pumping all of her baby's milk and feeding it by bottle instead of nursing. It may be that the baby has been unable to latch on to the breast, or even that the mother prefers to feed her baby this way. Many women have managed to produce enough milk to meet their babies' needs for a year or beyond while pumping exclusively.

Pumping full-time for a baby requires dedication and discipline. Unlike a baby, a pump does not signal for attention, and for most women pumping is more a chore than a pleasure. To feed your baby entirely or mostly on your own milk, however, is to give him an extra-special gift.

If you are exclusively pumping, frequent and effective expression during the first week after birth is critical for establishing an abundant milk supply. Read "Expressing Milk for a Baby Who Cannot Nurse" (page 258), and make sure you have a high-quality, comfortable pump. Starting out with a clinical-grade rental pump is the best way to bring in a full milk supply—about 24 ounces (720 ml) per day during the first month. Since clinical-grade pumps are expensive, women who use them rent them rather than buy them. If your income is low or modest, you may qualify for a rent-free clinical-grade pump through the WIC program (see page 280). In any case, long-term pump rental is much less costly than buying formula.

A double collection kit, for collecting milk from both breasts at once, makes pumping quicker and is usually more effective in establishing and maintaining milk production. Unless you are given a collection kit in the hospital, you will need to buy one when you rent a clinical-grade pump.

It is essential to pump often—every two to three hours during the day and at least once in the night, or at least eight times in each twenty-four hours. You must also spend enough time at each pumping to drain both breasts completely, since it is the frequent, thorough drainage of the breasts that signals them to increase milk production and keep it high. Some women can completely drain the breasts by pumping for ten minutes or less, but others need a longer time. Until you're sure how much time you need, pump until the milk stops flowing and then a couple of minutes longer.

Pumping shouldn't hurt. A properly fitting pump flange allows for the pull and release of the nipple without the nipple's swelling against the side of the tunnel. If the tunnel is too narrow for your nipple, your breast won't drain completely and pumping may be painful. For help in determining whether you need a larger flange, see page 256.

Once you have established a generous milk supply—at least 24 ounces (720 ml) per day—you might invest in your own personal-use pump. See "A Review of Breast Pump Models" on page 275. Some mothers, however, are unable to maintain high production with these pumps and continue to require a clinical-grade rental model.

After the first month, most women are able to maintain their production level with seven pumpings in each twenty-four hours. With less frequent pumping than this, however, most women find that their supply

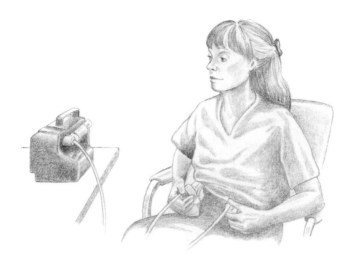

You can use a fully automatic breast pump with a double collection kit to pump breast milk more quickly and efficiently.

drops below the baby's needs. A very small proportion of women produce excessive milk while pumping only five or six times in each twenty-four hours. If you are an overproducer, you can freeze the extra milk for later use.

Mothers who are exclusively pumping especially appreciate products that allow hands-free pumping (see page 36, Other Purchases You Might Consider).

Your milk supply will need to grow as your baby does. From the fifth day after birth until about three months, babies generally gain about 1 ounce (28 g) per day. After three months of age, their weight gain typically slows to about ½ ounce (14 g) per day. They require 20 to 24 ounces (600 to 720 ml) of milk per day in the first month, and their intake gradually increases thereafter to 28 to 32 ounces (840 to 960 ml) per day. Their intake stays at about this level until other foods slowly begin to replace breast milk in the diet.

Bottle-fed babies often drink more than they need for normal growth, even when they're fed breast milk rather than formula. Since overfeeding a baby can lead to obesity later, you may want to keep track of how much milk your baby is taking. These guidelines may be helpful: During the first month, offer about 1 ounce per hour, or 3 ounces

(89 ml) every two and a half to three hours. After the first month, offer as much as 1½ ounces (45 ml) per hour, or 4½ ounces (135 ml) every three hours. If your baby seems to want more milk than this, try to keep in mind that babies often fuss when they are overstimulated, tired, or uncomfortable. A breastfeeding mother may put her baby to the breast hourly when he is tired or cranky, but he doesn't get a large meal at each comfort feeding. Carrying your baby or offering a pacifier between feedings may help in calming him. (If your baby is very fussy, see page 219, Fussiness, Colic, and Reflux.) Learning how to do "paced" bottle-feeding can also help your baby take a more normal volume of milk by bottle (see page 273 for information).

If you're pumping out of necessity rather than choice, it may be helpful to know that many babies become able and willing to take the breast despite weeks or even months of bottle-feeding. If your baby has been unable to latch on and suck well, it is still worthwhile to try nursing periodically. A lactation professional may be able to help you.

Increasing Your Milk Supply while Pumping

Some women who exclusively or frequently pump struggle with low milk production. If your production is lower than the norms specified here, you can take measures to increase it. Be sure that you are not pregnant or using estrogen containing birth control (combination birth control pills or the vaginal ring with estrogen), which typically lessens milk production. The progestin-only "mini-pill" is usually fine.

1. Consider using a clinical-grade pump and a double-pump kit, if you are not doing so already.

2. Pump or nurse *at least* eight times a day—more if you can manage. Distribute the pumping or nursing sessions more or less evenly during the baby's waking hours. If your baby sleeps a long stretch at night, pump just before you go to bed or very early in the morning. If you work away from home, nurse or pump right before leaving the baby and as soon as you return.

3. If you're not sure whether your pump is draining your breasts completely, try pumping fifteen to twenty minutes after a prior pumping. If you get ½ ounce (15 ml) or more at the second pumping, the collection kit, or even the pump itself, may be doing an inadequate job.

4. To be sure your pump is working efficiently, give it a checkup. Check the tubing, connections, rubber diaphragms, and filters. If the diaphragms get small tears, the pump will not work efficiently. If the filters get wet, the suction will stop entirely. A lactation professional may be able to check the pump's vacuum, which should reach 240 millimeters of mercury. Some pumps are simply not capable of reaching these vacuums.

5. Be sure the pump's nipple flanges fit you right (see page 256).

6. Pump at the highest suction possible without discomfort, and at a speed of about 50 times a minute.

7. Practice "hands-on pumping," as described on page 260.

8. Consider using Pumpin' Pal Super Shields (see page 256), which might help you express more milk, especially if your pump has adequate suction.

9. Consider taking herbal products that stimulate milk production, such as fenugreek or blessed thistle capsules, More Milk Plus tincture or capsules, or Go-Lacta (see page 392).

10. If your periods have resumed and you find that your milk production dips when you are mid-cycle until your period begins, consider taking 500 to 1,000 milligrams of calcium and 250 to 500 milligrams of magnesium daily. Take this from the time of ovulation until the day of your heaviest flow.

Collecting and Storing Your Breast Milk

Regardless of whether you have a healthy baby or one who is premature or sick in the hospital, you will always want to take special care when expressing and storing your milk.

A study of bacteria found in the mouths of infants compared those fed stored expressed breast milk with those infants who recently breastfed. Infants who drank stored breast milk had significantly more bacteria in their mouths than those who were tested right after being breastfed. This suggests that parents may need to be informed about the best practices for collecting and storing breast milk.

Using a "closed system" breast pump instead of an "open system" pump is one way to help limit the amount of bacteria found in pumped milk. A true closed system pump is designed to keep milk out of the tubing and filters of a breast pump. An open system pump can allow milk to enter the tubing and/or filters. If you are considering purchasing a pump or getting one through insurance, you can review the common pumps at the end of this chapter to see if they are open or closed system pumps.

The Centers for Disease Control and Prevention (CDC) have guidelines in the handling and storing of breast milk. Following these guidelines are important in limiting the growth of bacteria in your breast milk.

HUMAN MILK STORAGE GUIDELINES			
	STORAGE LOCATION AND TEMPERATURES		
TYPE OF BREAST MILK	Countertop 77°F (25°C) or colder (room temperature)	Refrigerator 40°F (4°C) Freezer 0°F (-18°C) or colder	Freezer 0°F (-18°C) or colder
FRESHLY EXPRESSED OR PUMPED	Up to 4 Hours	Up to 4 Days	Within 6 months is best Up to 12 months is acceptable
THAWED, PREVIOUSLY FROZEN	1–2 Hours	Up to 1 Day (24 hours)	NEVER refreeze human milk after it has been thawed
LEFTOVER FROM A FEEDING (BABY DID NOT FINISH THE BOTTLE)	Use within 2 hours after the baby is finished feeding		

1. Wash your hands thoroughly with soap and water. Alternatively, you may use a hand sanitizer that contains at least 60 percent alcohol.

2. All pump parts that come in contact with the milk or your breasts should be thoroughly washed after each use, with hot soapy water and separately from family eating utensils and food preparation equipment. Use a bottle brush, one with a smaller brush on the opposite end, to reach all the nooks and crannies of the pump parts. (Some mothers buy a second collection kit so they can do the washing at their convenience.)

3. Your daily bath or shower will cleanse your breasts sufficiently.

4. You can store your milk in plastic or glass feeding bottles or in plastic bags made for milk storage. Plastic bags take up less space in the freezer than bottles do, and you may be able to express your milk directly into the bags. Some mothers use disposable bottle liners, but these can break when the milk freezes and leak when it thaws. Bags designed for storing breast milk are made of thicker plastic, come sterilized, and have a place for writing the date. The main disadvantage of milk storage bags is that they are not reusable. Also, you should not add fresh milk to a bag of frozen milk or feed the milk to the baby directly from a defrosted bag. The bags are more prone to leakage than bottles, but you can minimize this problem by putting the filled bags into freezer-weight food storage bags. For information on popular brands of milk storage bags, see Appendix A, page 386.

5. Unless you are collecting 1- to 2-ounce (30 to 60 ml) bottles for practice feedings, store your milk in quantities of 3 to 4 ounces (90 to 120 ml). According to the CDC, breast milk can be stored in the back of the refrigerator, not in the door, at 34 to 40°F (1 to -15°C) for up to four days (ninety-six hours). Unless your refrigerator has a thermometer, purchase a small one from most any hardware store for under $10. Freshly refrigerated milk is better for your baby, as it retains more of its live cells than frozen milk. If you wish to add more milk to some that is already bottled, chill the new milk in the refrigerator for about half an hour before adding it.

If you will not be using your expressed milk within four days (ninety-six hours), store it in the freezer. Even milk that has been refrigerated for four days can be safely moved into a freezer.

Breast milk looks different from dairy milk, especially after storage in the refrigerator or freezer. Your fresh milk may be yellow, white, bluish, or even greenish, depending on what you have eaten and what medicines or vitamins you have taken. Frozen breast milk is usually yellow. Your milk will naturally separate in the refrigerator; the fat will rise to the top. After warming the milk, gently swirl it to mix the layers.

Fresh or thawed breast milk typically has a mild, slightly sweet smell. Occasionally a mother finds that her expressed milk has an unpleasant smell or taste. Certain vitamin or mineral supplements can cause this, and so can steroidal nasal sprays. In either case, the affected milk is harmless.

Breast milk can take on a soapy smell if the fat has broken down, freeing fatty acids. Apparently, some women have an excess of lipase, the enzyme that breaks down the fat in milk. Usually they notice the soapy smell after the milk has been refrigerated or frozen, but in some cases the smell develops immediately after expression. Most babies will take such milk without complaint, but the peculiar odor and taste can usually be lessened or eliminated either by chilling the milk before freezing it or by putting it directly into the freezer, and then thawing it in the refrigerator before warming it in a hot-water bath. If these methods fail for you, you can inactivate the enzyme by scalding the milk on the stove—that is, by bringing the milk almost to a boil—and then immediately refrigerating or freezing it. Do not let the milk boil; doing so would destroy its anti-infective properties.

Although freezing destroys the white blood cells found in breast milk, it preserves the many other antimicrobial properties and inhibits the growth of bacteria. Freezing does not affect the nutritional composition of breast milk.

You can safely store your milk in the freezer compartment of a refrigerator for three to six months, provided that the freezer compartment is separate from, not inside, the refrigerator, and that the temperature stays at −4°F (-20°C). Store the milk toward the back of the freezer, away from the door. If the freezer automatically defrosts, keep the milk away from the walls.

Again, if your refrigerator does not have a thermometer, purchase one. Freshly refrigerated milk is better for your baby, as it retains more of its live cells than frozen milk. If you wish to add more milk to some that is already bottled, chill the new milk in the refrigerator for about half an hour before adding it.

Because the entire amount must be used once breast milk is thawed, you will want to store small amounts, probably 3 to 4 ounces (90 to 120 ml). Regardless of what kind of container you use, leave some room at the top to allow for expansion and to avoid leakage. If you want to add fresh milk to some that is frozen, chill the fresh milk first to keep the top layer of frozen milk from thawing.

Date your containers so that you use the oldest milk first. While bottles are often recommended, you may find that bags made especially for breast milk will take up less space. Using other types of bags is not recommended due to leakage problems. If you will be taking the milk to day care, write the baby's name on the bags as well. Placing the bags in a plastic container will also help keep them safe from breakage.

Better yet, store the milk in a freestanding deep freezer, where the milk will be good for twelve months when the temperature is −4°F (-20°C). If you don't have a freestanding freezer and you are running out of space in the freezer section of the refrigerator, you might invest in a small one or find a friend or relative who has one that you can store your milk in.

Collecting Milk for a Premature or Sick Baby

If you are expressing milk for a premature or sick baby, you should not only wash the pump parts in hot, soapy water, you should also sterilize them every day. You can boil them in water for fifteen minutes or run them through a dishwasher's sanitizing cycle, or you can sterilize them in special bags in a microwave oven: Place all of the parts that come in contact with milk in one of the bags with 4 ounces (120 ml) of water, and microwave for the time recommended on the bag, usually between one and five minutes. For more information about Medela's Quick Clean Micro-Steam Bags, see Appendix A, page 386.

After collecting your milk, pour it into a sterile container; ask the hospital nursery staff what type they prefer. To avoid wasting milk, ask your baby's nurses how much to put in each container. Freshly refrigerated milk is better for your baby, as it retains more of its live cells than frozen milk, so try to provide fresh milk for your baby whenever possible. Milk for a premature or sick baby can be safely stored in the refrigerator for up to forty-eight hours (ask the nursing staff for their specific limit).

When transporting your refrigerated or frozen milk to the hospital, pack the containers in ice, or surround them with refreezable ice packs, inside a small cooler. If you're traveling a long distance, keep your milk frozen with dry ice.

Milk for a premature or sick baby should not be frozen or refrigerated after it has been thawed or warmed. Whatever is left over after the feeding must be thrown out.

Feeding Your Expressed Milk

Take your milk out of the refrigerator shortly before your baby is due for a feeding. Gradually, over five to ten minutes, warm the milk to room temperature in a container of warm water. Never warm or defrost milk in a microwave oven or on the stove. Microwaves do not heat evenly, and uneven heating can burn a baby's mouth. Bottles can explode in microwave ovens. In a microwave or on a stove, excess heat can destroy the immunological substances, proteins, and vitamins in breast milk.

When taking milk out of the freezer for feeding, choose the oldest milk; this way you're less likely to end up throwing away outdated milk later. Thaw the milk in any of three ways: hold the container under warm running water; swirl it in a bowl of warm water; or let it thaw overnight in the refrigerator. Do not thaw milk by letting the bottle sit at room temperature.

When breast milk thaws, the fat separates and rises to the top. Gently shake the bottle to blend the fat back in with the rest of the milk. Use thawed milk within twenty-four hours. Do not refreeze it.

Mothers often ask whether they can reuse breast milk left over after a feeding. Although there have been no scientific studies on this question, most lactation professionals believe that warmed or defrosted milk can be refrigerated, reheated, and used for the next feeding so long as the baby isn't sick or premature and the milk has not been left out for longer two hours.

Getting your baby used to a bottle is important if she will be fed by someone else while you are apart. It is best to wait until she is two to four weeks old before introducing a bottle. By this time nursing should be well established, so the bottle should not interfere with the baby's interest in the breast. Paced feeding is important so the infant does not rely on the fast flow of the bottle and then become impatient at the breast. Many babies refuse the bottle if it is first offered much after they are one month old.

Many kinds of bottles and nipples are on the market, and no one bottle or nipple is best for breastfed babies or more likely to be accepted over another. The best bottles are easy to clean and have accurate measuring indicators. Angled bottles are supposed to make it easier to keep the nipple filled, so the baby doesn't suck in air, but this is just as easy with straight bottles and actually unnecessary (see page 273, Baby-Led or Paced Bottle-Feeding). Bottles molded into unusual shapes or split down the middle for self-feeding are nearly impossible to keep clean. Some bottles come with disposable liners, which are supposed to cause less air swallowing. They don't.

Most bottles come in two sizes: 4 ounces (120 ml) and 8 ounces (240 ml). Four-ounce (120-ml) bottles make more sense for babies who are taking only 2 to 4 ounces (60 to 120 ml) at a feeding. You can buy 8-ounce (240-ml) bottles later, if your baby begins drinking 4 to 5 ounces (120 to 150 ml) at a feeding.

Nipples are made of latex or silicone. Silicone nipples are definitely preferable. Latex has a taste and odor and deteriorates faster than silicone. Latex also tends to break down in the dishwasher and so should be washed by hand. Silicone nipples *can* be washed in the dishwasher.

To introduce a bottle, manually express or pump your milk instead of nursing, and then, if possible, have your partner or someone else feed the milk to the baby. If you do this about three times a week until you go back to work, your baby should continue to accept a bottle. Offering a bottle periodically will also give you the opportunity to practice manual expression or become proficient with your pump.

Parents who stop offering a bottle once the baby has taken it sometimes find themselves struggling with the baby and bottle weeks later. Giving the baby 1 or 2 ounces (30 or 60 ml) of breast milk by bottle every few days is very important if you want to avoid problems later.

Should your baby refuse to drink from a bottle, keep trying. The following suggestions may help:

- To avoid wasting your milk, practice with just 1 or 2 ounces (30 or 60 ml) in the bottle.

- Don't substitute formula for your milk in these practice sessions. Most babies prefer sweet-tasting breast milk to formula.

- Try a variety of bottle nipples. Look for one with a faster flow. Try a tasteless silicone nipple instead of a latex one. Different mothers swear by different brands, including Avent, Playtex, Mimijumi, and Dr. Brown's.

- Try offering the bottle while walking with the baby. Hold the baby facing away from you, and bounce her gently as you walk. This will be easier if you put the baby in a front-facing carrier.

- Try nursing the baby for just a few minutes, and then unlatching her and slipping the bottle into her mouth. If she objects, try again after a few minutes more of nursing.

- Have someone else try; frequently a baby is more confused and upset by a bottle when her mother tries to persuade her.

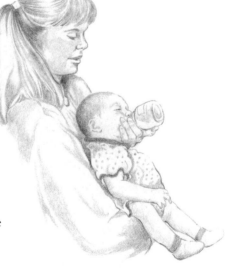

A baby may more easily accept the bottle if you hold her facing outward and walk.

- As long as the baby is refusing the bottle, offer it a couple of times each day, both when the baby seems hungry and when she is not.

- Do not allow these sessions to become too upsetting for the baby or for you. Trying to force a baby to take a bottle is distressing for everyone and rarely successful. Also, "starving" the baby until she accepts a bottle is somewhat abusive and rarely effective.

Although you want to know before you are apart that your baby will drink from a bottle, the baby who won't take a bottle from Mom may do well when the caregiver offers it. At the age of three months, my daughter, Kate, screamed bloody murder whenever I approached with a bottle, but her caregiver had no problems feeding her when I was away.

The baby who refuses a bottle may do surprisingly well with an ordinary, unspouted cup, particularly if she is nearing six months or older. A sippy cup may be too much like a bottle for a baby who is continuing to refuse one.

Baby-Led or Paced Bottle-Feeding

When you are feeding your baby your milk by bottle, always hold him in your arms. Let him control the feeding in the ways he does when you nurse him: Wait for him to open his mouth instead of pushing in the nipple. Be patient when he pauses in sucking; don't stimulate him to suck continuously. Even if there is breast milk left in the bottle, let your baby stop drinking when he signals that he has had enough.

A full bottle-feeding should take seven to fifteen minutes. If the feeding takes longer, the nipple flow may be too slow. If the baby chokes frequently, the nipple flow is too fast.

Breastfed babies, in most instances, control the flow of breast milk as they nurse. When you're breastfeeding, the milk may spray as it lets down, and the baby may let go of the breast to prevent himself from choking. After the first letdown, the baby then controls the flow of milk by sucking and pausing when needed. In contrast, some babies fed from a bottle, particularly those younger than four months, struggle to keep up with the rapid flow of milk. If your baby seems to be gulping down the milk as fast as he can, you may think he is very hungry, but actually he may be swallowing quickly just to avoid choking. You may see signs that the baby is feeling stressed: He may tense up, and his eyes may open wide. Milk may leak from the corners of his mouth. He may spread out his fingers. He may try to pull away from the bottle or "shut down," pretending to fall asleep in an attempt to end the feeding. A baby who manages to chug his milk from a bottle may end up taking more than he needs.

You (or whoever is feeding the baby) can avoid this problem by making sure that the baby is comfortable, that he can pause to take a breath between swallows, and that he can end the feeding himself when he has had enough. This is known as "baby-led" or "paced" bottle-feeding. Use a slow-flow nipple, and sit the baby almost upright. Touch the bottle nipple to the baby's lips to stimulate him to open his mouth wide, as he does when he seeks out the breast. Then place the nipple in his mouth. Hold the bottle horizontally to slow the flow of milk through the nipple. There will be air in the nipple, but try not to worry about the baby swallowing it; you can burp him periodically. If he is sucking without pause but showing facial signals of stress, lower the bottle while keeping it in his mouth. This will give the baby the chance to rest and to begin sucking again when he is ready. When the baby stops sucking, do not jiggle the nipple in his mouth to get him to resume. Assume that he has had enough even if there is still milk in the bottle. You can view Jessica Barton's video on "Paced Bottle-Feeding for the Breast-Fed Baby" on YouTube.

Some final words on bottle-feeding: Never prop a bottle for a young baby or allow an older baby to bottle-feed himself. A baby needs an adult in close contact not only to monitor the amount of milk taken but also to provide the pleasure of her arms and attention.

A Review of Breast Pump Models

- Clinical-Grade Rental Pumps
- Multiuser Loaner Pumps Through the WIC Program
- Clinical-Grade, Multiuser Double Electric Breast Pumps for Purchase
- Personal Use Double Electric Pumps
- Wearable Breast Pumps
- Milk Cups
- Personal Use Single Electric Pumps
- Manual Pumps
- Silicone Squeeze Pumps

It is important to understand the terms used when deciding which pump is best for you at any given time, as sometimes the terms can be confusing and misleading. For example, some pump manufacturers may use the term "hospital-grade" to convince mothers that these pumps are the highest possible quality when, in fact, they may not be. Instead, the term "hospital-grade" actually refers to the electrical standard of breast pumps, not their quality. Technically, a "hospital-grade" pump has a three-prong plug for use in an electric outlet found in hospitals.

Mothers who need the highest quality pump to bring in, maintain, or increase milk production do best by using what I describe as a "clinical-grade" pump. These pumps are also often referred to as "rental-grade" pumps or "multiuser" pumps. These pumps are intended for mothers who need an excellent pump for exclusive or nearly exclusive pumping, often due to a breastfeeding complication or a baby who is yet to latch on well and effectively drain the breast.

"Personal use" pumps are intended to be used by a mother for occasional or even daily pumping. This type of pump may be provided through insurance providers or purchased by mothers to use for upcoming separations, such as the return to work or school. These pumps are not intended for mothers to share.

Many new mothers who experience breastfeeding issues may think that the pump they received from their insurance provider will be fine if the baby is not nursing well or there are other feeding issues early on. This may not be the case. If advised by a lactation professional to secure a clinical-grade rental pump, or multiuser pump, don't pass up this advice. Rental pumps cost only a few dollars per day and may very well bring in and protect a milk supply much better than a personal use pump either purchased or obtained through insurance.

Historically, pumps have been divided into those that are considered "closed system" pumps and those that are considered "open system" pumps. Closed system pumps are ideal, as they do not allow milk or condensation to enter into the tubing, filters, and/or motor. Open system pumps are less desirable because they may allow milk to enter the tubing, the filters, and, for some, the pump itself. If milk is able to get into tubing or the pump itself, it may become contaminated. As of this writing, there are just a few breast pumps on the market that are not closed system pumps.

Clinical-Grade Rental Pumps

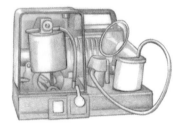

Clinical-grade pump

Medela Classic Electric Pump. A sturdy machine weighing over 20 pounds, this internal-piston pump is no longer being manufactured but is still available through a few rental stations. This pump is an open system pump and should be used with a filter that keeps milk from entering into the pump. If you can find this great pump, it cycles at about 50 times per minute and generates suction of at least 240 millimeters of mercury. When you rent the pump, you must purchase a milk collection kit, at a cost of about $60. To locate a rental station near you, call Medela at 800-435-8316 or check www.medelabreastfeedingus.com.

Medela Symphony Pump. The Symphony is probably the most popular rental pump in the U.S. and has been ever since its launch in 2003. The Symphony pump was designed to be a lightweight rental pump for mothers needing to express their milk because of various feeding issues.

Symphony, a diaphragm pump, was the first fully automatic pump with a two-phase sucking pattern.

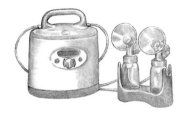

Medela Symphony Pump

The first phase, lasting about two minutes, has rapid cycling that stimulates the milk to release; the second phase has slower cycling and higher suction and keeps the milk flowing. If the milk lets down before the first phase is up, the mother presses a button to switch to the slower, deeper phase. It is not possible to adjust suction and speed independently, as can be done with other pumps. Still, many women report that the Symphony is gentler and more comfortable to use than other clinical-grade pumps. This may be important if you are pumping because of sore or injured nipples. Symphony is not a closed system pump and milk can enter into the tubing.

Medela's own research showed that the Symphony was ineffective in bringing in a full milk supply for mothers who were exclusively pumping for premature or term newborns.

Because many hospitals provide Symphony pumps for mothers expressing milk for their non-nursing newborns, Medela and Rush University's Director for Clinical Research and Lactation, Dr. Paula Meier, designed a special program of sucking patterns known as the Symphony PLUS program. The Symphony PLUS program is designed to bring in, as well as maintain, a full milk supply. A micro-processor chip on a program card located in the back of the pump, creates this two-phase sucking pattern. The PLUS program card creates a more rapid sucking and pausing pattern so the pump will more closely mimic a baby's sucking pattern.

Studies show that mothers using the Symphony with the new Symphony PLUS card installed in the pump have collected more colostrum in a shorter period of time than without the card. Most, but not every, hospital or rental station have the new cards for their pumps. You can find out which circuit board is in the pump by asking the hospital staff or rental station if they are using the "PLUS" program card. There should also be a sticker on the pump that shows mothers how to start the PLUS program.

Once the pump is turned on, prompts on the screen will help you set up the one of the two programs: initiate or maintain. The initiate program is used for the first few days. When the baby is six days old or the mother begins pumping 20 milliliters, three pumpings in a row—whichever comes first—she should switch over to the maintain program. This pattern switches back and forth between milk stimulation and expression modes with several pauses in between. If you will be exclusively pumping, and the hospital or rental station pump does not have Symphony pump with the new card, Symphony PLUS, I recommend you either spend time hand-expressing after pumping or secure another clinical-grade pump as soon as possible.

Rental rates for the Symphony may be higher, about $75 per month more, than for most other rental pumps. As with other rental pumps, you must buy a collection kit, unless you received one at the hospital. The pump normally comes without a rechargeable battery. To locate a rental station near you, call Medela at 800-435-8316 or check www.medela.com. For more information, visit www.mybreastpumprental.com.

Ameda Platinum Breast Pump. Weighing just under 10 pounds, this internal piston pump is used in hospitals and is available at some rental stations. The speed and suction levels are displayed on the front of the pump. Speeds that increase to as high as 80 cycles per minute help stimulate milk letdown, and a suction that reaches an effective 240 millimeters of mercury promotes breast emptying. All Ameda pumps are closed system pumps, meaning that mothers won't need to worry about milk, condensation, and mold getting into the tubing and pump. When you rent the pump, you must purchase a milk collection kit, at a cost of $60. See Appendix A, page 386, for more.

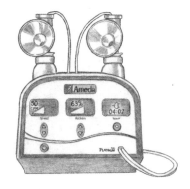

Ameda Platinum Breast Pump

Ameda Elite Pump. Intended for rental use, the fully automatic external-piston Elite weighs only 7 pounds, and mothers can vary the rate and the strength of suction with separate dials. For women who will be pumping where there is no electric outlet, one model comes with a built-in battery pack. The Elite reaches a weak suction strength of only 220 millimeters of mercury with double pumping, which may affect the pump's efficiency. I recommend finding a stronger suctioning pump. Long-term rental rates of $30 to $60 per month are available through a few rental stations. You will need to purchase your own milk collection kit. Some WIC programs have this pump available for their mothers who need one.

Ardo Carum Pump. This Swiss-made, internal-piston pump is used at some hospitals and through just a few Ardo rental stations in the U.S. It has a sleek, lightweight design and a very quiet motor. A range of vacuums and speeds are available, all independent of one another, so that mothers can choose their own pumping patterns with both stimulation and expression modes. One creation of Carum is the

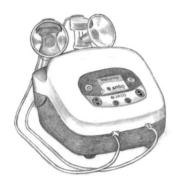

Ardo Carum Pump

"drop zone," a pattern that actually holds the vacuum momentarily at the height of the suck, similar to that of a nursing infant. Also, this pump has a special "sensitive setting" for mothers experiencing sore nipples. Carum has a large color display and is also available in a battery-powered version. A closed system pump, milk cannot get into the tubing or the pump itself. In my opinion, the Carum is one of the best pumps on the market today. The personal-use double kit necessary for pumping is about $50 and is also available as sterile versions for immediate use in NICUs that use Ardo pumps. To find a rental station, contact Ardo or a hospital or local lactation consultant. Visit www.ardo-usa.com or call 1-844-411-ARDO (2736).

Multiuser Loaner Pumps Through the WIC Program

Women, Infants, and Children (WIC) programs across the U.S. often have breast pump loaner programs for participant mothers who require one because of separations from their babies due to work or school commitments or babies that are not feeding well from the breast.

Medela Lactina and Lactina Select pumps. Weighing just 4 pounds, these external-piston pumps are capable of strong suction. The Lactina Select has a variable speed control, which many mothers prefer. These pumps are no longer manufactured by Medela but many WIC agencies that work with low-income mothers may still have the pump available as a loaner.

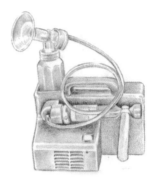

Medela Lactina Pump

Hygeia EnDeare Pump. The EnDeare, a lightweight, external-piston pump, is identical to Medela's Lactina Select. EnDeare pumps also have variable speed control that reaches up to 60 cycles per minute and suction levels of 250 millimeters of mercury. There are separate dials for selecting both suction strength and pumping speed. This pump is almost exclusively available as a loaner pump through some WIC agencies.

Clinical-Grade, Multiuser Double Electric Breast Pumps for Purchase

These "clinical-grade" multiuser pumps are typically higher quality pumps than most "personal-use" double electric pumps. This category of pumps may be of interest to mothers who want or need a high-quality pump of their own or would like to share a pump with another mother. It also could be an economical choice to purchase a great pump and use it with any subsequent babies. When comparing the price of a very nice pump with that of infant formula, a year of formula feeding is estimated to be between $1,200 and $1,500—three to four times the price of the very best pumps on the market today!

Some mothers decide to exclusively pump and bottle feed, including a newborn having problems latching on to the breast. In that case, purchasing a higher-quality pump might be worthwhile.

These pumps may also work well for mothers who would like to share a pump with friends or family members, and are thus considered "multiuser" pumps. Other mothers may simply want to own one of the best pumps on the market!

The pumps in this category need to be very durable to withstand the demands of multiple users or the test of time.

When sharing a pump, keep in mind that there may be bad feelings if the pump breaks down and leaves one of the users empty handed. The following pumps are true multiuser pumps but mothers must still purchase their own personal use kit.

ARDO Calypso Pro. This small, 1-pound, near silent multiuser breast pump is a Swiss-made model from ARDO designed for some loaner and rental programs. ARDO pumps are the quietest on the market. Mothers can purchase this pump for $499, which includes an eighteen-month warranty. Visit www.ardo-usa.com or call 1-844-411-ARDO (2736).

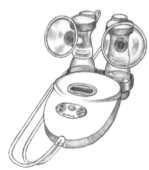

Ardo Calypso Pro

Unimom Opera Pump. Relatively new to the market, Opera is a small, lightweight, quiet, multiuser clinical-grade pump powered by two motors. The pump has high vacuum capability and includes massage and expression phases. What is unique is that, because of the two motors, the vacuum strength and cycle speeds can be adjusted manually and for either breast, enabling a more personalized experience. Another exclusive part of Opera is the four modes that enable mothers to experience sucking patterns that mimic a nursing infant.

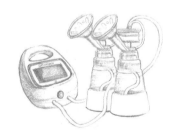

Unimom Opera Pump

This pump gives mothers a choice between alternating or synchronized pumping and the ability to create and save custom settings for future use. Opera has an LCD touch screen, a rechargeable battery, and a nightlight with three levels of brightness. Flange sizes include 24 and 28 millimeters with sizes 20 and 32 millimeters available for purchase separately. A USB port with a cable for connecting to a power source is standard with all Unimom models. This pump costs $599 with a full three-year warranty. To find Opera, contact Unimom at 954-858-5588.

Melodi One Advanced Pump. The Melodi is an ultra-small, well-built, double electric model resembling a thick cell phone. This multiuser pump is very different from most other pumps. Instead of a speed control, it has a pattern of sucking six times in a row with a long pause, mimicking a baby's sucking and resting pattern. The pump suction levels reach a

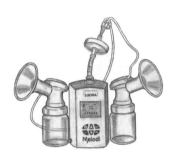

Melodi One Advanced Pump

strong 250 millimeters of mercury. While there is a standard flange size that will fit most mothers, the company also offers larger sizes, as well as silicone inserts. In addition to being a closed system, the Melodi also has a hydrophobic filter to prevent airborne viruses and bacteria from entering the pump. The pump runs with AC power and an internal battery holds a charge for up to six running hours. This pump includes a Shabbat mode and is available through some rental stations. Very few insurance carriers cover the purchase of clinical-grade pumps, but as of this writing, some insurances may offer the Melodi One with a prescription from a doctor for mothers with sick or premature babies or those newborns with certain feeding problems. This pump comes with a one-year warranty. The pump is sold by Lucina Care for $399, and their customer service can be reached at 888-809-9750.

Limerick "Joy" and "PJ's Comfort" Pumps. These Limerick pumps are lightweight, 1.5-pound multiuser pumps that share the same expression method—compression and vacuum, instead of pull and release present on every other pump on the market today. Some mothers find this sucking pattern uncomfortable.

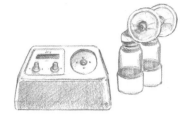

Limerick Joy

The Joy has a digital display and affirmations to encourage mothers as they pump. There is also a "favorite settings" option. Both the Joy and PJ's Comfort have timers, as well.

Limerick pumps are not closed system pumps. Because it is possible to get condensation in the tubing and filter of the pump, there is a mode that allows the pump to run for ten minutes to clear out moisture and lessen the possibility of growing mold.

These pumps are warrantied for three years. Joy ranges in price from $600 to $850, depending on the accessory package. PJ's Comfort ranges in price from $450 to $600, depending on the accessories included. Some insurances may cover the cost of Limerick pumps.

Visit www.limerickinc.com or call 818-566-3060.

Personal Use Double Electric Pumps

The number of available models of personal use, fully automatic double electric pumps, either purchased by mothers or received through insurance, are now at an all-time high. In recent years, more and more breastfeeding mothers consider a pump as a necessity, regardless of whether they are returning to school or the workplace.

Many of these pumps, or downsized versions, are offered by insurance carriers through the Affordable Care Act (see page 246 for information on getting a pump through the Affordable Care Act).

Some of the pumps in this category are quiet, some are quite loud. Most all of them are closed system models. A closed system pump is one that does not allow condensation or milk to enter into the tubing or into the pump motor. Personal use pumps are not intended for sharing, even with a new kit. (See page 280 for multiuser pumps for purchase.) They should also come with flanges that will fit your nipple or offer other size flanges that are available. See more on getting the right size flange in earlier in this chapter.

Other important features include vacuum levels and cycles per minute. Breast pumps with a low vacuum may not do a good job of draining the breast and, depending on how often a mother uses a pump, can lead to overall low milk production. Most pumps offer two phases of cycling: an initial rapid, shallow sucking pattern and then a slower, deeper one. Ideally, vacuums should reach at least 240 millimeters of mercury during the slower expression phase.

If your insurance covers the cost of a breast pump, find out from them which Durable Medical Equipment (DME) providers they work with. Next, contact each DME to find out which pumps they offer. Then, learn more out about each of these pumps by reading the descriptions and reviews of each one offered to you before ordering a pump.

Some of the pumps you may be interested in could have helpful YouTube videos explaining the pros and cons of each model. Since breast pumps cannot be returned if the box has been opened, it is important to be 100 percent sure which model you want to purchase. These videos can be very insightful.

If you will be purchasing a breast pump yourself, you can probably find it for much less if you compare prices online. Even very expensive models can often be found for much less on Amazon.com or other sites such as Target.com or Walmart.com. If you have coupons for any discount stores, you may even be able to save more.

ARDO Calypso Breast Pump. Ardo Calypso looks just like the Ardo Calypso Pro, but this Swiss manufactured pump is one of Ardo's personal-use models. Ardo pumps are known for being the quietest pumps on the market, and similar to other Ardo electric pumps, Calypso allows for independent vacuum and cycle adjustments with up to sixty-four possible settings.

This pumps weighs in at just one pound, but depending on the package, it may come with accessories, including a breastfeeding bag and several flange sizes. The soft "Optiflow" inserts (26 millimeters) actively massage the breast and ensure efficient and gentle expression

There is no single pump that is perfect for every mother, even if the pump is from a popular brand. Keep in mind that insurances will generally only cover one pump every two to three years or, in many cases, just one pump for each baby. If you will be purchasing a pump instead of receiving one through your insurance, you may be able to use your HSA or FSA funds. Deciding what kind of pump is best for you depends on many factors:

- **How often do anticipate using a pump?** Pumping just a few times a week or only on occasion means you may not necessarily benefit from a pricey model. And the opposite may also be the case: A rental-grade or multiuser pump is recommended for mothers who are dependent upon a pump for full-time or near full-time pumping—especially during the early weeks after giving birth.

- **Are you pumping for a newborn or a baby with medical issues or hospitalization?** Using a multiuser/rental pump, even just temporarily, may be critical in both bringing in and maintaining a healthy milk supply.

- **Will you exclusively pump to provide milk for your baby, rather than directly nursing?** Having a sturdy, dependable model is recommended to have an abundant milk supply.

- **Will your medical insurance cover the purchase of the pump you are interested in or will you need to purchase it yourself?**

- **Do you need a pump that does not require an electrical outlet?** If so, consider a pump that is battery operated or, better yet, has a rechargeable battery.

- **Would you benefit from a hands-free "wearable" pump?** If you prefer to be mobile while you express milk, the extra expense of these models may be worth the investment.

- **Does the pump kit have just one standard flange size or are other sizes available?** There is no one size that fits every mother.

- **Do you need a quiet pump for more discrete use?**

for mothers with smaller size nipples. Calypso works on AC power or AA batteries and comes with either a 400-hour warranty or a one-year warranty, whichever is better for the mother. This pump retails between $150 and $200. Visit www.ardo-usa.com or call 1-844-411-ARDO (2736) for more information.

ARDO Alyssa Pump. This small double electric pump offers a digital screen with several phases of both pumping and pauses with strong vacuum capability. As with all other ARDO pumps, this model is nearly silent. Alyssa includes a rechargeable battery and costs $249, including a one-year warranty. Visit www.ardo-usa. com or call 1-844-411-ARDO (2736).

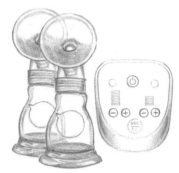
ARDO Alyssa Pump

Medela Pump in Style Max Flow. One of Medela's newest pump offerings, this lightweight model has strong vacuum with "micro vibrations" that assist in increasing milk flow. Additionally, the new "PersonalFit Flex" oval-shaped flanges have a soft, comfortable outer rim, which gently compresses the breast and can be rotated to the best position that helps milk flow. These flanges retail for $18.99, as they are a supplement to the two sets of flanges that come with the pump—sizes 21 and 24 millimeters. Pump In Style Max Flow runs on AC power or AA batteries.

There are only four buttons on the motor which makes use easy, and the pump automatically changes from "stimulation" to "expression mode" at two minutes. However, the pump lacks any further customization, including setting up speed settings.

This model also comes with a new pump connector, which covers the top of the five-ounce bottle, meaning milk can leak out if the bottle is overfilled or if mothers don't sit up straight while pumping. Using larger bottles

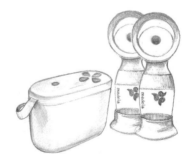
Medela Pump in Style Max Flow

can help eliminate this problem. The bottle and connector piece are also top heavy, so it is quite possible milk will spill out if these pieces fall over. Therefore, when pumping is over, it is recommended to place the bottles and connectors in the holders that come with the pump.

Some versions of this pump include a nice bag with a separate cooler case and re-freezable blocks to keep milk cool; however, there is no LCD screen, timer, or memory feature on the pump. Lastly, the pump is pretty loud and gets even louder when the vacuum is increased, in addition to an intermittent "knocking" sound.

While the warranty on this pump motor is one year, the estimated lifespan for the model is about 45 minutes per day for one year. The "MyMedela" app helps keep track of pumping sessions and other infant information. The price of Max Flow is $249.99, though it may be offered through some insurance plans.

Medela Sonata. This $400 pump from Medela is intended for mothers who pump on a daily or near daily basis. It is fairly large and weighs two and a half pounds, though it does have a handle to help move it around.

Sonata includes an AC power cord and a rechargeable lithium-ion battery that allows for one hour of pumping time. Also included is a nice tote, a cooler bag, and an ice pack.

The LCD screen on the pump's face is somewhat blurry and may be a bit hard to read. In addition to a count-down timer and a "pause and resume" button, there is also an "air leak alert," which will appear if the pump is not correctly assembled. While the pump starts out in the rapid stimulation phase, it automatically changes into

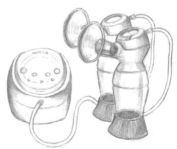

Medela Sonata

the slower, deeper expression mode at two minutes or sooner if the expression button is pressed. There is also a "mute" button, though it doesn't seem to lower the noise of this already fairly quiet pump.

Like other Medela pump models, Sonata is compatible with the soft-rimmed, oval-shaped "PersonalFit Flex Flanges" (see page 286). Otherwise, two flange sizes—21 and 24 millimeters—are included. Additional sizes for mothers with larger nipples can be purchased separately.

Once the milk lets down and is flowing well, mothers are offered a choice of two rhythm options: "Signature" and "Lifestyle." The Signature mode is supposedly similar to the Symphony model's sucking pattern. The LifeStyle mode makes the pump quieter with a slower drain of the battery. Mothers report that they do not notice much difference between these two rhythm choices. Sonata reaches high vacuum levels and some mothers complain of an uncomfortable mechanical pull that is long and drawn out.

The Sonata comes with a new connector piece, which has similar issues to those written about in the Pump in Style Max Flow review (see page 286).

Sonata also connects to the "MyMedela" app to easily track of pumping sessions and other infant information. While this pump is expensive, there is lower pricing at third-party online stores. The warranty is for one year on the motor.

Medela Freestyle Flex. Medela's Freestyle Flex model replaces the original Freestyle model and is an expensive, ultra-small pump, weighing less than a pound. Featuring two sets of Medela's new "PersonalFit Flex" flanges (see page 286)—sizes 21 and 24 millimeters—mothers will be able to pump nearly 12 percent more milk, according to the company. A USB charging cord is included with the pump, which is powered by a built-in rechargeable battery which holds a two-hour charge. The suggested

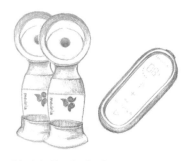

Medela FreeStyle Flex

lifespan of this pump is only 250 hours, which could come quickly for mothers who exclusively pump. Included also is a very nice travel bag with a milk cooler pouch and ice pack.

Freestyle has a simple touch screen which lights up and displays the battery charge. Touch areas on the screen also allow mothers to choose the modes for stimulation and expression, in addition to the new "pause" option, which can come in handy when a mother needs to briefly interrupt pumping. Freestyle starts out with a ten second start delay, which is helpful for the few moments it takes to adjust the flanges on the breast.

On the downside, the flexible membrane that is used in the pump is fragile and may need to be replaced often, depending how often the pump is used. And this pump is not leakproof. Should a mother lean sideways or forward, milk can spill from the large connector piece which has a slit on the side. The connector also presents similar issues to those described in the Pump in Style Max Flow review on page 286.

Whenever the pump is not attached to the breast, Freestyle is somewhat noisy, but it quickly gets quieter once the flanges are put in place. And the pump itself vibrates quite a bit and can actually "travel" on a hard surface, such as a table top. This pump, which connects to the "MyMedela" app (see page 287), includes a one-year warranty on the motor and retails for $379.99.

Medela Swing Maxi Double Electric Pump. This small, portable pump is operable either by rechargeable battery or by electricity from a wall socket or USB port. Designed for either single or double pumping, the Swing Maxi has slower cycling and stronger suction for expression—just like other Medela models. The adjustable suction reaches high levels, and there are nine pre-programed settings that mothers can choose from for optimal milk output. Unfortunately, this pump is loud and increases in noise as the vacuum is turned higher.

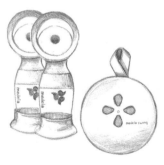

The flanges on Swing Maxi are small—21 and 24 millimeters—but

Medela Swing Maxi Double Electric Pump

they are the new "flex" flanges which may help mothers pump more milk (see description on page 286). Other size flanges can be ordered separately.

Like other Medela models, this one also includes the new connector piece, which may occlude the top portion of the collection bottle. See issues on page 286. Also included is small draw string bag to use as a carry case.

This model connects to the Medela "Family App" (see page 287) and retails for $279.00.

Ameda's Mya Joy. This ultra-small, quiet pump with an LCD screen has two phases of sucking, including both stimulation and expression modes, along with lots of settings for speed and vacuum. The pump goes into the expression phase whenever it reaches two minutes of pumping or sooner when the mode button is pushed. Mya Joy has strong suction, reaching up to 240 millimeters of mercury. Powered by AA batteries, Mya Joy also includes

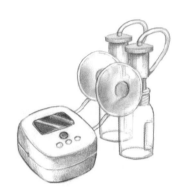

Ameda's Mya Joy

three sets of flanges (25, 28.5, and 30.5 millimeters). Two unique features include a built-in clip which allows the pump to attach onto clothing and the ability to convert into a hand pump. Mya Joy comes with a two-year warranty is priced around $145.00. The Ameda Mya Joy Plus, which sells for $159.99, includes a rechargeable battery, a USB-C charging cord, and a lanyard for "wearing" the pump. Call Ameda customer care at 1-866-992-6332 or visit www. ameda.com.

Unimom Minuet Double Electric Breast Pump. This multiuser, ultra-small, quiet pump resembles a

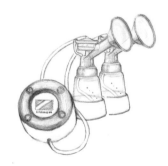

Unimom Minuet Double Electric Breast Pump

cupcake. Minuet is a closed system pump with an LCD display. The Minuet has several modes of milk stimulation and expression. There are also two patterns of pauses that mimics the way a real baby feeds.

Minuet has a rechargeable battery, and a ninety-minute charge via the USB port and standard cable allows for two and a half hours of pumping time. Flange sizes 24 and 28 millimeters are included with the pump and sizes 20 and 32 millimeters are available separately for purchase. This pump is nearly silent, and another plus is the included lanyard, which helps turn this pump into a near hands-free portable model when used with a pumping bra. Minuet has a two-year warranty and sells for $189. Reach Unimom by phone at 954-858-5588.

Hygeia Evolve. The newest pump offering from Hygeia, this double electric model reaches strong vacuum levels and is both quiet and effective. Separate speed and vacuum controls can be adjusted independently and the pump includes a rechargeable battery for pumping without an electrical outlet. The only flange included with this pump is size 28, which will be too large for mothers with small nipples. More flange sizes are available for an additional $12.99. This lightweight pump is available through some insurance providers or online for $199.99. Contact Hygeia at 714-515-7571.

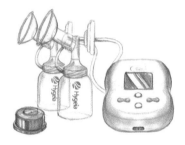

Hygeia Evolve

Spectra S1 Plus and S2 Pumps. Spectra has certainly become one of the most popular pump companies in the U.S.—especially with its two best-selling models, the Spectra S1 and S2. The Spectra S1 not only plugs into a wall socket, but also has an internal rechargeable battery that will hold a charge for up to three hours. These pumps tend to be on the loud side,

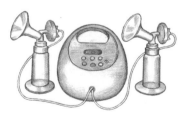

Spectra S1 Plus and S2 Pumps

especially with increasing vacuum levels, but placing them on carpeting or a towel helps. Both models have an LCD display to show timing, suction, and speed. The handle lights up for nighttime pumping and one bottle can be nestled into a holder on the back of the motor.

Contact Spectra

S1 and S2, 9+, Synergy Gold (S-G), Cara Cups

1-855-405-0993 or **855-44-MOMBABY**

www.spectrababyusa.com

Spectra pumps offer unique sucking patterns, but there is a definite learning curve. For example, these pumps start out in the expression phase of longer, slower pumping—which is the opposite of most every other pump on the market, as well as actual nursing babies. And since the pump begins on the same vacuum level the previous pumping session ended on, mothers could be off to an uncomfortable start if the pump starts on a high vacuum level. There are ten settings for suction levels and the speed/cycling rates are between 38 to 70 times per minute. The pump automatically shuts off at thirty minutes.

Two pairs of flanges, sizes 24 and 28 millimeters, come with the pump, as do soft silicone "massagers" that work with the flanges. Purchasing other size flanges (20 and 32 millimeters) will cost $12.99 apiece and the massagers for those cost an additional $9.99 each. A new addition to the popular Spectra pumps, "Cara Cups" can be purchased separately for hands-free pumping. See page 308 for more. A car adapter can also be purchased for $8.99.

The S1 pump retails for $200 and the Spectra S2 for $159. Both are covered by a two-year warranty.

Spectra Synergy Gold (S-G). This large, heavy multiuser pump from Spectra has a sleek new design, including a touch screen. The main selling point for this pump is the two motors that allow for independent vacuum

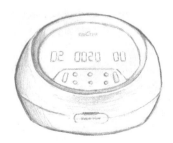

Spectra Synergy Gold (S-G)

and cycling settings for each breast. Otherwise, for a retail price of $325, there are really no other reasons that this pump is a better choice over the Spectra S1 or S2. The S-G must be used with a wall adapter and comes with both size 24 and size 28 flanges.

The suction reaches a strong 280 millimeters in the expression mode. The pump sounds like a purring cat that does get quite a bit louder as the vacuum increases, though there is a "mute" button to help quiet the sound. Like the S1 and S2 models, the last vacuum setting used on this pump will automatically be the first setting when pumping the next time. Spectra S-G comes with a two-year warranty.

Spectra 9+ Pump. Weighing less than 1 pound, this model offers multiple pumping speeds of up to 60 cycles per minute. The pump works on AC power or rechargeable battery. Some mothers say that their milk supply declined with the frequent use of this pump. Spectra technical staff suggest that mothers

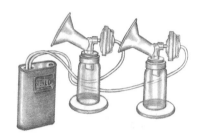

Spectra 9+ Pump

who require a pump for regular or frequent pumping select another pump like the Spectra S1 or S2. The price of this pump is about $180.

Pumpables "SuperGenie" Hospital Grade Breast Pump. This company has come out with three pumps, but this is their high-end model. While the term "hospital grade" technically refers to having a three-prong plug, this pump does not have one. Instead, it has a rechargeable battery or works with an included USB charger. The battery life is nearly three hours and one charge takes about four hours to complete.

The vacuum for SuperGenie reaches up to a very strong 330 millimeters of mercury with variable cycles per minute. Mothers should start on a very low suction rate and then increase it to whatever feels most comfortable. The best part of this pump may be that it is totally programmable, including through an optional app, which is great for mothers who prefer certain cycle settings or suction levels. Some mothers like that they can also program pauses to then start a second pumping session, attempting to stimulate another letdown. There is also a "pause" button if the mother needs to briefly stop pumping.

Perhaps the next best part of this pump is the "liquid shield" flange system for incredibly comfortable pumping sessions. They can be ordered in sizes 17, 21, 25, and 29 millimeters.

SuperGenie has a moveable handle with a light for nighttime pumping, though the pump does emit a loud groaning sound. Weighing two and a half pounds, this pump can be ordered on www.pumpables.co for $249. Two other models include the "Genie Advanced" and the "Genie Plus," which each cost $150.

Lansinoh Signature Pro. This pump has been around for quite some time and has both stimulation and expression modes, as most other pumps do. The Lansinoh pump also offers three pumping patterns, as well as adjustable suction levels that reach a strong 280 millimeters of mercury. The pump can run on either AC power

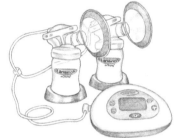

Lansinoh Signature Pro

or with AA batteries and has an LED display for timing and setting speeds, patterns, and suction levels. Lansinoh pumps are loud.

Signature Pro comes with just one set of size 25 millimeter "Comfort Fit" pump flanges, which have a soft outer rim that may provide more comfort and form a secure seal. Many mothers will need other sizes to fit their nipples more comfortably and for optimal milk flow. Sizes 21, 30.5, and 36 millimeters can be purchased for about $10 per set. The third-party company Nenesupply offers 17-, 19-, 24-, and 28-millimeter flanges that will also fit this model, but they do not have the soft outer rim. (See Appendix A.) The bottles used with this pump are specific only to the Lansinoh brand, but you can also pump directly into Lansinoh bags.

Lansinoh does not sell pumps or accessories on their website or by phone. Retailers include Walmart, Target, and Amazon. Signature Pro and the Lansinoh "Smart" Pump (see below) can be ordered through some insurance plans. If you want to try and get this pump through your insurance, go to Lansinoh.com and click on "Free Breast Pump" and follow the prompts. This pump, which comes with a tote bag, is priced at a very reasonable $86. The pump motor is warrantied for one year; parts are warrantied for 90 days. Reach customer service at 800-292-4794 or www.lansinoh.com.

Lansinoh Smart Pump 2.0. This model has a new look, including an updated pump body with a carrying handle. It has very strong suction capability of 280 millimeters of mercury and there is also a battery option. This lightweight model is also loud. The purchase also includes a tote bag, a cooler, and an ice pack.

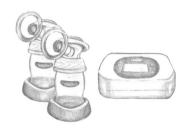

Lansinoh Smart Pump 2.0

The pump comes with only two flanges (sizes 25 and 30.5 millimeters), which may not fit all mothers. Additional sizes (21 and 36 millimeters) can be purchased for about $10 per set. Mothers with Smart 2.0 can download the Lansinoh 2.0 app via Bluetooth to automatically track pumping sessions and other details about your baby. The motor for this pump, which costs $159.99, is warrantied for 12 months. See the Signature Pro review for details about pumping into bottles vs. bags, retailer options, and steps for securing a pump through your insurance. Visit www.lansinoh.com or call 800-292-4794.

Evenflo Advanced Double Electric Pump. This pump offers four speeds and eight suction levels, and with this new version, the suction reaches strong levels of 240 millimeters of mercury. This model can run pretty much anywhere—on AC power, with AA batteries, or with a car adapter (sold separately). On the downside, there is no screen to easily time sessions and it is loud. Because this pump does not automatically switch over from the

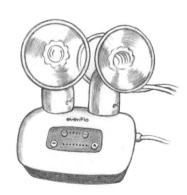

Evenflo Advanced Double Electric Pump

stimulation mode to the expression mode, it needs to be done manually when the milk begins flowing.

The pump comes with two hard flanges size 30.5 millimeters and two pairs of silicone inserts (sizes 25.5 and 28 millimeters). Additional sizes (21, 30.5, 33, and 36 millimeters) are sold separately. Unfortunately, the suction decreases quite a bit when using the soft inserts, making the pump less effective. Evenflo has designed the pump so that mothers can comfortably sit back to pump without spilling milk. However, some mothers have reported that milk can get into the tubing, which means this is not a closed system pump. If the tubings are not quickly cleaned out, mold can grow in the tubes and motor. The pump costs about $99 and is available through big-box stores, online, and many insurance plans. A "Deluxe" model ($140) comes with additional items, including a shoulder bag and a smaller milk cooler bag.

These pumps come with a three-year warranty but only after registering them with Evenflo. Customer service can be reached at 855-334-2229.

The First Years Quiet Expressions Double Breast Pump. This inexpensive pump ($66) has only one speed and eight suction levels, reaching a very weak 180 millimeters of mercury. It works on both AC power and AA batteries. Some mothers complain that the stiff silicone flanges are uncomfortable and difficult to position with the unusual "handlebar" that holds the flanges and bottles together for one-handed pumping. Visit www.thefirstyears.com or call 800-704-8697.

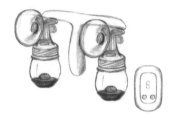

The First Years Quiet Expressions Double Breast Pump

Philips Avent Double Electric Breast Pump. This lightweight pump offers two phases: a lighter, quicker pattern for stimulating milk letdown and a slower, deeper one for milk expression. The pump offers three suction levels, with the highest reaching a strong 240 millimeters of mercury. There is also a timer as well as a "pause" button to allow for mothers to walk away and return without needing to enter their pump settings again.

This new model is fairly quiet and has both a USB adapter and a rechargeable battery option. When the pump is fully charged, mothers can pump for about three sessions. Included is a unique "pumping belt," which allows mothers to have mobility when the battery is charged. Pumping bras typically don't work with this model unless the opening of the bra

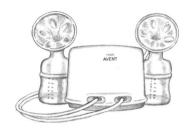

Philips Avent Double Electric Breast Pump

is very large. Mothers might consider using "milk cups" (see page 308) with this pump to make it more hands-free and portable.

While the pump includes a nice carrying bag, it only comes with two bottles, and bottles from other companies do not fit. Also included are a set of hard flanges and a pair of 25 millimeter soft silicone inserts that will adapt to most nipple sizes. Smaller 19.5 millimeters soft inserts are also available for $10.95 per pair. The pump is $269.95 and comes with a 24-month warranty (30 months, if registered with the company). For more information, call 800- 54-AVENT or visit www.philips.com.

Rumble Tuff Breeze. This is one of seven electric pumps available through the company. Breeze is a quiet model with strong suction. The pump has a built-in rechargeable battery and records and recalls pumping prefer-ences. A timer lets you know how long you have been pumping. Breeze costs $159 and the motor is warrantied for

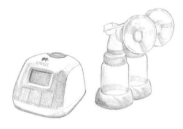

Rumble Tuff Breeze

two years. Rumble Tuff pumps are sold through the company, online, and through some insurance plans. Breeze can also be turned into a manual pump. Contact Rumble Tuff at 1-855-228-8388.

Rumble Tuff Whisper Electric Breast Pump Duo. Another quiet breast pump from Rumble Tuff is the "Whisper" double electric breast pump. This pump offers a selection of stimulation phases that initiate milk letdown, after which there are several other vacuum levels—including those that are very high—to choose from to help empty the breast. However, there is a rather annoying beep after each pull. The standard hard plastic flange size is a very large 28 millimeters, though soft inserts decrease the size to 25 millimeters. This model also turns into a hand pump and comes with a two-year warranty. Whisper can be purchased through Rumble Tuff for $84.99 or received through some insurance plans. Contact Rumble Tuff at 1-855-228-8388.

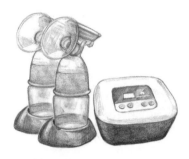

Rumble Tuff Whisper Electric Breast Pump Duo

Tommee Tippee "Made for Me" Double Electric Breast Pump. Like most other pumps, this small, quiet British model has two-phase technology, offering both stimulation and expression modes. Unfortunately, this pump reaches unnecessary high vacuum levels of 350 millimeters of mercury, nearly twice the usual, which could easily cause painful nipples. Mothers who have this pump will want to start out pumping on the lowest vacuum levels and then turn up the suction slowly until the best level is reached. The pump offers five levels of suction. The one flange size, 27 millimeters, will fit many but not all mothers. The model is USB rechargeable and comes with soft cushioned inserts and two bottles—other bottles will not work with this model. "Made for Me" comes with a one-year warranty, two if the pump is registered with the company, and retails for $159.99 (lower at big box stores and Amazon). Visit www.tommeetippee.com.

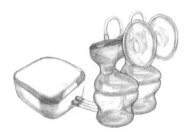

Tommee Tippee "Made for Me" Double Electric Breast Pump

Unimom Zomee 1 and 2. These Zomee double electric breast pumps are small, lightweight, quiet breast pumps that include a durable lithium rechargeable battery providing more than two hours of pumping time. Two flange sizes (24 and 28 millimeters) come with the pump, though 20- and 32- millimeter shields are available separately through Unimom. These

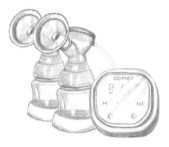

Unimom Zomee 1 and 2

flexible shields not only make pumping more comfortable but may also make pumping a bit quicker. A USB port with a cable for connecting to a power source is standard with all Unimom pumps, which is useful both at home or when traveling.

Zomee 2 features an LCD screen, a nightlight, three different suction patterns, and nearly twenty suction levels. Zomee 1 offers a one-year warranty and is priced at $159 while Zomee 2 includes a two-year warranty and costs $189. Visit www.zomee.com or call 954-858-5588.

Dr. Brown "CustomFlow" Double Electric Breast Pump. This 2-pound pump from Dr. Brown, maker of the popular feeding bottles, features a two-phase pattern for stimulation and expression. One of the best parts of this pump may be the large, lightweight, motor body, which includes an LCD screen display, a grip for carrying the pump, and three silicone stretch storage areas along its sides—great for holding pumping bottles, breast pads, or even a cellphone.

The flanges are stiff silicone, which may not feel comfortable when coupled with the very strong suction of this pump. Mothers should begin pumping on the lowest vacuum level to avoid a painful start to their pumping session. While the website says that flanges that are included with the pump are size "B" or about 25 millimeters, they are actually much, much larger—possibly too large for most mothers. You can order smaller size "A" flanges for $9.99 a pair, or consider ordering "Beaugen" breast pump cushions (see page 257) to get a better fit.

This pump is loud, perhaps in part because of the strong vibrations when the pump is placed on a hard surface. The pump includes four of the popular Dr. Brown bottles and retails for $159.99, including a one-year warranty after registering the pump with the company. Also available for purchase are a rechargeable battery pack ($29.99), a car adapter ($24.99), and a pumping bra in black or beige ($29.99). Excellent customer service can be reached at 800-778-9001 or www. drbrownsbaby.com.

Motif Duo. This pump is also an ultra-small, closed system pump. Duo comes with an AC adapter and also works with rechargeable battery. Included are three different flange sizes—21, 24, and 27 millimeters—that will fit most every mother. Size 32 millimeter flanges are available separately for purchase.

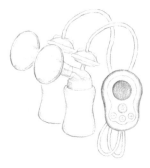
Motif Duo

Duo also has an LCD screen with a timer. There is a bit of a learning curve setting up and managing the features of the pump, but it does include a memory feature. Unfortunately, the pump's vacuum is very weak unless only one breast is being pumped at a time. The membrane and the stem of the backflow protector is fragile and must be handled with care. Duo, priced at $200, may be covered by some insurance plans and is warrantied for twelve months.

Motif Luna. Luna is sleek, attractive, lightweight, double electric pump which has become a favorite of mothers. This model with two-phase technology works off of AC power and the newer version includes a rechargeable battery that lasts for up to two hours of pumping time. The vacuum on this model is low, but the suction has an increased number of cycles per minute as well as "micro" pulsations or vibrations, the sounds of which can certainly be heard while pumping. Perhaps these vibrations may be part of the reason this pump is so effective.

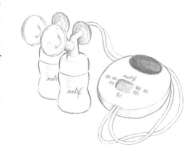
Motif Luna

The pump can also be customized for independent cycling on each breast. This feature is really only beneficial if a mother requires a different suction or speed levels on either breast. As of this writing, only a handful of other pumps—including Unimom Opera and Spectra Synergy Gold (S-G)—offers this option and most of these are more expensive. Luna also has a memory feature for mothers who have certain preferred settings and automatically shuts off after thirty minutes.

Contact Motif

Duo, Luna, Twist

1-844-272-8390

www.motifmedical.com

An LED screen and a backlight may allow for easier pumping during the night. The collection kit includes two flange sizes—24 and 28 millimeters—that will accommodate most nipple sizes. Other flange sizes—21 and 32 millimeters—are available separately for $13.99 per pair.

Luna costs $259 for the standard model and $299 for the version with the rechargeable battery. Both models include a one-year warranty. Luna is available through some insurance providers as well as online sellers, often at a lower price.

Motif Twist. This small, 1-pound pump is powered by either AC power, via the included USB cord, or AA batteries, which allow up to four hours of pumping time. Twist, unlike other Motif models, has strong suction capability. It includes three flange sizes—24, 28, and 32 millimeters—that will accommodate most mothers'

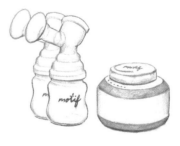

Motif Twist

needs. This model, which is loud, costs about $120 and is warrantied for 12 months. Twist is available through some insurance providers and online vendors.

BabyBuddha. Another ultra-small, portable double electric pump known for its very strong suction is the BabyBuddha. The suction capability is so strong, well over 310 millimeters of mercury, it could easily cause painful pumping or even bruising to a mother's nipples if the vacuum is close to or at its highest level. (Typical strong suction is usually 240 millimeters of mercury.) The suction on this pump also has a long pull, which may be too intense for some mothers. It is important that mothers who have this pump start pumping on the lowest settings and increase the vacuum slowly. A tiny rollerball is used to change the vacuum settings while the time lapsed is displayed on the motor. BabyBuddha has five stimulation and nine expression modes for more customized pumping sessions, though, like many small pumps, this one is loud.

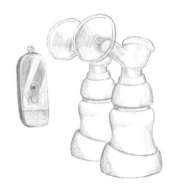

BabyBuddha

The pump comes with a long USB charge cord. Once the battery is fully charged, about four hours, the pump will allow for about four to six 15-minute sessions. Buddha comes with a set of size 24-millimeter flanges. Other styles and sizes of flanges, including 21, 24, 28, and 32 millimeters, are also sold for $19.99.

Unlike most every other small portable pump on the market, a lanyard is included that allows a mother to wear the pump around her neck. When used with a pumping bra, or with milk cups, this pump allows for near complete mobility.

Buddha can only be purchased at www.babybuddhaproducts.com, which also has a guide to determining the best flange size. The pump is normally $299 but is often on sale. BabyBuddha comes with a two year or 800 to 1000 hour warranty, whichever comes first and only for the original owner. You can contact BabyBuddha on their website or at 201-500-9745.

LactaMed breast pump lanyard. This lanyard clips to an included connector piece, which attaches to the top of almost any portable pump that weighs up to 2 pounds. It costs $8.99 and can be ordered through LactaMed.com or by phone at 1-866-322-2471.

Wearable Breast Pumps

The newest category of pumps is known as "wearable" pumps. Arguably, most any small, portable pump can be considered wearable with the use of a pumping bra and lanyard, belt, or clip, but as of this writing, there are really only a handful of pumps that are truly hands-free. These self-contained pumps fit into any bra and pump on their own without limiting cords and/or tubing and allow for complete mobility.

The first wearable pump models were the "Elvie" from the United Kingdom and the "Willow" from California. A second model from Elvie, the Elvie "Stride," followed. These pumps are used with an app that allows for the functioning of the motor and settings. Each one of the wearable pumps has different pros and cons.

Freemie Independence II and Liberty II Pumps. Perhaps the very earliest "near wearable" model was the Freemie pump, invented by a physician who needed something portable in her work environment. Now we have two updated Freemie models.

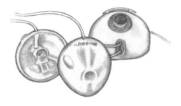

Freemie Independence II and Liberty II Pumps

This very small, portable pump comes with milk "cups" instead of flanges and bottles. Cups make it a bit easier to pump discreetly, compared to pumping using a standard setup—although the cups do protrude forward quite a bit. The cups are centered over each nipple and are held in place by almost any roomy bra. Tubings go from the milk cups into the small pump motor, which can be clipped onto clothing, providing a near "hands-free" experience. This pump and cup system is far cheaper than the other wearable brands, such as Willow and Elvie.

Many mothers report that they like the feel of the cups compared to typical pump flanges. And each cup can hold a whopping 8 ounces of milk! On the other hand, some mothers complain that, because the cups are opaque, it can be hard to center the nipples or see how much milk is being pumped. Mothers with very large breasts may have difficulty using this pump system. It is also possible to spill milk during pumping if the pour holes are not centered at the top of the breast, or if the mother is in any position in which the cups are level with or below the pour holes, such as bending over.

The milk cups can be ordered in one of two sizes, depending on nipple width. The two cup sizes—25 and 28 millimeters—that come with both Liberty II and Independence II Deluxe are suitable for small and medium-size nipples. Independence II Standard only includes the 25-millimeter flanges. Additionally, several optional inserts, known as "fitmies," are available. These inserts, which can be purchased for $22.99, come in sizes 15, 16, 17, 18, 19, 20, 21, 22, 23, 24, 25, and 26. The milk cups can also be ordered separately for $90 or less, along with a conversion kit to be used with some Spectra, Medela, Philips Avent, Melodi Prime, and Ardo Calypso pumps. However, using the cups with other pumps may very well lower the suction levels.

Unfortunately, and perhaps most importantly, the vacuum on Independence II and Liberty II is quite low unless it is used with typical flange and bottle or, interestingly, with other cup brands such as Spectra and Legendairy cups. See pages 308 to 309. There is also some difficulty connecting the tubes to the pump. Also note that the assembly order does affect the cups' suction—always place the barriers onto the flange backs first.

Both Freemie models are fairly quiet, have a rechargeable battery, and are warrantied for 12 months. The pump and cups are sold online directly from freemie.com. Liberty II has a small LCD screen and Independence II. The vacuum on both pumps depends on the rate of frequency. Lower speed settings achieve a higher vacuum.

The Liberty II, which has a small LCD screen, sells for $179.99 with size 25 millimeter and 28 millimeter collection cups. The Independence II pump, which features only buttons that input vacuum and speed, includes 25 millimeter collection cups and sells for $139.99. Visit www.freemie.com for more information or call 916-339-7388.

Willow Gen 3 Breast Pump. The Willow pump is one of three truly "wearable" self-contained, cup-style pumps. This pump was first introduced in 2017 and the Gen 3 has some new features. The Willow app, once downloaded to a smartphone, sets up the pump and displays the milk volume, pumping time, and past pumping sessions. The app also has a video with instructions on how to use the model. Mothers simply center the pump cups over the nipples and, when turned on by the Willow app, milk flows into the cups. Willow flanges are transparent, so centering nipples is relatively easy and mothers can also see the milk flowing. If pumping into reusable collection containers, it is possible to spill milk if not sitting upright, but pumping directly into disposable milk bags makes things spillproof.

Like most other pumps, Willow has two-phase technology, the faster stimulation mode, as well as the slower, deeper sucking pattern. The pump senses when the milk lets down and automatically changes into the slower, deeper sucking pattern. In addition, it allows the mother to increase or decrease the suction level throughout the pumping session. This pump is quite loud during the early stimulation mode but gets much quieter during the expression mode once the milk begins flowing.

Mothers need to order a certain size milk cup—either 21, 24, or 27 millimeters, depending on the size of the nipple. It is very important that mothers use Willow's online style guide before ordering the pump. Inserts to improve the fit of the pump cost $19.99 each. This pump cannot be returned if the package is opened.

When the pump is purchased, it includes twenty-four disposable, single-use, plastic milk bags. Additional milk bags in packs of 48 sell for $23.99. There are also spill-proof, reusable collection containers that are not included with the pump and cost an additional $49.99 each. Willow does not sell single pumping cups.

Willow continues to be a work in progress. We struggled with getting the pump to change from the stimulation mode to the expression mode. Happily, that issue was eventually resolved by the Willow staff.

Willow includes a rechargeable battery. The battery will be fully charged for two hours, which allows for about five pumping sessions. The life of this model is about 275 hours of use. Willow costs $499.99 and is available through the Willow website at www.willowpump.com or on Amazon for the same price. If you sign up for the Willow emails, you will see sales quite often. There is also a financing option available. The warranty on the pump is twelve months. Information about getting a Willow pump through insurance can be found on Willow's website.

Reach Willow at www.onewillow.com or by phone at 1-888-WILLOW3. Willow customer service is quite helpful.

Elvie. Another wearable pump, Elvie is from a British company and was the first wearable pump introduced in the U.S. Both lighter and smaller than Willow, the Elvie pump is silent. It comes pre-assembled, which can help mothers learn just how the pump needs to be put together. The Elvie app or buttons on the hub (the motor) are used to work the pump. When downloaded, the app not only allows mothers to have remote control of the pump, but also tracks pumping sessions. A video on the app is also helpful in learning more about the important details of this pump.

Elvie has two phases, both stimulation and expression, with seven variable suction levels. The pump switches from stimulation into expression mode when it detects letdown and pauses when the cup becomes full. Both pumping cups come with rechargeable internal batteries that hold a charge for up to two and a half hours of pumping time or about five pumping sessions from the two USB cables.

Elvie pretty much comes with everything you need, including two sizes of flanges—24 and 28 millimeters. For an additional $29.99, 21-millimeter flanges can be purchased. The pump includes four 5-ounce milk containers, though mothers who want extra containers can purchase two-packs for $34.99.

Some mothers struggle getting a strong enough vacuum, which can occur for a variety of reasons, including low battery or if the pump is pushed into the breast too tightly. For that reason, the pump includes four bra extenders to help create more space. Additionally, lines on the flanges help center the breast and nipples near perfectly for adequate suction. Suction can also be affected if pump parts are not completely clean and dry before assembly or if warping occurs after parts are sanitized. Some mothers complain that this pump leaks.

The "hub" of the pump comes with a two-year warranty while the washable parts have a ninety-day warranty. The purchase price is $499. Elvie offers the option of purchasing just one pumping cup for the price of $279, which may work fine for some mothers. Shipping is free. Visit Elvie at www.elvie.com or call 508-300- 9989.

Elvie Stride. The Stride is the second wearable model from the British company, Elvie. This motor weighs less than 1 pound, is hands-free, and can be controlled remotely by the Elvie app (in addition to using the settings on the pump motor). Worn inside a bra, it connects to the small motor with tubing and allows for complete mobility with the included clothing clip on the motor.

With just four parts, this pump is fairly simple to use. Like most every pump, mothers can double or single pump.

While the Stride is quiet, it's not quite as quiet as the original Elvie wearable pump. However, it is capable of suction up to 270 millimeters of mercury, which is stronger than the original Elvie model. Stride has two pumping modes, both expression and stimulation, which automatically change at two minutes, as well as ten settings for vacuum levels. There is also a default setting for mothers who have a favorite setting, along with a timer, and a pause button; however, there is no digital screen and it is not possible to change the speed level. Included with the pump is a USB charging cable. A two-hour charge allows for up to two and a half hours of pumping time. The pump automatically shuts off at 40 minutes.

Size 24 millimeter flanges come standard with this pump, but sizes 21 and 28 millimeter can be ordered separately for $29.99 per two-pack. Inserts for this pump can be purchased from other companies, such as Maymom, Freemie, Beaugen, and Willow.

A pour spout on this pump makes it essential for mothers to be in an upright position so milk does not leak while pumping, though mothers may want to lean a bit forward before ending the pumping session to collect every drop of the milk. Pump parts must be completely dry when assembling, or suction could be low. Visible lines inside the flanges help center the nipple and mothers can peer through the pour spout to double check alignment. While each cup holds about five ounces of milk, there is not a great way for the cups to rest on a table top.

At $249, this pump is half the price of its predecessor and shipping is free. The Elvie Stride offers a two-year warranty on the motor. Visit www.elvie.com or call 1-508-300- 9989.

Milk Cups

Milk cups are a new option to collect milk while pumping instead of using standard flanges and bottles. Worn inside most any bra and connected to most any pump, cups offer more discrete pumping, in addition to being a hands-free option. As of this writing, there are three companies that manufacture milk cups: Freemie, Spectra, and Legendairy.

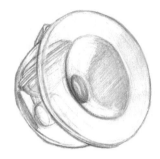

Milk Cups

All these cups are similar in size and shape, and include tubing to connect with almost any pump model. A flat bottom makes it easy to rest the cups on a hard surface until the milk is poured into a collection container.

Freemie Cups. Designed to work with the Freemie Independence and Liberty breast pumps, Freemie cups have been available the longest and can be used with almost any other pump. These cups come in flange sizes 25 and 28 millimeters but can also be sized down with Freemie inserts. Holding up to eight ounces of milk, these cups feature a well-placed pour hole, which make it easy to transfer milk.

On the downside, Freemie cups are very hard to see through and milk can leak out of the pour holes while pumping if a mother bends over. Unfortunately, these cups are not dishwasher-safe.

Most importantly, these cups do not provide strong vacuum. In some cases, the lower vacuum may be because the tubing is not pushed all the way into the motor. Freemie cups can be purchased for about $69.99.

Spectra Cara Cups. Offered in flange sizes 24 and 28 millimeters, Spectra Cara Cups hold about eight and a half ounces of milk each—more than either of the other two cup options on the market. Cara Cups are easy to assemble, include extra valves, and can be sized down with inserts from MayMom.

In addition to strong suction, these cups are clear for easy positioning and seeing the milk filling inside. Leaking is possible if a mother tilts while wearing the cups and also while transferring milk into a bottle, as there is no pour spout. However, a quick fix is to simply place the flange of the cup into the mouth of a bottle and pour the milk that way. Spectra Cara Cups can be purchased for about $75.

Legendairy Cups. These cups stand out because of their silicone flange, which may be more comfortable against the breast. Flanges in sizes 24 and 28 millimeters are included, though mothers can purchase sizes 19- and 21-millimeter inserts for just $10 more. Legendairy cups are sold for $59.99 on www.legendairymilk.com.

Personal Use Single Electric Pumps

Although few mothers are interested in purchasing a single electric breast pump, some do prefer to pump one side at a time. Single pumping allows mothers a free hand to massage the breast being pumped or to manage other tasks like eating, drinking, or reading. For mothers who rarely pump, buying a single pump may be a better option than purchasing a more expensive double electric model. While there are models of single electric breast pumps, nearly every double electric pump can be set up to express milk from just one side at a time. The models listed here are sold exclusively as single electric pumps.

Tommee Tippee "Made for Me" Single Electric Breast Pump. This single electric pump reaches high vacuum levels and offers both stimulation and expression modes, along with nine levels of suction. Also included is just one flange size (27 millimeters), which will fit most mothers. The pump comes with a one-year warranty, two if the pump is registered with the company. It sells for $99.99 but can be found at lower prices online.

Evenflo Advanced Single Electric Pump.
Powered by AC power or three AA batteries,
this handheld, fully automatic pump cycles
at about 57 times per minute and reaches
suctions of 250 millimeters of mercury.
Intended for mothers who only pump on
occasion, this model does have a slouch-free
design, meaning you can lean back while
pumping. This pump is loud and, because
it is top heavy, using a bottle stand after
pumping is advised. The Advanced Single
costs about $45 and is only warrantied for
90 days. For more information, visit www.
evenflo.com or call 855-334-2229.

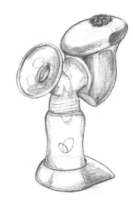

Evenflo Advanced Single
Electric Pump

Manual Pumps

For mothers who rarely pump, manual pumps are inexpensive, and
sometimes more comfortable and less tiring to use than others. Manual
options are also great backup options for mothers who use electric
pumps, in case of breakage or power outages.

Medela Harmony Pump. With a soft
flange and a squeeze handle, this manual
pump offers two basic settings, one to stimulate letdown and the other for after the
milk starts flowing, depending on how the
handle is turned. In place of a hard plastic flange is a soft, flexible silicone one;
but its 24 millimeter nipple tunnel may be
too small for some mothers. Other sizes
can be purchased from the company. The
Harmony is available, with a 30-day warranty, for about $49. Contact Medela at 800-
435-8316 or visit www.medela.com.

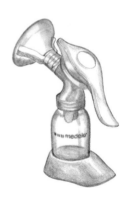

Medela Harmony Pump

Philips Avent Comfort Manual Breast Pump. This pump is a favorite among nursing mothers. It has a similar look to the Medela Harmony. When you squeeze the handle, a soft silicone cover over the hard, plastic flange gently compresses the areola to stimulate milk flow, but the silicone insert may be too small or short for some mothers. The pump is available for about $45. Visit www.philips.com or call 800-54-AVENT.

Ameda One-Hand Pump. With this pump, you create suction by squeezing a hand grip. The One-Hand is available for about $40. For more information, call 877-992-6332 or go to www. ameda.com.

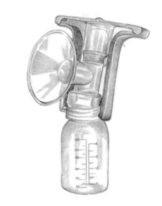

Rumble Tuff Sweet Assist Manual Breast Pump. The squeeze handle on this pump can be held in any position, which may mean more comfortable hand motions. It comes with a soft silicone flange insert. This model has a higher slot to provide a short, quick sucking pattern to stimulate letdown, and then a lower slot to provide deeper, slower sucking at good pressures of 240 millimeters of pressure. On the top of the pump, there is a dial to turn the suction higher or lower. This pump sells for about $38. Rumble Tuff's customer service is available at 855-228-8388 or www.rumbletuff.com.

Ameda One-Hand Pump

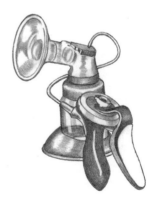

Rumble Tuff Sweet Assist
Manual Breast Pump

Silicone Squeeze Pumps

Last but not least are the new, inexpensive, one-piece, milk pumps and silicone milk collectors. The original pump is known as the "Haakaa" pump and was designed by a mother in New Zealand.

While these are referred to as "pumps," there is really no pumping involved. Most mothers use the pump to collect "drip" milk on one side, while nursing their baby on the opposite breast. By taking advantage of the baby stimulating the letdown response, they can effortlessly collect milk on the opposite breast. This milk may be somewhat lower in fat, but is still nutritious for the baby.

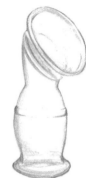

Silicone Squeeze Pumps

The silicone pump can easily slip off in certain situations. When placing the pump onto the breast, turn the flange inside out before centering it over the nipple. Also, squeeze the pump body on the front and back, instead of from side to side before centering it over your nipple. As the pump fills, it may need to be momentarily removed and squeezed again. Nursing using the football hold may prevent a baby from kicking the pump off. Another option for preventing the pump from falling and spilling is to purchase the inexpensive Haaka Silicone Breast Straps, which will help prevent the pump from falling if it loses suction.

As of this writing, there are many pump companies that label this pump as their own. Some may not be the same quality as the original Haakaa brand. There are also new generations of these silicone pumps, which, in some cases, have changed the design, and, in other cases, not for the better. Features that are worthwhile include the models with a base and a stopper to avoid spilling. Haakaa can be found on Amazon for about $13 to $33.

Silicone "milk collectors," also known as breast shells, are different from silicone "pumps." Collectors are squeezed and then placed over the breast inside the bra. Collectors can collect milk throughout the day or while nursing and be emptied whenever needed or desired.

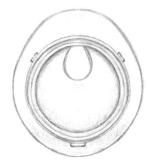

Silicone "milk collectors"

Haaka Ladybug. Sold in both single ($18) and twin ($35) packs, there are currently two sizes: 2½ ounce and 5 ounce. Haaka's collector features "feet" at the bottom so that the container will stand upright without spilling.

Milkies Milk Saver and Milk Saver On-the-Go. Milk Saver ($28) collects up to 2 ounces of milk while a mother nurses on the other side. Milk Saver On-the-Go is intended for mothers who leak in between nursings and holds just 1 ounce of milk per cup. Two cups cost $17.95. Visit www.mymilkies.com or call 800-367-2837.

Lacti-Cups. Two cups are included in each box, each capable of holding up to 2½ ounces of milk. Drip milk can be worn in the cups for up to four hours (but only two hours if saving milk for a premature or sick newborn). The price is about $27. Visit www.lacti-cups.com.

Elvie Curve. A bit different than most other milk collectors, Curve is a 1-ounce silicone pouch that is pressed before placing into the bra. It also features a one-way valve to control the suction level. Curve can be re-pressed from time to time and removed whenever desired. Curve can be purchased for $49.99. Visit www.elvie.com.

Elvie Catch. Worn inside the bra, Catch consists of two slip-proof cups that collect drip milk any time a leak occur during or in between feedings. Catch costs $34.99. Visit www.elvie.com.

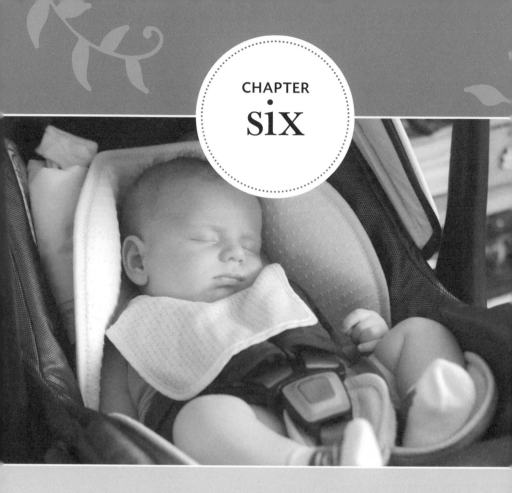

TRAVELING TOGETHER, BEING APART

TAKING THE BABY ALONG

BEING APART

- Occasional Separations

RETURNING TO WORK OR SCHOOL

- Work Options
- Choosing a Caregiver
- Planning Your Return to Work
- Instructions for the Caregiver
- Back at Work

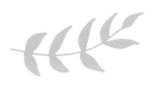

T ODAY'S NURSING MOTHER IS OUT AND ABOUT, taking care of business, enjoying the company of friends, returning to work or school, taking time out for fun. In many ways, nursing simplifies life considerably. With the increasing acceptance and popularity of breastfeeding, more and more mothers are able to nurse their babies while participating in a wide variety of activities.

TAKING THE BABY ALONG

Your nursing baby can go with you almost anywhere—and with a lot less hassle than you would face if you were fussing with formula and bottles.

You may feel comfortable nursing in the presence of family or friends you are visiting, or you may be a bit uneasy. You can always retreat to the bedroom, of course, but that's not much fun. Learning to nurse discreetly and without embarrassment will put most people at ease. You might want to practice ahead of time getting the baby on your breast with a blanket or shawl draped over your shoulder and the baby's head. If you wear a shirt or a sweater you can pull up, or if you unbutton your blouse from the bottom, you will expose less of yourself. Most maternity shops carry a line of attractive tops and dresses designed for discreet nursing. Try nursing in front of your partner or in front of a mirror so you'll know what others will see. There are also nursing covers available for purchase that cover the baby but allow you to look down at him while feeding.

If you are going out for the day or spending a few hours in town, you may want to nurse just before you leave. A couple of diapers and a few moist wipes in a zipper-top bag, and you're off. If you are using a cloth baby carrier, you may find it easier to put it on before you go.

After a couple of hours out, look around for a comfortable place to sit with your baby. Many mothers feel comfortable nursing in public places and are hardly noticed when they do so. Some stores and restaurants have dressing rooms or pleasant restrooms where you may prefer to feed the baby.

Many first-time mothers worry about being asked to cover up or leave when they are nursing out of the house. You may have heard of others who have been harassed when they nursed their children in public. But know that every state, the District of Colombia, and the Virgin Islands have laws protecting the rights of nursing mothers in public. South Dakota, Idaho, and Virginia exempt breastfeeding mothers from public indecency laws. Visit http://www.ncsl.org/research/health/breastfeeding-state-laws.aspx for an up-to-date review of state breastfeeding laws. You can find your state's laws at www.nursingfreedom.org.

Mothers appreciate the ease of taking long trips with their nursing babies. Most young infants travel well in a car. (Of course, the baby should always ride in a car seat approved for safety, no matter how short the trip.) You will want to stop every few hours for nursing and a diaper change. As the baby's car seat faces backward, you may be able to manage nursing while sitting in the back seat next to her.

The older baby may be less happy in the car seat for long periods. Whenever possible try to start long stretches in the car just before naptime. Try hanging some of the baby's toys on her car seat or keeping a bag of toys and other fun things in the back seat.

Flying with your baby means knowing the rules ahead of time. Airlines have regulations regarding how old babies must be to fly, as well as information on necessary identification. You will also need to decide whether to fly for free with the baby on your lap or purchase a ticket for the baby instead. This option is generally not available if you will be taking an international flight.

You might try to reserve bulkhead seating next to a window; this will give you extra space and more privacy. Similarly, try to choose a flight that is lightly booked for more room and, again, more privacy. Avoid getting a seat next to a bathroom, which may be noisy. Nursing during takeoff and landing will help the baby's ears adjust to the changing air pressure. If you must fly when the baby has a cold, give her a safe decongestant an hour before takeoff. Visit www.babycantravel.com for more helpful tips.

In 2018, Congress passed legislation that all medium- and large-size airports are required to provide a clean, private non-bathroom space in each terminal building after the security check point for the expression of breast milk. It must include a place to sit, a table or other flat surface, and an electrical outlet. Airports must also provide a baby changing table in one men's and one women's restroom in each terminal building.

You can carry breast milk with you through security so long as the amount in each bag of fresh, cold, or frozen milk is less than 3½ ounces (104 ml) per container. In general, you should only carry the amount of milk you will need for the day or for the flight. Additional milk should be carried in checked luggage. Milk that is put through the x-ray machine will not be harmed. You can carry milk in a cooler and the cooler should not be considered a third carry-on item. Carrying breast milk in other countries may mean different regulations. For more complete discussion of carrying milk on a plane, visit https://www.verywellfamily.com/breast-milk-on-airplanes-431745.

BEING APART

Occasional Separations

Any number of situations may come up in which you must be separated from your baby—an evening out, a family or career obligation, or a stay in the hospital.

When you plan to be away from the baby for just a few hours, you can manually express or pump some milk for him ahead of time (see Chapter 5). If you will be separated from the baby for a day or longer, you may be able to store enough milk for him ahead of time. If not, you can substitute a commercially prepared formula. While you are away, try to pump at least once every three hours. A clinical-grade rental pump or a double personal use breast pump may be more convenient than other kinds, and also most effective for keeping up your milk supply. If possible, keep the milk you pump cold while you are apart so that it can be frozen and used later.

Hospitalization of a nursing mother rarely necessitates weaning. Many hospitals have electric breast pumps available for nursing mothers. If your hospital doesn't, you can rent a pump and take it with you, or have one brought in. You may be able to arrange for the baby to be brought in for nursing visits, or even for the baby to stay with you (providing that you, a family member, or a friend can care for him). Try to express your milk frequently to maintain your milk supply. Ask the nursing staff to refrigerate your milk so that it can be taken home for your baby. After surgery, mothers can safely nurse or express milk and save it for the baby, as once you are awake from anesthesia, there is not enough left in your body to be a problem for the baby. See Appendix D, page 402, for more information on anesthesia.

Questions may arise about the safety of medications you need to take in the hospital. Although most medications pass through into the breast milk, the majority are safe for nursing babies. If you or your doctor is unsure whether a given medication is safe for a baby, check the safety of the drug yourself in Appendix D. If a drug is not considered safe for a nursing baby, you can continue to pump your milk, discarding it until the medication is no longer required.

Ship Your Milk

Milk Stork is the first service of its kind to help get a traveling mother's breast milk back home safely. Special refrigerated boxes which hold 34 or 72 ounces of milk can be carried back home with a tote or shipped overnight through Fed Ex. Go to www.milkstork.com to see how it works and find pricing.

RETURNING TO
WORK OR SCHOOL

Not so long ago, a new mother planning to return to work might never have considered nursing her baby or would have decided to wean near the end of her maternity leave. Today, with the growing number of working women and the increasing awareness of the many benefits breastfeeding offers, more and more mothers are choosing to nurse their babies while continuing with their careers.

Your extra efforts to continue nursing are well worth your while. The cost of formula aside, breastfed babies are generally healthier. The less your baby is sick, the less time you must spend away from work or school. Nursing also saves you time and energy, which is especially important when you are combining the responsibilities of employment and family. Perhaps most important, nursing helps you maintain the close, loving relationship you have with your baby. Many mothers who work outside the home or attend school feel that breastfeeding offers emotional compensation for the hours that must be spent apart. The security of your breast comforts the baby and helps make the time you are together special and rewarding for both of you.

Work Options

Although there may be no question in your mind that you will be returning to work or school after your baby is born, you are lucky if you have some flexibility in determining the length of your maternity leave. Your time at home after giving birth is important for both you and the baby: It is the time in which you will get to know each other and form a special bond. It will also be a time for you to rest and recover from the physical stress of the birth process. Some women need a little while, and some need a long while, before they are ready to add the demands of work or school. Breastfeeding experts have noted that mothers who stay home for sixteen weeks or longer experience fewer difficulties maintaining their milk supply once back at work.

Because you cannot know just how you will feel after you deliver, explore what options may be open to you ahead of time. Depending on your financial situation and your work demands, you may be able to arrange for an extended leave, beyond the usual six to eight weeks. In 1993, the United States enacted the Family Medical Leave Act (FMLA), which requires employers with fifty or more employees to allow twelve weeks unpaid leave each year for any employee who needs to care for a dependent. Taking unpaid leave may be helpful to you, or it may not be financially feasible. As of this writing, there are now nine states and Washington, D.C., that offer mothers paid family leave for twelve weeks. Visit https://babygate.abetterbalance.org/know-your-rights/state-local-rights/ to learn if your state offers paid family leave.

For other options, you may be able to arrange to work at home, return to work part-time, or share your job with another person. Each of these options has worked well for many mothers. If you are a student, perhaps you can take fewer classes for a term or take some classes online.

Part-time work offers many advantages to the nursing mother. Fewer hours apart means fewer missed feedings, lower childcare costs, and generally less stress for both mother and baby.

An employer also benefits by agreeing to shorter hours. You might agree to come in for fewer hours each day, or have fewer full-hour days. Both arrangements have advantages and drawbacks for the nursing mother.

Still, a somewhat flexible arrangement may be possible. With a "flex-time" schedule, you might work eight hours a day but remain free to start earlier or later than normal. This system could allow you to spend a leisurely morning with the baby and perhaps get a few chores done. If your partner also has a flexible schedule, you might be able to minimize the number of hours that the baby must be left with someone else.

Some mothers arrange to take their babies to work with them. Although this is not possible for most women, it can be managed in some work settings. Another option is childcare at the work site. Some employers and employees have found this to be an ideal arrangement. If you work with other parents of infants or small children, you might together explore this possibility. As of this writing, four states—Arizona, Kansas, Nevada, and Washington—have Infants at Work programs.

State employees can bring their babies to work until the infant is six months old or crawling, whichever comes first.

Another possibility is having the baby brought to you for nursings, or going to the baby yourself during your lunch hour. Usually, the major obstacle in having the baby come to your workplace is finding someone willing and able to bring her. If instead you'll go to the baby, you will want to find childcare as close as possible to your workplace. If you have a full hour for lunch and your baby is nearby, you may have enough time to leisurely manage travel, nursing, and eating.

Choosing a Caregiver

Finding just the right person to care for your baby can make all the difference in your state of mind while you are away. If you will be shopping for a caregiver, be sure to start early so you can take your time. You may prefer someone who will care for your baby alone, or you may be willing to share the caregiver's services with others. Finding a caregiver who lives close to your workplace or school will help you minimize the time you and your baby are apart even if you decide against nursing during your lunch breaks.

You may be fortunate enough to have a partner or another relative who is able and eager to provide childcare. Childcare with a loving relative can make the separation easier on both mother and baby and is usually inexpensive, if not free. Working out differences in philosophy about napping, feeding, and the like, however, may be more difficult with a family member.

Some families decide to hire a nanny. This is usually the most expensive option for childcare, but it also has some great benefits: The baby has one-on-one attention and is less exposed to infectious disease, and the nanny may offer more flexible scheduling and may also be willing to take on household duties besides infant care. Special arrangements may need to be made, however, if the nanny gets sick. Some nannies commute to the family home each day, while others live in. You can find a nanny through a local or Internet-based agency or through private advertisements and word of mouth. If you plan to hire someone without the help of an agent, you will want to not only interview the nanny but also check her references and perhaps order a criminal background check.

The U.S. Department of State authorizes agencies for au pairs, college-aged men and women who come to the United States from other countries to live with a family and care for the family's children for a year. This program is a cultural exchange program through a J1 Exchange Visitor program. Visit https://j1visa.state.gov/programs/au-pair to learn more.

Au pairs speak English, have at least 200 hours of child-care experience, and have received instruction in child safety and child development. The family provides meals, a private room, and $500 toward six credits of college classes. The agency that sets up the relationship also monitors it. An au pair costs approximately $13,000 for the year, less than a typical nanny. For more information about the Au Pair Program, visit www.iapa.org.

Family day care is the most popular childcare option, partially because it's usually less expensive than one-on-one care. For older babies and toddlers, family day care also offers the benefit of getting to know other children. In most states, family day care providers are licensed, unless they are caring only for their own children and one other child, and are legally limited in the number of infants and older children they can care for. Family day care providers aren't required to have had formal instruction in child development, and some states don't even require health and safety certifications. Like nannies, family day care providers seldom offer alternative care when the provider gets ill or goes on vacation, although parents may be expected to pay for vacation time.

Lastly, there are day care centers, which care for large numbers of children and are usually licensed by the state. Many day care centers have numerous employees with education in childhood development. If one employee gets sick or goes on vacation, there is always another to fill in. There are disadvantages to day care centers: The children generally get less one-on-one care than those with a nanny or au pair or in family day care; there may be much more sickness when large groups of children are kept together; and hours at a center are usually strict, so you may have to pay extra if you are late picking up your child. Also, some

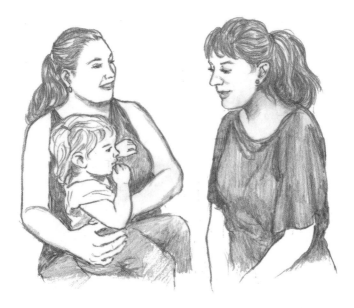

centers do not take infants. Often, the best centers have waiting lists; you may need to get on one months before your baby is born.

Let each prospective caregiver know about your nursing relationship and your own particular style of baby care. Ask for the names and telephone numbers of other families whose children she has cared for in the past or is caring for now, and call the families to hear about their experiences with the caregiver. If she is caring for other children now, plan to meet with her at a time when they will be present and awake. This way you'll be able to not only see the environment but also observe her style, and judge whether she would give your baby enough individual love and attention. As you chat with the caregiver, try to find out if she can make a long-term commitment to your baby; having to find a replacement suddenly could be upsetting for both you and the baby. Discuss arrangements for illness (either your baby's or hers) and vacations (your family's or hers), who would be called in an emergency, how much advance notice would be necessary if the baby were to be absent or late, and fees and when they would be due. Ask to look at any written agreements before you're expected to sign them. In making your final choice of who will care for your baby, trust your intuition. If something doesn't feel quite right, look elsewhere.

Consider having the baby spend several hours or a full day with the chosen caregiver a week or so before you go back to work or school. Such a "trial run" might be reassuring for you, or you may feel, as many mothers do, that the first separation should occur only when the situation demands it.

Planning Your Return to Work

If you will be missing one or more feedings while you are away at work or school, you should plan to express your milk. This will help prevent engorgement and, more important, maintain your milk supply. The milk you express can be used later to feed your baby while you are away.

See Chapter 5 for information on:

- expression methods
- types and brands of pumps
- other purchases you may want to consider
- pumping at home in preparation for your return to work or school
- expressing milk in the workplace
- increasing your milk supply
- storing your expressed milk
- feeding your milk to the baby.

Besides finding a caregiver for your baby, choosing a pump, and learning to use it, your main task in planning a return to work is to identify a place to express your milk. For some mothers, this can be difficult. Working out this problem ahead of time can help reduce the stress once you are back at work or school.

In 2010, the Affordable Care Act amended the Fair Labor Standards Act to require employers with fifty or more employees to provide a "reasonable" break time for employees who need to express breast milk for their nursing children. They are required to provide this until the baby turns one year old. Employers must also provide a place for the employee to express the milk, other than a bathroom. This area must be shielded from view and free from intrusion from co-workers and the public.

Employers are not required to pay an employee for any work time spent for expressing breast milk. However, employees who already receive compensated breaks may use that time to express milk.

State laws override this federal law if they provide greater protections to employees. For example, some states may mandate providing paid break time or providing break time beyond the baby's first birthday. As of this writing, twenty-four states, the District of Columbia, and Puerto Rico have additional laws regarding breastfeeding in the workplace. If you have additional questions about this law, visit www.usbreastfeeding.org.

Ideally, the place where you will pump will be quiet and private, with few distractions. A women's lounge with a comfortable chair (and preferably a sink and a refrigerator) or your own private office might be perfect. Other possibilities include a lighted storage closet, a conference room, or a borrowed office. If your workplace has a break room that both male and female employees use, you might be able to schedule your break at a time when you can have the privacy you need.

You may find that the only available place for you to express milk is a bathroom. It may be adequate as long as it is clean and has a chair, or room for one to be brought in.

If your job requires a good deal of travel, you can express milk in your car or in comfortable restrooms on your route. Medium- and large-size airports now have rooms specifically mandated by Congress for the use of mothers for the expression of breast milk set up in each terminal after the security check point. Each room must include a place to sit, a table, and an electrical outlet.

If you are returning to school, you may be able to find a private place there, as well. Locker rooms, empty classrooms, and health centers are all possibilities.

You may have an easier time identifying a pumping place if other mothers have worked this out before you. Otherwise, you may need to make a special trip to your workplace or school to search out a site that could work for you.

Once you're sure of your rights, discuss your need for a pumping place with your supervisor or human resources manager. Do so by letter or email if you fear your boss will be uncomfortable discussing your breasts in person or over the phone. You might consider including a letter from your doctor or your baby's doctor (you can find a letter to download and have your physician sign at www.workandpump.com/letter.htm). You might also refer your boss to two good sources of information about why employers should support nursing mothers in the workplace. One is the United States Breastfeeding Committee website, at www.usbreastfeeding.org; the other is the Office on Women's Health website, at www.womenshealth.gov. The latter site includes an excellent printable brochure called "The Business Case for Breastfeeding." Your boss may be more supportive knowing that by facilitating breastfeeding, the company will be reducing medical costs, absenteeism, and employee turnover.

Your boss may want to know whether you'll be using work time to express your milk. Your regular breaks will probably be adequate. If you need extended breaks, you can deduct the time from your total hours or perhaps be able to make it up at the end of the day.

You will also need a cool place to store your milk. Investigate whether a refrigerator is available. Note that breast milk is not considered by the U.S. Centers for Disease Control and Prevention (CDC) or the Occupational Safety and Health Administration (OSHA) to be a "biohazardous material," which would require storage in a refrigerator where no other food is kept. If it makes you or your co-workers more comfortable, of course, you can put your milk containers in an opaque sack or lunch bag.

If no refrigerator is available, you can plan to bring a small cooler with plastic ice packs inside. Milk stays cold for several hours in a cooler, which is also handy for transporting milk home or to the caregiver.

Instructions for the Caregiver

Whether your baby goes to day care, has a nanny, or stays with a friend or family member, it is important for you to communicate exactly what you expect. Reviewing your expectations with your baby's caregiver before your return to work can help prevent misunderstandings and disappointments.

There may be many other matters that you wish to discuss, but when it comes to feedings, the first and most important rule should be that your baby always be held while being fed. Your baby may be capable of holding his own bottle, but he would miss out on important human contact if he were left to feed himself.

Your baby's caregiver will also need to know how to defrost and warm breast milk. You can write these instructions out so she won't forget them. Be sure to say what to do with milk that is left in the bottle.

Give the caregiver general guidelines on how often the baby should be fed and how much he will need at each feeding. When a baby fusses, it's easiest to respond first with a bottle. Without guidelines, a caregiver may feed a baby as much milk during an eight- to ten-hour period as he would normally take over an entire day! Explain that most breastfed babies need to be fed about every two to three hours and need no more than 1½ ounces (44 ml) per hour. This means, for example, that a typical baby needs about 3 ounces every two hours or 4½ ounces (133 ml)

Refrigerated Milk

Use refrigerated milk within seventy-two hours. Take the milk out of the refrigerator just before the feeding. Over five to ten minutes, warm the milk to room temperature in a container of warm water. Do not warm the milk in a microwave or on the stove. If the baby doesn't take all the milk at once, you can return the leftover milk to the refrigerator and use it at the next feeding.

Frozen Milk

Use milk within three months if it has been stored in the freezer compartment of a refrigerator. Milk stored in a deep freezer is good for six months or longer. Always use the oldest milk first. Thaw the milk either in the refrigerator, where it can remain for up to twenty-four hours, or in water just before feeding, gradually increasing the temperature to warm. Do not defrost the milk in a microwave or on the stove. Whatever milk the baby does not take must be discarded. Breast milk should not be refrozen.

every three hours. You might also describe to your care provider how to feed your baby using "paced" bottle-feeding (see page 273).

Underfeeding can become a problem, too. A baby who enjoys sucking on his fingers or a pacifier much of the time may not give clear feeding cues and end up not taking enough milk during the time mother and baby are apart. The general rule of 3 ounces (89 ml) every two to two and a half hours should prevent this.

Ask the caregiver to plan feedings so that the baby is hungry when you return for him. This generally means that the baby's last bottle-feeding of the day should be two to three hours before you are expected. If the baby seems hungry after that, the caregiver might offer a partial feeding.

When you pick up the baby at the caregiver's house, you can leave milk, labeled with the date, in her refrigerator for the next day. Fresh refrigerated milk is best for the baby, since it retains more antibodies than frozen milk. If the milk will not be used during the following three days, it should be frozen.

A few caregivers express concern about the safety of handling breast milk; they apparently fear that diseases might be transmitted through it. You can assure your caregiver that, according to the CDC and OSHA, people handling and feeding breast milk need not wear rubber gloves nor store the milk in a refrigerator where no other foods are kept.

Back at Work

Once you are back at work, you will discover what routines work best for you, your baby, and your milk supply. It will help if you can nurse as much as possible when you are with the baby and express milk frequently when you are apart. Some mothers keep their milk plentiful by encouraging their babies to nurse frequently during the evening and night. You may find that bringing the baby to bed with you, if she isn't already there, and nursing an hour or so before getting up works well. Nursing twice in the morning before you leave the baby is ideal. You can nurse again just before you leave home or when you arrive at the caregiver's. While you are at work, try to express milk about as often as you would be nursing at home. Ideally, if you will be missing three feedings, you should express milk three times. Your goal should be to drain both breasts as completely as possible, by either nursing or expressing milk, at least seven times in each twenty-four hours.

While some mothers need to concentrate on the task at hand while they are expressing milk, others take this time to simply relax, and some mothers use the time to get work done. For mothers who use a pump, pumping both breasts at once not only increases the amount of milk collected but cuts the time of expression in half. You can probably learn how to hold both flanges to your breasts using just one arm so you can use your free hand to massage your breasts, turn pages of a book or magazine, or hold the phone to your ear. You might also try a "pumping bra," which holds both flanges in place so that a mother can express her milk and have both hands free (see page 388 and Appendix A, page 386). The latest category for mothers who express milk at work are the cord/tubing free, "wearable" breast pumps. See Wearable Breast Pumps in Chapter 5 (page 303). Another option is to wear "milk cups" instead of bottles and flanges to collect milk. See page 308. Label your milk with your baby's name and the date before storing it in a refrigerator or placing it in a cooler for transport.

Some mothers leak milk while they are at work. You may need to wear thick pads in your bra; keep an extra supply of them with you. Or try silicone nursing pads, which don't absorb milk but instead apply pressure to prevent leakage (see Appendix A, page 386). Some mothers prefer to use plastic breast shells to keep their clothes dry. Although they usually serve the purpose, these plastic shells can also encourage further leaking. Finally, wearing printed blouses or keeping an extra jacket or sweater at work will help hide any wetness.

After work, you may want to nurse when you arrive at the caregiver's, before going home. Many mothers find this provides a welcome opportunity to relax and talk with the caregiver about the baby's day.

Some women find that they are unable to express as much milk as they would like, especially after three to four months postpartum. At this point you may notice a drop in the amount you can pump, but this doesn't necessarily mean you can't meet your baby's needs. Many women overproduce in the first few months; after about four months, milk supply is determined by demand. If you had previously been pumping excess milk, you might now find yourself producing only as much as the baby drinks while you are away. This means that your body has adjusted to the baby's needs. Normal milk production is about 1½ ounces (44 ml) per hour, so if three hours have passed since you last pumped, you should get 4 to 5 ounces (118 to 148 ml) combined when you pump both breasts.

If your milk production is good but your caregiver is running out of the milk you save, find out just how much milk your baby is taking while you're away. A baby in day care for eight hours needs no more than 12 ounces (355 ml) of milk during that period. If you are able to nurse when you drop your baby off, or shortly before that, and again when you pick her up, she needs only about 8 ounces (237 ml) while you're gone. Your baby is being overfed if she is taking much more than this. If the caregiver requests more milk to feed your baby, say that your doctor recommends that the baby have no more than 1½ ounces (44 ml) per hour. You might have the baby's caregiver try a slow-flow bottle nipple so the baby can suck for a longer period of time without taking more milk. Although babies do not require fluids in addition to breast milk, you might suggest a bottle of water to soothe your baby when she has been recently fed but is fussy, especially if you are expected to arrive shortly.

Your caregiver may say that your baby needs more milk because she is getting bigger. In fact, researchers report that the amount of breast milk needed over a twenty-four-hour period by an exclusively breastfed baby changes little between the ages of one and six months. As they get older, babies utilize breast milk more efficiently.

If a baby begins taking less milk at home because of longer sleep stretches at night, however, she may want to make up for it with more milk during the day, at least until she begins eating solid foods. In this case, try to nurse more often in the evening and early morning.

If you think that your milk supply truly is too low, be sure to read page 264, Increasing Your Milk Supply while Pumping, in Chapter 5.

If you follow all of the other recommendations here and in Chapter 5 and still cannot express milk as often as necessary at work, you may find that the baby needs supplemental formula when you are away.

Combining nursing and working takes a great deal of time and energy. Aside from the responsibilities of your job, the baby, and the rest of your family, it is very important that you take time to care for yourself. Nursing mothers need to eat well. Although it may be tempting to skip breakfast or lunch, most women who do this find they have little energy to meet the many demands of the day. Get up a little earlier, if you must, to fix a nutritious breakfast. Bring snacks such as yogurt, cheese, nuts, and fruit to eat throughout the workday. Some mothers find that brewer's yeast gives them an energy boost and helps keep up their milk supply. To avoid constipation and plugged milk ducts, you will also need to drink plenty of fluids while you are at work. Finally, rest is essential. Most working and nursing mothers find that they must go to bed earlier than they once did. If you can, take an hour's nap just before dinner, and nap on your days at home with the baby.

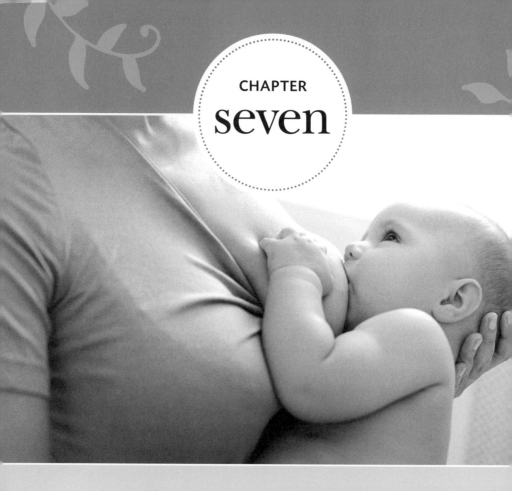

THE REWARD PERIOD: FROM TWO THROUGH SIX MONTHS

- Caring for Yourself
- Resuming Sexual Activity
- Nursing Your Baby
- Scheduled Feedings
- Distractibility
- Night Waking
- Starting Solid Foods

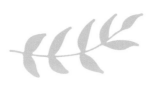

Two to Six Months

THE PERIOD BETWEEN THE BABY'S SECOND AND SIXTH months is exciting and rewarding. With the newborn stage behind, most mothers feel relaxed and confident. The baby is more predictable, his needs easier to interpret. By three months, his crying lessens considerably. Day by day, the baby becomes more sociable and attuned to the people and things around him. Still, nursings are an important part of his day, intervals for nurture and nourishment at the breast.

Caring for Yourself

During this time, I hope, you are beginning to feel more like your usual self. Napping whenever possible is still important, especially if your baby is waking at night for feedings, if your energy seems low, or you are back at work. Your intake of food and drink continues to be essential to your well-being. Neglecting your need for fluids could lead to constipation and, possibly, recurrent plugged milk ducts. Skipping meals or substituting "empty calorie" foods for more nutritious ones could result in fatigue. If you are overweight, limit your weight loss to 1 pound (.5 kg) per week; crash dieting could decrease your milk supply. Most nursing mothers lose weight gradually without worrying about snacks or calories, but others find that eating three regular, satisfying meals and limiting high-calorie snacks and beverages, such as juices and soft drinks, helps them achieve their weekly goal.

If you have your cholesterol levels checked during these months, keep in mind that it's normal for some women to have very high levels of both "good" and "bad" cholesterol during pregnancy and lactation.

Levels as high as 200 and 325 milligrams per deciliter are normal for pregnant and nursing women and do not require treatment or weaning.

Resuming Sexual Activity

After the birth of a baby, most couples need time to readjust to each other sexually. You can probably resume intercourse by the sixth-week postpartum exam. In the meantime, you and your partner can enjoy physical loving such as cuddling, kissing, massage, and fondling. If your perineum feels fine and you want to have intercourse at three or four weeks postpartum, there is no reason to wait. But you may not yet feel ready even when your doctor, nurse, or midwife gives you the go-ahead.

You may be worried that intercourse will be painful. If you have had an episiotomy, you may feel some initial tenderness and tightness, but your stitches should be completely healed after one month. Relaxing as much as possible will help make lovemaking more comfortable the first few times. A warm bath, a glass of wine, and extra time with foreplay may be helpful. You may also want to experiment with different positions, especially if you have had an episiotomy. Some women prefer to be on top so that they control the degree of penetration. Others find that a side-lying position feels best at first.

Most new mothers experience some vaginal dryness during lovemaking because of the hormonal changes that occur after giving birth. The vaginal secretions will increase again once regular ovulation resumes, but ovulation is generally delayed during nursing. Until your periods resume, a lubricant can make intercourse more comfortable and pleasurable. Use a generous amount of lubricating gel, such as K-Y, Astroglide, or a contraceptive gel, in and around your vagina. (I don't recommend tablets or creams containing estrogen, which when absorbed can diminish milk production.)

Your breasts need not be off limits when making love. Some women, however, find them less sensitive to stimulation during the nursing period; they may also feel tender during the early weeks, and later on just after nursing. Breast stimulation and orgasm may cause the milk to letdown and leak or spray. If leaking milk is bothersome for you or your partner, you might nurse shortly before you make love, or wear a blouse, a bra, or a nightgown during lovemaking.

For some time after having a baby, many women find they have less interest in making love than formerly. There are a variety of reasons for this. Estrogen, which influences a woman's sex drive as well as the amount of vaginal secretions, is produced in lower levels after she gives birth. Sometimes having so much skin-to-skin contact with the baby all day dampens a woman's desire for more physical contact. A new mother may also fear another pregnancy—whether or not the recent one was planned. At the end of the day, too, a mother may be just too tired for lovemaking.

Co-parents also suffer from overwork and night wakings. Like their partners, they may be too exhausted to make love, and they may also worry about having another baby too soon.

It is important that your intimacy as a couple continue. As with most other changes in life, talking over your feelings and making some adjustments will make this period easier.

Finding the time to make love can be difficult, especially when you are tired. You may need to plan times to be together when you are rested and when the baby is likely to be asleep. Making love early in the morning or when the baby is napping may work the best. Perhaps you can take a nap in the afternoon so you will have more energy for your partner in the evening. Having the baby sleep in another room may help you to feel more comfortable.

But if neither you nor your partner is much inclined to have frequent intercourse, your physical and emotional intimacy can continue without it. Passionate feelings will probably come more easily as the baby gets older. Remember, you have a lifetime ahead of you to share your love.

Contraception

If you are concerned about the possibility of getting pregnant again, talk over birth control options with your partner and your healthcare provider. Foam and other spermicides, condoms, an IUD, a diaphragm, a cervical cap, a female condom, and surgical sterilization are all considered safe during nursing. If you used a diaphragm or cervical cap before your pregnancy, you will need a refitting now.

A spermicide is a chemical that you put deep into your vagina right before sex. It prevents pregnancy by blocking the entrance to the cervix so sperm can't swim to your egg. Spermicide can be used by itself, or combined with other birth control methods like condoms, an IUD, a diaphragm, and a cervical cap. Using spermicide plus a condom gives you extra protection from pregnancy and also prevents sexually transmitted diseases. Women who use diaphragms and cervical caps should always use a spermicide.

Many women want reliable and convenient birth control in hormonal form. Although "the pill" and other hormonal birth control products apparently do no direct harm to the nursing baby, pills containing estrogen, even in low doses, often reduce a mother's milk supply and may thereby lead to poor weight gain in the baby. The vaginal ring (NuvaRing) and the contraceptive patch (Ortho Evra and Xulane) both contain estrogen and can lower milk production. These products are best avoided during breastfeeding.

Fortunately, not all types of hormonal birth control interfere with milk production. The progestin-only pill, also known as the "mini-pill," usually has no effect on milk supply. Nor do progestin-only injections, like Depo-Provera, which give three months' protection against pregnancy. IUDs that contain small amounts of progesterone or progestin are also considered safe and should not have any effect on milk production. All of these products are considered safe during breastfeeding.

Some healthcare providers offer hormonal contraceptives just hours or days after birth. This practice may interfere with the onset of lactation and should be postponed for at least four to six weeks.

Whichever birth control method you use, its reliability is increased by the fact that you are breastfeeding. For now, in fact, breastfeeding may be the only birth control method you need. That breastfeeding affects fertility is a truth that has been largely ignored in an era when partial breastfeeding and early weaning have been the norm. But breastfeeding has provided more contraception worldwide than all other methods combined. Frequent nursing, especially during the first several months after birth, suppresses ovulation in most women. In fact, if a woman hasn't yet had a period since her pregnancy, exclusive breastfeeding provides her more than 98 percent protection against pregnancy in the first six months postpartum (Kennedy, 1989). But when her periods resume, when the baby is receiving any food or drink besides breast milk, or when the baby reaches six months of age, the mother's chance of getting pregnant again increases. If you want to rely on breastfeeding-as-contraception (which medical texts call the lactational amenorrhea method, or LAM), nurse at least eight times in every twenty-four hours, with no more than six hours between nursings and a cumulative sucking time of at least sixty minutes per day. For best results, don't feed formula or solids or even use pacifiers.

Once your periods resume, you may prefer to track your natural menstrual cycle, abstaining from intercourse around the time of ovulation, instead of relying on birth control pills or devices. If you want to use "natural family planning," try to get personal instruction in it. Learn to keep track of all three basic body measures: basal body temperature, cervical mucus, and length of menstrual cycle.

Nursing Your Baby

As your baby quickly grows and develops, you will notice that her nursing pattern also changes. You can expect two more appetite spurts during this period, the first at about two and a half to three months and the second between four and a half and six months. As with the earlier appetite spurts, the baby will nurse more frequently for a few days to stimulate an increase in milk production. Most mothers produce 28 to 32 ounces (828 to 946 ml) of milk each day during this period, about a 30 percent increase over the first month.

By three or four months of age, many babies have dropped a feeding or two and are nursing seven or eight times a day. Nursing less often than seven times a day may result in decreased milk production and slowed weight gain for the baby. This most commonly occurs when a baby spends much of her day sucking on her fingers or on a pacifier, or when she begins sleeping long stretches at night but isn't nursed more often during the day. It can also happen when a working mother expresses milk infrequently while she is away. Your baby should continue gaining about 1 ounce (28 g) a day until she is three months old. Between three and six months of age, a breastfed baby normally gains about ½ ounce (14 g) each day.

During this period, some women begin to fear that their babies aren't "getting enough." You may find that your breasts feel less full, that you leak less or not at all, and that the sensations of the milk letting down are less intense than before. None of this necessarily means your supply is low or your baby isn't getting enough milk. If your baby is taking the breast at least seven times in twenty-four hours, has plenty of wet diapers and yellow bowel movements, and seems content after feedings, you probably have no cause for concern. Your breasts may feel less full simply because they have adjusted to your baby's needs and now produce only as much milk as she wants.

However, if your baby does not suck well or take the breast often enough, if you are using a birth control product containing estrogen, or if you are taking a medication that can interfere with milk production (such as a pseudoephedrine-containing decongestant like Sudafed or an antihistamine like Benadryl), your production may truly be low. The baby's weight gain is the best gauge of adequate milk production. A quick weight check at the doctor's office may help you feel more confident.

Some babies prefer to nurse from just one breast at each feeding. So long as the baby seems content and is continuing to gain enough weight, this is normal.

You may notice that your baby is nursing for shorter periods. She can now get a large quantity of milk quickly because both she and your breasts have become so efficient.

Most three- to six-month-old babies are chubby; some may be quite plump. Parents and sometimes even doctors may become concerned about the baby who gains weight above the norm. These babies slow their growth during the second half of the first year and typically begin to slim down during toddlerhood. It is not advisable to restrict the baby's nursing because of her weight.

Doctors have long charted babies' growth according to standards based on infants chosen without regard to what or how they were fed. Because formula-feeding alters a baby's normal growth pattern, old growth charts are inaccurate for breastfed babies. In 2006, the World Health Organization (WHO) released findings from a study of breastfed babies in Brazil, Ghana, India, Norway, Oman, and the United States. The children were exclusively breastfed for several months, and their growth and development were monitored for several years thereafter. In accordance with the findings, WHO introduced new universal growth standards for infants and children.

The study showed that healthy children from around the world grow within the same range for both height and weight. For the first time, we have charts showing how all children naturally grow, beginning during six months of exclusive breastfeeding. These charts are useful tools for monitoring children and identifying those who are under- or overfed or in some other way malnourished. The new charts show that breastfed babies tend to be slightly leaner and somewhat taller after the first six months than the old charts showed. I have included the weight charts for your use in Appendix C (see page 399).

Scheduled Feedings

Some parenting books and classes have promoted a philosophy of scheduled breastfeeding. Called "Parent Directed Feeding," the program teaches parents to feed babies on a rigid three- to four-hour schedule and to eliminate nighttime feedings at an early age. The purpose is to relieve parental anxiety and instill a sense of order and discipline in the infant. Although most parents like the idea of predictable, widely spaced nursings and full nights of sleep from the early weeks on, Parent Directed Feeding can cause some problems. See page 185 for more information.

Distractibility

Between three and five months, a baby starts to become more aware of the world around her. When she can see clearly across the room and interact more with her family, she becomes easily distracted while nursing. At any new, sudden, or interesting sight or sound, she pulls away from the breast to look around. Older siblings are a common distraction. At around this age the baby may also start to play nursing games; she may stop sucking, for instance, to pat Mom's face and smile. Although these antics can be adorable, you may become frustrated if nursing sessions become longer and longer because the baby seems never to want to get down to the "business" of nursing.

This behavior does not mean the baby has lost interest in nursing. Of course, you'll want to rule out any contributing problem, such as a low milk supply or painful reflux. But if the baby is generally content, you needn't worry about her distractibility. It may help to nurse while lying down in a quiet, semi darkened room. Some mothers reserve for nursing sessions a special toy—a blanket or necklace that the baby likes to hold and stroke—to keep her from being distracted by other things.

After several weeks of interrupted feedings, your baby will no longer have to let go of the nipple to check out what's going on around her. Instead, she'll turn her head with the nipple still in her mouth.

Night Waking

Although some babies start sleeping in stretches of up to ten hours as early as six weeks of age, most continue to wake at night until they are six to twelve months old or older. Most babies, especially those under six months of age, can be expected to wake up to nurse at least once each night, and as often as every three hours.

Night wakings may frustrate you, especially if your older child or a friend's baby slept long stretches at an early age. If you are tempted to give the baby formula or cereal in a bottle just before bedtime in the hope of encouraging him to "sleep through," keep in mind that night waking is normal for a baby this age. Besides, as many studies have shown, feeding cereal early has no effect on when a baby starts sleeping through the night. In fact, one study suggested that when parents supplement their babies' last nursing of the day with infant formula, babies sleep even less at night.

Babies who sleep long stretches during the first few months typically begin waking again around three to four months of age. Perhaps teething is to blame. Other signs of teething may include general fussiness, drooling, changes in nursing patterns, biting, and finger sucking. Giving the baby a cold washcloth or a chilled water-filled teething ring to bite on may make her more comfortable. For babies who are at least six months old, some doctors recommend the use of gum gels, acetaminophen drops (Infants' Tylenol), or ibuprofen drops (Infants' Motrin, Infants' Advil) for teething pain. Amber necklaces are used in some European countries for teething pain and are gaining popularity here. Worn against the baby's skin, the amber beads are thought to have an anti-inflammatory effect. Although scientific evidence is lacking, many parents swear that amber beads ease teething pain. At night, they can be wrapped around the baby's ankle and covered with a sock.

A baby may also wake more at night when daytime nursings decline, because Mom is away during the day, because he gets distracted during daytime feedings, or because he spends too much time sucking his fingers or a pacifier. To encourage your baby to get more of his milk during the day and evening, try offering the breast in a quiet, darkened room, nurse whenever he begins sucking his fingers, and limit or eliminate the use of a pacifier.

Waking every one to two hours all night long is *not* normal for a baby this age. If your baby starts waking very frequently, perhaps teething, an ear infection, or another illness is to blame. If he has recently had a cold or an ear infection, his ears may be the problem now, even if he has no fever and isn't pulling on them. If the baby has never been a good sleeper, reflux or a low milk supply might be causing the problem. For more information, see page 219, Fussiness, Colic, and Reflux.

If your baby wakes frequently at night, for whatever reason, taking him into your bed for all or part of the night may make nursing easier and lessen your own sleep disruptions. For information on bed sharing, see page 40, A Place to Sleep.

For additional information on babies and sleep, I recommend the book *The No-Cry Sleep Solution* by Elizabeth Pantley and William Sears (see References & Reading, page 423).

Starting Solid Foods

Probably no area of infant development attracts as much confusion and range of opinion as the starting of solid foods. Your family, friends, and childcare advisors probably all have different ideas on when and how to begin giving solid foods to your baby.

Solid foods are best introduced when a baby becomes developmentally ready for them and is able to benefit from the nutrition they offer. Although this does not happen until a baby is six months of age or older, many mothers feel pressured to begin solids earlier. Some think of feeding solids as a sort of status symbol, something to brag about.

Some doctors suggest that when babies are very large, they need solids sooner than six months. This is certainly not the case. Very big babies are large mostly because their mothers have abundant milk supplies. These babies are growing very well on mother's milk.

The AAP, as well as many other health organizations, now recommends that breastfed babies not be fed solid foods until they are at least six months old. Rest assured: Your milk provides all the nutrients your baby needs for at least the first six months of life.

There are many good reasons to delay solids until this time. Offering solids prematurely means replacing breast milk, which is nutritionally perfect, with foods that are nutritionally incomplete.

Surprisingly, babies who are started on solid foods before six months of age do not receive additional calories. This is because most of the solids fed to babies are relatively low in calories, and these foods tend to displace higher-calorie breast milk in the diet. Besides, when solids are given, breast-milk production typically lessens. Decreased milk production all too often leads to early weaning.

Babies who are exclusively breastfed for the first six months of life experience slower weight gain but faster growth in length and head size than babies fed solids earlier. After exclusively breastfed babies begin eating other foods, at about six months of age, these children tend to be leaner than the national average. They are less prone to become obese than are their peers who started on solid foods before six months (Wilson, 1998; von Kries, 1999; Kalies, 2005).

Holding off on offering solids may contribute to your baby's health in another way. In the Wilson study, babies who were offered solid foods before six months of age had more colds and other respiratory infections, wheezing, and ear infections than babies who were not given solids until six months. Starting solids early is also associated with food allergies (Fiocchi et al., 2006).

Delaying the introduction of solids is beneficial for mothers as well. Women who exclusively breastfeed for a full six months are more likely to return to their pre-pregnancy weight, as compared with mothers who offer solids prematurely, and have a lower risk of long-term obesity.

Mothers who nurse exclusively are also less likely to resume their periods in the first few months postpartum. One advantage of not having periods is the opportunity to rebuild one's iron stores, which are often depleted during pregnancy and birth.

You'll know that your baby is developmentally ready for solid foods when he can sit with support, control his head and neck movements, and tell you he is hungry (by leaning forward with an open mouth) or full (by pulling away and turning his head). He may indicate his readiness for solids by grabbing food off your plate or out of your hand.

At this time, he will also begin to lose his tongue-thrust reflex, which causes him to push anything in his mouth forward and out. This means he will be better able to eat from a spoon, move the food to the back of his mouth, and swallow. The baby's digestive system will also be mature enough to handle solids at this time. His kidneys will be able to excrete the waste products of solid foods. His iron stores will lessen, so the iron from solid foods will be beneficial for him.

Holding off on feeding solids is also practical: The closer to six months you introduce them, the more likely it is you'll be able to skip the "baby food" stage and start with table foods. Guidelines for offering solid foods are discussed in Chapter 8.

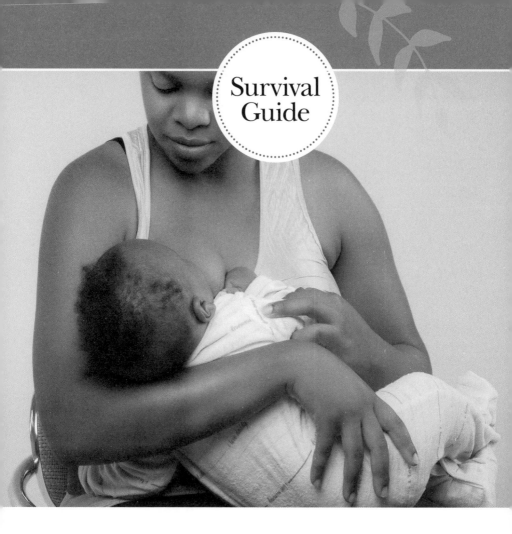

MONTHS TWO
THROUGH SIX

CONCERNS ABOUT YOURSELF

- Recurrent Plugged Ducts and Breasts Infections
- Overabundant Milk

CONCERNS ABOUT THE BABY

- Slow Weight Gain
- One-Sided Nursing
- Sudden Refusal to Nurse

CONCERNS ABOUT YOURSELF

Recurrent Plugged Ducts and Breast Infections

Some nursing mothers experience recurrent plugged ducts or breast infections. If you are suffering from either at the moment, carefully review the information in "Survival Guide: The First Two Months," starting on page 194. If you have had more than two occurrences, the following suggestions may be helpful in preventing future episodes.

Treatment Measures for Recurrent Plugged Ducts and Breast Infections

1. Be sure that you are nursing the baby frequently, and that at least one breast is emptied well at each feeding.

2. Avoid skipping or delaying feedings. Pick a quiet place to nurse if your baby gets distracted during feedings. Wake the baby at night if your breasts feel too full. If your baby routinely sleeps for long periods at night, consider pumping before you go to bed, after the first morning feeding, or both. This way you'll ensure that your breasts are completely drained at least once or twice a day.

3. To encourage complete drainage of the milk ducts, gently massage your breasts while nursing.

4. Change nursing pads whenever they become wet.

5. Get as much rest as possible. Nap whenever you can. Consider sleeping with the baby if you aren't already.

6. Make sure you are getting plenty to drink every day.

7. Check that your bra and other clothing are not too restrictive. If you use them, consider getting rid of underwire bras.

8. If you use a Medela, Ameda, Lansinoh, Spectra, Avent, or Hygeia breast pump more than once a day, try Pumpin' Pal Super Shields. These elliptical shields inserted into pump flanges gently milk the breast instead of pulling on just the nipple and areola (see Appendix A, page 386, for more information).

9. Consider taking nutritional supplements. Many lactation consultants believe that vitamin C supplements may prevent recurrences of breast infections. Some suggest that taking supplemental lecithin may prevent plugged milk ducts; start with one 1,200-milligram capsule three or four times a day, and reduce the dosage after a few weeks without another episode. (Note that these dosages of lecithin are relatively low; higher doses of lecithin can lead to depression for those who have a history of it.) If you are anemic, take a daily iron supplement.

10. If your periods have resumed, try limiting your salt intake before your period is due. A high salt intake may increase susceptibility to breast infections, and some women seem to be prone to breast infections premenstrual. This may have to do with the fact that they retain water just before their periods.

11. Try to reduce the amount of saturated fats in your diet.

12. If a plugged duct or breast infection does not go away within two or three days, consult your physician.

13. If your doctor prescribes antibiotics, take the entire course. A ten- or fourteen-day prescription may be needed. If an infection recurs in the same part of the breast shortly after antibiotic therapy has ended, the antibiotic may be ineffective. Some antibiotics do not penetrate breast tissue as well as others. Discuss this possibility with your doctor (see page 203).

14. Recurrent mastitis can also be a sign of methicillin-resistant *Staphylococcus aureus*, or MRSA (see page 204). Ask your doctor whether this might be the case.

15. Mothers experiencing recurrent plugged milk ducts may find using the "Leaf" vibrator quickly dislodges them. See Appendix A (page 386) for more.

Overabundant Milk

Some mothers continue to be bothered by an oversupply of milk after two months postpartum. You are not necessarily producing too much milk, however, if you leak or become engorged during the baby's long sleep stretches. Only if you are still feeling uncomfortably engorged most of the time should you consider decreasing your milk supply.

Treatment Measures for an Overabundance of Milk

1. Continue drinking plenty of fluids. Decreasing fluids does not decrease milk production.

2. Nurse your baby at just one breast per feeding. Let him suck as long as he likes on one side. If you become uncomfortable, express a small amount of milk from the other breast. Switch breasts with each feeding.

3. Should you be caught in a routine of expressing milk while nursing full-time, gradually decrease the amount of milk you take until you are no longer expressing any.

CONCERNS ABOUT THE BABY

Slow Weight Gain

A two- to three-month-old baby is considered a slow gainer when he is putting on less than 1 ounce (28 g) a day over a period of a few weeks. A slow-gaining three- to six-month-old is gaining less than ½ ounce (14 g) per day over a period of a few weeks.

A baby who is gaining weight slowly, not gaining at all, or losing weight may be nursing too infrequently—that is, fewer than seven times in a twenty-four-hour period. Between three and four months of age, most babies find their fingers or become avid pacifier users. Some babies stop letting their mothers know when they are hungry and instead suck away at fingers or a pacifier, decreasing the number of nursing a day. The baby who sleeps eight or more hours at a stretch each night may fail to get enough milk if he doesn't nurse at least seven times during his waking hours. A baby may also slow his weight gain if juices or solid foods have been introduced prematurely, especially if they have replaced nursing.

Parents who have decided to use "Parent Directed Feeding" or "scheduled" feedings (see page 185) often find that their babies who typically do not nurse a minimum of seven times each twenty-four hours fail to gain weight as expected.

Slow weight gain may occur, too, when a working mother fails to express her milk often enough while she is away from the baby or is using an ineffective pump, causing an overall decrease in her milk supply. Estrogen-containing birth control pills, even the low-dose kind, often decrease milk production. Occasionally, a baby who has never had normal weight gain suddenly becomes a worry to his physician and parents. This happens because health professionals do not always identify a newborn who gains less than 1 ounce (28 g) a day during the early weeks as being underfed. Eventually such a baby may become obviously underweight. This is unfortunate, since a low milk intake can be much more easily remedied if the problem is recognized early on. A milk supply that has been low for two, three, or even four months can be very difficult to improve without the help of herbs and/or medication.

Treatment Measures for Slow Weight Gain

1. Devote at least two or three days to nursing the baby and doing little else. Put the pacifier aside, and offer the breast each time you notice the baby beginning to suck a finger. You may find yourself nursing every hour or so, although increasing feedings to eight or more per twenty-four hours is usually sufficient to quickly increase milk production. If your baby is sleeping through the night, try to include at least one late-evening feeding. You might also consider waking the baby for a feeding after he has slept for five or six hours.

2. While the baby is nursing, listen for swallowing. As soon as you notice the swallowing taper off, switch breasts. Continue switching back and forth for as long as the baby is willing to continue, ideally at least ten minutes. If the baby is easily distracted, nurse in a quiet, darkened room.

3. Should your baby refuse to nurse as often as every two hours or resist switching back and forth, consider expressing or pumping

milk after each nursing to stimulate an increase in milk production. After two or three days of this regime, both the baby's nursing pattern and your milk supply should begin to improve.

4. If your baby has been losing weight or has never gained weight adequately, consider giving him supplemental formula while you work on increasing your milk supply. For instructions on estimating the amount of milk you are producing and the amount of milk your baby needs, see page 233, Underfeeding.

5. Consider taking herbs that stimulate milk production or perhaps even a pharmaceutical medication to help increase your milk production (see page 84).

6. If you are working away from the baby, try to spend two or more consecutive days at home following the above recommendations. If you can't stay home from work, express milk as often as possible.

7. After two or three days of stepped-up nursing, you should notice that your breasts feel fuller and that the baby swallows over a longer period during feedings. Continue nursing frequently, at least eight times a day. Have the baby's weight checked after a week of frequent nursing, and again a week after that. If the baby still isn't gaining well, supplementation with an ounce or two of formula after some of the feedings may be necessary.

Adding solids to a baby's diet is not a good way to deal with slow weight gain. Most solid foods are less calorie-dense than breast milk, and low-calorie foods can displace some of the milk in a baby's diet. So, feeding solids tends to slow rather than speed a baby's weight gain.

One-Sided Nursing

Occasionally a baby develops a preference for one breast over the other. Perhaps the favored breast produces more milk or lets it down more rapidly. Sometimes there is no apparent reason—the baby simply prefers one side. Twins usually choose opposite sides.

Sometimes a mother unknowingly nurses the baby more at one breast than the other, increasing milk production on that side. Some mothers prefer nursing on one side only; in certain cultures, one-sided nursing is common.

One breast can fully support a baby's nutritional needs. However, the less used breast may become noticeably smaller. After weaning, the breasts will equal out in size.

Treatment Measures for One-Sided Nursing

1. Offer the baby her least favorite side first. After she has nursed on both sides, encourage her to nurse on the first side again.
2. Should the baby totally refuse one side, try changing positions. Use the football hold, or nurse while lying on your side. The baby may be more willing when she is sleepy or actually asleep, or when you nurse in a darkened room.
3. Increase the milk supply in the less-used breast by manually expressing or pumping milk after each nursing for a few days.
4. If all else fails, simply accept your baby's preference.

Sudden Refusal to Nurse

Occasionally a baby under six months old suddenly refuses to nurse. A "nursing strike" usually lasts for a few days but sometimes for as long as two weeks. It rarely means the baby is ready to wean; weaning seldom occurs this suddenly. See page 374, Nursing Strike, for the reasons behind this problem and suggestions for coping with it.

Some babies who suffer from painful reflux may refuse to nurse. Often, though, they will take their mother's milk by bottle. See page 222, Colic and Reflux.

If your baby suddenly refuses one breast but is happy to nurse at the other, see "One-Sided Nursing" above.

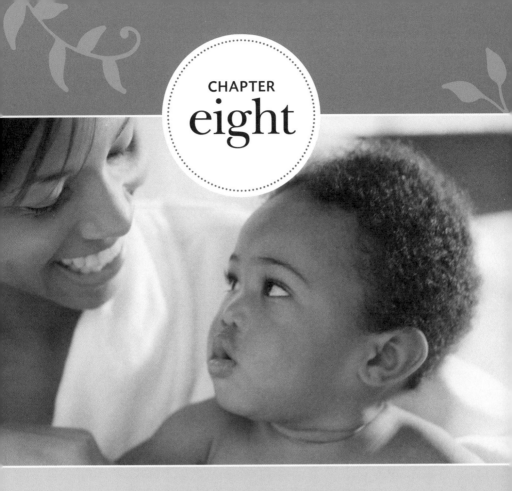

eight

NURSING THE OLDER BABY

- Caring for Yourself
- Nursing Your Six- to Twelve-Month-Old
- Coping with Night Waking
- Coping with Teething
- The Transition to Table Food
- Considering Weaning

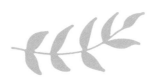

As breastfeeding progresses to six months and beyond, the nursing relationship continues to change. Although the baby is busy exploring the world around him and has probably shortened most of his nursings, breast milk continues to be his primary source of nutrients until he is well established on table foods. Breastfeeding also continues to provide protective antibodies against illness.

For you, nursing provides the opportunity to sit down for a few minutes and just enjoy your baby. Nursing may also become your main tool to help your baby fall off to sleep at naptime and bedtime.

Caring for Yourself

You may sometimes feel tired and run-down during your baby's second half-year. Becoming more active and getting overtired seem to be especially common among mothers around six months postpartum. Certainly, eating poorly and losing too much weight can contribute to a loss of energy. Taking it a bit easier, getting some extra rest, and paying attention to your diet can do a lot to improve your overall well-being. Taking brewer's yeast or a vitamin B-complex supplement may also be helpful.

Resuming Your Periods

If your periods haven't resumed yet, they may well do so during your baby's second half-year. Although some women see the resumption of their monthly cycles as early as six weeks after birth, most women's periods resume as their babies begin eating regular meals at the table.

Other women, especially those who nurse frequently, don't start menstruating until twelve to twenty-four months postpartum. Your initial periods may be lighter, heavier, or less regular than normal.

In most cases, fertility returns before menstruation. If you don't want to become pregnant again soon, you should be using some form of birth control even if your periods haven't resumed.

Both nursing mothers and their babies may feel out of sorts around the time of menstruation. Some mothers report that their babies fuss for a couple of days, or even refuse to nurse for a short time, when periods resume. Other women experience sore nipples for a few days between ovulation and the start of menstruation.

Often, a nursing mother experiences a dip in the milk supply a few days before her period starts. Although this dip tends to be greatest during the first few cycles, some women have low milk production just before their periods for as long as they continue nursing. Calcium and magnesium supplements may help; try taking 1,000 milligrams of calcium and 500 milligrams of magnesium each day from mid-cycle until your period starts. If your periods are very regular, you can also try taking fenugreek capsules or other herbal preparations in the days before you expect your period to start (see page 125, Underfeeding and Weight Loss).

Nursing Your Six- to Twelve-Month-Old

The typical baby of this age is venturing out on his own and seemingly becoming more independent, but he often scampers back to the safety and reassurance of his mother's arms. By eight to ten months, in fact, he probably cannot bear to have his mother out of his sight for even a minute. This is known as separation anxiety. Until the baby learns to trust that his mother will return, out of sight means gone forever.

During the first four months, both babies and their mothers tend to be captivated by nursing; they give it all their attention. After the first four months, babies are easily distracted; if anything catches their interest, they may pull off the breast momentarily. As your baby passes six months and develops more motor skills, he may still be somewhat distractible, and he will probably become more active during nursings.

This is a normal stage of development and a healthy part of the nursing relationship. Your baby may play with his foot and smile at you as he nurses. He may adopt some really annoying behaviors—pinching the breast, pulling or twiddling the nipple, or doing acrobatics while nursing. You can put an end to these antics by holding your baby's hand or giving him something else to hold—a beaded necklace, for instance, or a soft blanket.

When your baby is between six and twelve months of age, you should strive to be nursing about seven times a day, on average, and offering him solids only after nursing. Some people might tell you that four or five feedings a day are sufficient, but this number typically applies to formula-fed babies, who take more at a feeding and tend to eat more solids than breastfed babies of the same age. You may also hear that you should expect your baby to go longer between daytime feedings. In fact, as your baby begins to sleep longer stretches at night, he may need to nurse more frequently during the day—as often as every two hours—to get as much breast milk as he needs.

Crawling and cruising babies can be so busy that they may not "ask" to nurse as often as they should. If your baby goes longer than three hours during the day without expressing a desire to nurse, take him to a quiet, dark room and offer your breast, or put on a brightly colored scarf or beaded necklace before picking him up. Some mothers reserve a special toy just for nursing sessions.

At around seven to nine months of age, many babies go through a stage in which they seem to lose interest in nursing. The parents may be told that their babies are "self-weaning." In truth, babies rarely wean themselves without cause before one year of age, and most babies will happily nurse for two to four years without initiating weaning. In most cases of "self-weaning" in seven- to nine-month-old babies, what actually happens is a nursing strike (see page 374). Usually, the baby's normal distractibility results in infrequent nursing, which in turn causes a low milk supply. If the mother takes measures to rebuild her supply, the baby will happily return to nursing. Even if the milk supply is abundant, it's best to assume that when a baby under twelve months loses interest in nursing, he does so because of a problem that can be corrected.

Teething pain, a sore throat, a stuffy nose, and an ear infection are all possible reasons that an older baby might temporarily refuse to nurse.

Many women notice that it takes longer for their milk to letdown in the second six months of nursing. This may be a sign of a dwindling milk supply. Delayed letdown may contribute to a baby's loss of interest in the breast, especially at nine to ten months of age.

Many parents and physicians worry when weight gain in a healthy breastfed baby dramatically slows in the second six months after birth. Keep in mind that most U.S. babies are totally weaned to formula and solids by six months of age, and that formula-fed babies tend to gain more weight between six and twelve months than breastfed babies. The charts still used in most doctors' offices reflect this growth pattern. Normal weight gain for a breastfed baby between six and twelve months is 1 to 4 ounces (28 to 113 g) per week. Babies with small parents fall in the lower end of this range.

The World Health Organization's new growth charts are based on a multinational study of children who were exclusively breastfed for six months. These charts show that breastfed babies are slightly leaner and taller in later months than the old charts would lead you to expect. See the new charts in Appendix C, page 399.

Coping with Night Waking

Although some older babies and toddlers sleep well at night, most wake frequently, night after night. Your baby may in fact be waking more at night and napping less during the day than she did in the first few months. You may have thought that when your baby reached six months of age or older and started taking solid food that her nighttime wakings would diminish. You probably even know someone whose baby "sleeps through the night." But such a baby is atypical. When health professionals talk about sleeping through the night, they are referring to a six-hour stretch. Although some babies sleep a six-hour stretch, waking one to three times a night is entirely normal for babies as old as two years. Many babies who slept long stretches in the early months wake more frequently later.

You may think something is wrong if your baby doesn't sleep through the night. Well-meaning family members may say that night waking is not normal. Pediatricians may point out that a baby this age does not "need" to nurse at night. You may wonder if your baby wakes because of teething, illness, digestive problems, wet diapers, chilling or over-heating, superior intelligence, upcoming developmental milestones, or separation anxiety. Although any of these might perhaps contribute to night waking, the basic cause may simply be your baby's need for a cuddle and a snack or drink. Six- to twelve-month-olds may actually wake at night out of thirst or hunger.

As you may suspect, breastfed babies are less likely than formula-fed babies to sleep through the night. Chances are your friend's sleeping baby is already fully weaned or never nursed. One study found that whereas weaned babies slept a median of nine to ten hours at a stretch at every age after four months, nursing babies slept in bouts of four to seven hours to the end of the second year (Elias et al., 1986).

Not only do breastfed babies sleep in shorter bouts than do bottle-fed babies, nursing babies also sleep less overall. In the Elias study, weaned babies slept a median of thirteen to fourteen hours per day throughout the first two years, but nursing babies gradually lessened their total hours of sleep from a median of fourteen to a median of eleven hours.

Why do bottle-fed babies sleep in longer stretches than breastfed babies? Marsha Walker (1993), a lactation consultant, points out that babies formula-fed from birth have poor "vagal nerve tone"; that is, their autonomic nervous systems are measurably disordered. This makes them sleepier and less alert than breastfed newborns.

Babies who are weaned after several months of breastfeeding may start sleeping through the night for other reasons. They certainly have waking episodes, as everyone does, but these babies fall back into deep sleep without any intervention from parents. Most have probably learned to go back to sleep alone—through the use of a thumb, pacifier, or bottle, through their parents' ignoring them, or perhaps with a sophisticated method such as scheduled awakenings, whereby a parent rouses a child in time to prevent spontaneous awakenings, until both spontaneous and scheduled awakenings are gradually eliminated. In most of these cases, the parents' desire for separation has overcome the baby's natural urge to be close to other human beings.

No one knows for sure why weaned children sleep more overall than those who are still nursing. It seems that babies often nurse during light sleep; they release the nipple when they fall into deep sleep. This may be why a child who was obviously tired will, instead of falling asleep after a long nursing, come off the breast seeming completely refreshed. If nursing in a light-sleep state were counted as sleep, the average total hours of sleep might not vary at all between nursing and weaned children.

A baby's night wakings can be handled in a variety of ways. Some mothers find that sleeping with their babies disrupts their own sleep less, while others prefer to get up, nurse, and return the baby to a crib. If a baby wakes very frequently, it's best to figure out why. Teething, an ear infection, separation anxiety, stomach problems, an allergy, a chill from kicking off the covers, or a low milk supply are all possible causes.

For advice on getting a baby to sleep longer at night, see page 367, Survival Guide: Months Six through Twelve.

Coping with Teething

By six months of age, most babies begin teething. This can affect their nursing patterns. Some babies are less interested in nursing when their gums are tender, and others want to nurse more often, especially in the night. To soothe your baby's aching gums, give him things to bite on during the day, such as a cold, damp washcloth or a teething ring. You might freeze and slightly thaw the wet washcloth or teething ring before offering it to him. If he fusses during nursing sessions, you can rub his gums with a cold washcloth or apply Baby Orajel just before nursing. If your baby is very uncomfortable, acetaminophen drops (Infants' Tylenol) or ibuprofen drops (Infants' Motrin, Infants' Advil) may help. Check with your baby's doctor before using ibuprofen, an anti-inflammatory, and ask for the correct dosage.

Some mothers swear by amber necklaces to help their babies with teething pain. When worn against the skin, amber is believed to be a natural pain reliever and anti-inflammatory. While there are no studies on the effectiveness of amber, these necklaces have been used by

European mothers for quite some time and are now popular in the United States. The necklaces are not recommended to be worn at night, so some parents wrap them around the baby's ankle at night and cover with a sock.

Many mothers worry that the eruption of teeth means that nursing must come to an end. But babies and toddlers with teeth can and usually do nurse without causing pain to their mothers' nipples. While the baby is sucking, the tongue protects you by covering the lower teeth. In other words, so long as a baby is swallowing milk, she cannot bite. If your baby does bite you, you can take measures to make sure it doesn't happen again (see page 368, Biting).

Some mothers find that their nipples get sore during teething even though their babies aren't actually biting. When babies are cutting teeth, they may adjust their latch on the breast to put pressure on sore areas of their gums. This can make your nipples sore. To avoid the problem, ease the baby's pain before nursing with one or more of the remedies I've just described. If you feel tenderness while nursing, adjust the baby's position at the breast (see page 368, Nipple Soreness from New Teeth).

The Transition to Table Food

Around the age of six months, your baby will begin to show readiness for solid foods. You'll know he is ready when he can sit up with some support, when he reaches for food at the table, when he explores his world by grabbing objects and placing them in his mouth, and when he generally acts interested in eating what the rest of the family eats.

By six months of age a baby begins to require more nutrients than his body stores and his intake of breast milk can provide. He needs more protein and, especially, more iron and zinc. Even in a healthy, full-term baby, iron stores sometimes fail to last beyond the first months, and when this happens, a baby becomes at risk for developing iron-deficiency anemia. Babies born prematurely may need additional iron even earlier than six months. Iron-deficiency anemia is common in infants between nine and twelve months of age who do not receive iron-rich foods. If the anemia continues unabated for long, it can cause long-lasting harm to mental, motor, and behavioral functioning. Zinc-rich foods are also important, for growth and development as well as for proper immune functioning.

Throughout the twentieth century, the first foods usually recommended for babies were commercial infant cereals, followed by pureed fruits and vegetables. Most parents started feeding their babies cereal at four to six months of age. Made from refined grain, infant cereal lacks some of the nutrients of whole grain, and the iron and zinc added to the cereal are poorly absorbed by the baby's body. Because cereal is very filling and digested slowly, it tends to replace breast milk and other solids in the baby's diet, especially if the cereal is fed by spoon. When breast milk is replaced with cereal, the baby's protein intake declines.

Recently, nutritionists have developed new guidelines for starting the breastfed baby on solid food. They now recommend introducing foods rich in protein, iron, and zinc as well as fruits and vegetables at around six months of age, and whole-grain cereals and breads, rather than infant cereal, a little later.

Breast milk will continue to be your baby's most important food until he is eating three daily meals of table food, at around nine months of age. Until then, you should always nurse your baby shortly before offering him any solid foods.

Your baby's first solids need not be pureed. Pureed foods require spoon-feeding, which sometimes leads to food battles. Besides, babies always fed pureed rather than more textured foods don't learn to chew at the appropriate stage of development and may have more trouble learning later. And babies can chew with their gums.

Just as a baby learns to walk by trying, he can learn to feed himself as part of his natural development. To help him, you need only place him in a high chair or on your lap at the family

Babies born earlier than 36 weeks' gestation may not be ready for self-feeding at six months, but they may well need extra iron at this age. Some health professionals recommend spoon-feeding prematurely born babies pureed high-iron foods, such as meat, beginning at the age of six months. Others recommend giving liquid iron supplements until these babies are ready for self-feeding.

table, with a sheet or mat on the floor to make cleanup easier, and offer him appropriate foods from the family meal. Let him grab handfuls of food, transfer them to his mouth, and chew them. If your baby takes charge of what he eats and how much he eats, he will be able to feed himself regular meals by the time he is a year old.

The British midwife and breastfeeding counselor Gill Rapley is the creator of a wonderful video about what she calls baby-led weaning. You can have a brief look at the video by following the link at www.nursing motherscompanion.com/resources. To purchase the complete video or the book *Baby-Led Weaning: Helping Your Baby to Love Good Food*, by Gill Rapley and Tracey Murkett, see Appendix A, page 386. Rapley also has an informative website, www.rapleyweaning.com.

Your baby will be a clumsy eater at first. A six-month-old is not able to purposely open his fist to place food in his mouth, so you'll need to offer large chunks or sticks of fruits and cooked vegetables that your baby can grasp while still having a portion available to chew on. The baby may seem to spit much of the food out at first; this is because he is not yet good at moving food to the back of his mouth to swallow it. A baby at this stage may also gag when eating. This is not choking but a normal part of learning to eat.

Note that certain foods do pose a choking hazard; these include raw vegetables, nuts, whole grapes, raisins, and dried fruits. But the baby who is being spoon-fed is actually at greater risk for choking than the self-fed baby, because the former has less control of the process of moving food to the back of his mouth and swallowing. Nevertheless, you should never leave your baby alone while he is eating.

Offering a wide variety of fruits and vegetables will allow your baby to pick what is interesting and tasty to him. These foods are useful more for the experience of self-feeding than for the nutrients they provide. Most babies enjoy the taste and texture of fruits such as apples, bananas, apricots, peaches, nectarines, pears, avocados, mangoes, plums, and melons. (Because citrus fruits are very acidic and can cause rashes and upset stomachs, some experts suggest waiting until a baby is ten to twelve months old before offering them.) Cooked vegetables such as sweet potatoes, potatoes, carrots, squash, asparagus, broccoli, cauliflower, snap beans, and beets are also good choices for babies just starting to learn to feed themselves. (Large quantities of green and orange vegetables can give a baby's skin a yellow tinge, but this is completely harmless.)

Babies do best with little salt, if any. If you are offering cooked vegetables for the family, salt them after taking out the baby's portion, because young babies are unable to handle large amounts of sodium.

As soon as a baby is managing small amounts of fruits and vegetables, you should offer meats or other foods high in protein, iron, and zinc. Meats, such as beef, pork, and poultry, especially dark poultry flesh, are especially good sources of these nutrients. Although chicken and fish (carefully boned) are fairly easy for a baby to manage, red meats may need to be slow-cooked and shredded or ground or minced. Avoid lunch meats, hot dogs, cured sausage, and ham, which are high in salt and sodium nitrate and are not the best sources of protein.

Good non-meat sources of protein and iron include scrambled eggs, semi-hard cheeses like cheddar and Monterey Jack, nut butters (such as almond), tofu and tempeh, and tahini. Peanut butter provides protein, iron, and zinc as well as fat, but be sure to choose a brand without added fat or sugar and preferably without salt. Beans, whole wheat, and oats are also rich sources of zinc.

If any of the baby's close blood relatives, however, are allergic to egg whites, cow's milk products, nuts, soy, wheat, or fish or shellfish, you will want to postpone offering these foods to your baby. Families with food allergies should introduce wheat after seven months of age, soy after eight months of age, cow's milk products after one year, egg whites after two years, and peanuts, tree nuts, and fish and shellfish after three years.

If your baby's blood relatives have no food allergies, you shouldn't worry about your baby's developing them. The American Academy of Pediatrics recently advised that feeding commonly allergenic foods need not be postponed unless specific foods have produced allergic symptoms in a family member.

Offering new foods a few days apart can help you identify any allergy your baby may have. Signs of allergy include diarrhea, gassiness, and redness around the anus; vomiting and increased spitting up; and rashes (especially on the face), wheezing, and a runny nose.

Should you prefer that your child have a vegetarian diet, you can feed him accordingly. If cheese and eggs are not included, tofu, tempeh, and cooked legumes, when combined with whole-grain cereals, can provide protein as well as iron and zinc. Winter squash, sweet potatoes, broccoli, and dark leafy vegetables such as spinach and Swiss chard are especially good sources of iron, and iron absorption is increased a great deal when foods containing vitamin C are eaten at the same time. Do take the time to learn all you can about vegetarianism and the nutritional needs of infants and toddlers. You might want to consult with a nutritionist, especially if you are considering a vegan diet for your baby. Young children on such diets are at substantial risk for B-vitamin deficiencies and, because of a lack of protein, general growth deficiencies. The federal Special Supplemental Nutrition Program for Women, Infants, and Children (WIC) or your local public health department can probably refer you to a nutritionist who can offer further guidance.

Once your baby is eating protein foods as well as fruits and vegetables, you can also offer whole-grain breads and cereals. These offer B vitamins, iron, zinc, and all the other nutrients of the grain in its original form. Refined grains—white rice, white breads, regular pasta, and dry cereals not made from whole grains—are less healthful. Whole-grain cereals of rice, corn, and barley are good first choices, as are corn tortillas and whole-wheat pasta (I've found tastier brands of whole-wheat pasta in natural-foods stores). Whole buckwheat flour contains more protein than any other grain flour and makes delicious and nutritious pancakes. Last but not least, most babies enjoy rice cakes, some of which are made with whole-grain rice.

When shopping for breads and cereals, check the ingredients. The first ingredient should be whole wheat or another whole grain. Do not accept products made with partially hydrogenated oils (or trans fats). Try to find breads and cereals that have little or no added sugar.

As your baby progresses with his self-feeding skills, you will gradually begin to see from his diaper that he is taking in more solid foods. His stools will begin looking and smelling more like adult bowel movements.

At some point after your baby's first six months, you may want to offer him a cup to learn drinking skills. Most babies are ready to begin learning how to drink from a cup by the time they are six or seven months old. You can begin with water. A cup is also useful for feeding semi-liquid foods like yogurt. Many parents offer fruit juice, but juice offers no nutritional advantage over fruit, and it often lessens a baby's appetite for milk and solid foods. "Juice abuse" is a common mistake in infant feeding that can lead to diarrhea, dental decay, and possibly childhood obesity.

If you give your baby juice, limit it to 3 ounces (89 ml) a day, and offer it only alongside a meal or snack. Be careful with citrus, tomato, and pineapple juices, which can cause reactions in babies. Avoid "fruit drinks"; they contain mostly water and sugar or corn syrup. If you buy juice in a metal can, transfer it to another container after the can is opened.

Once your baby begins drinking from a cup, be prepared for her to turn the cup over to see what happens—all part of the learning process. You can try a sippy cup, one with either a spout or a straw, which comes with a tight-fitting lid and therefore won't spill.

At around seven to nine months of age, your baby will be able to use his thumb and fingers to pick up both large and smaller pieces of food. He'll be able to eat brown rice, diced meat, or small pieces of pasta, fruits, and vegetables with his fingers.

Once the baby is doing well with different food groups, you can offer him more complex family foods, such as pasta, casserole dishes, and sandwiches. But try to minimize the salt in your cooking until the baby is at least a year old.

The baby will begin to use cutlery, if you let him, sometime between ten and eleven months of age. At this point he'll be able to spoon-feed himself yogurt and cooked cereals. By the time he reaches his first birthday, your baby will probably be proficient with a spoon and fork.

When your baby is eating table foods fairly well, you can give him regular meals and snacks. Offer three or four small servings of whole-grain cereal or bread per day and at least four daily servings of fruits and vegetables, at 1 to 2 tablespoons (15 to 30 ml) per serving. The baby also needs at least two daily servings of high-protein foods. A serving of meat, poultry, fish, or eggs is about 1 tablespoon (15 ml), or ½ ounce (14 g). The baby can have an egg three or four times a week. Should allergies be a concern, cook the egg until solid and offer only the yolk. Other high-protein servings for a baby of this age might be 1 ounce (28 g) of semi-hard cheese, ¼ cup (60 ml) of cottage cheese, or ½ cup (120 ml) of cooked shell beans or lentils.

While your baby may not always get precisely the suggested amounts of grains, fruits, vegetables, and high-protein foods every day, averaging close to these amounts over a week will ensure he is well nourished. But if by eight to ten months your baby will still take solids only sporadically at best, it may be time to give him a little extra encouragement. In this case, try nursing after meals, not before. If he is desperate for the breast, try to keep the nursing short, and then encourage him to return his attention to other foods. Always include him in family meals, but offer food at other times of the day if he refuses it at mealtimes. Never assume that because he spits something out in disgust one day he won't take it a week later.

One of the last transitions is postponing breastfeeding until after the meal; this encourages the baby to take more solids. I recommend making this transition at ten to twelve months.

After the baby is established on table foods, the final transition is serving cow's milk along with the meal. Ideally, this should be accomplished when the baby is around twelve months of age (a baby much younger than that can't digest cow's milk well). Use whole milk; low-fat milk does not provide the fat that the older baby or toddler needs. If the rest of the family drinks low-fat milk, you might feed the baby whole evaporated milk, diluted one to one with water. Because evaporated milk is treated with high heat, it is more digestible than whole milk, and it is no more expensive. If your baby is allergic to milk and is not yet one year old, use soy formula or hypoallergenic formula instead. If your baby does not like any milk but yours, offer plenty of cheese and yogurt, and try tofu—it is also very high in calcium.

After your baby's first year, you can feed him regular soy milk in place of cow's milk or formula, provided that the soy milk is whole, not low-fat or nonfat, because fat is important for brain development in children under two years of age. The soy milk you choose should also be fortified with vitamins A and D and calcium. Try to offer plenty of calcium-rich or calcium-fortified foods as well, because soy milk contains phytates, which can reduce the absorption of calcium and other minerals.

You may be wondering if we have just weaned your baby. In a sense, yes. Weaning is the process of expanding a baby's diet to include other foods. For another year or two or more, however, nursing may continue to be important and convenient for early morning feedings, snacks, naps, bedtime, and general soothing and comforting.

Considering Weaning

For any of various reasons, you may be considering giving up nursing altogether. If you truly resent breastfeeding, if you need to stop because of a serious illness, or if you are planning to get pregnant soon, you can wean completely and easily at this stage.

Perhaps there are other reasons you want to stop nursing. Maybe months ago you set a time limit for breastfeeding, or maybe you think your baby is simply too old to nurse. You may have heard that older babies bite or that weaning a toddler is just too difficult.

Or you may hope that ending breastfeeding will solve various problems like the shape of your body, fatigue, marital troubles, or sibling rivalry. Rarely does total weaning solve problems like these.

It is normal to feel ambivalent about nursing. Sometimes you may wish you could be free of this intense relationship, and other times you may adore putting your baby to your breast and watching him fall off to sleep there. Such ambivalence is a natural part of an intimate relationship. Simply recognizing this may help put your mind at ease.

Perhaps the problem is friends and relatives. If they have started asking when you plan to wean the baby, you may feel pressured to give up nursing. Our society seems to rush babies and toddlers toward independence. Keep in mind that nursing is still providing your baby with protective antibodies; even at twelve months, a baby has only 60 percent of an adult's ability to fight off infection. If a friend's baby weaned early and easily, remember that some babies need the comfort of the breast much longer than others. Babies who are allowed to wean themselves do so when they feel that their source of security will always be there when they need it.

Since your nursing older baby will soon be a talking nursing older baby, you might consider what word you'll feel comfortable hearing your baby use in public for breastfeeding. Words like booby might be fine at home, but they could cause you embarrassment elsewhere. You might choose a term such as *nursie* or *numnums* or use a word that your baby makes up.

You won't, of course, be able to hide your nursing relationship from your partner. If they are bothered by your breastfeeding, you can talk about its benefits to your baby's health and to your family's finances. If your baby is waking at night, you might invite your partner to take over night duty.

You can find support for your continued nursing by seeking out mother-to-mother support groups such as La Leche League. See Appendix A, page 386, to learn how to find a local group.

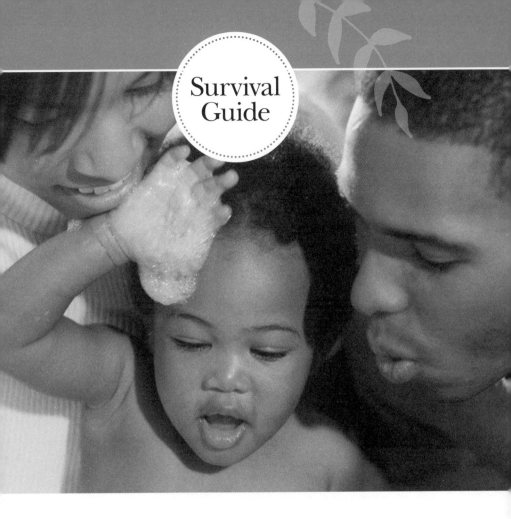

Survival Guide

MONTHS SIX THROUGH TWELVE

CONCERNS ABOUT YOURSELF

- Nipple Soreness from New Teeth

CONCERNS ABOUT THE BABY

- Biting
- Night Waking
- Nursing Strike
- Weaning the Older Baby

CONCERNS ABOUT YOURSELF

Nipple Soreness from New Teeth

Your nipples can become temporarily sore when the baby's new top teeth erupt. New teeth must be very thin and sharp to make their way through the tough gums, and this can cause you some discomfort until they thicken up after a few weeks.

Coping Measures for Dealing with New Teeth

1. Because the baby's mouth tends to drag down the breast tissue, it may help to lift her upward by using a pillow and lifting your breast upward.
2. Experiment with other nursing positions to see which positions are more comfortable.
3. If the baby is letting her chin rest on her chest, try to get her head tilted back a little more.
4. Offer your breast with the nipple pointing downward and wait for a wide-open mouth before latching.
5. After nursings, rinse your nipples with cool water and apply a thin coating of modified lanolin ointment.

CONCERNS ABOUT THE BABY

Biting

While not all babies bite, some do. In fact, some mothers actually decide against breastfeeding out of fear of being bitten, or may end breastfeeding prematurely when their babies begin to get teeth. Being bitten can be painful, and it can also make a mother tense for fear it will happen again. Some mothers may wonder if this is the baby wanting to be weaned, which is not the case. Most of the time, biting is a temporary problem, and babies can be taught not to bite. The behavior may continue for a few days, but it usually ends as suddenly as it began.

If your baby has bitten you, there are a few things you should know. Most importantly, babies don't do this intentionally, and they certainly don't understand that they are causing you pain. Second, babies cannot bite when they are actively sucking and drinking milk, as their tongues cover their lower teeth. But with that being said, they can certainly stop sucking, pull their tongue back, and bite down. Your baby is most likely to bite at the end of a feeding or when she is just snacking; she may have a playful look on her face and may push the nipple to the front of her mouth just before she takes a chomp. So, if you are bitten by your baby, do not nurse her again until you are sure she is hungry.

If you are bitten, there are a few ways to react. Biting hurts, and there is no reason not to let your baby know by responding with an unpleasant natural noise, like "No!" or "Ouch!" This doesn't work with all babies, however; some get so frightened that they go on a nursing strike. Others enjoy the reaction and want to continue the "game."

This is likely the first disciplining you will do as a mother. The goal is to teach your baby that biting is unacceptable behavior. I think that the most effective thing to do after being bitten is to simply end the nursing session so that the baby learns that biting is not allowed while nursing. If the baby bites down and does not let go, put your finger in between his gums to release the suction.

Many mothers are told to respond to biting by flicking their baby's cheek or pulling him in toward the breast so that he cannot take a breath and will let go. I am not a fan of either of these tactics, as both seem variations on hurting the baby back in some way. Babies are learning to trust in their first year, and I don't think it is an emotionally healthy response for the person that they love and depend on most in the world to hurt them in any way.

A baby most commonly bites before her teeth come in, often just before the top two teeth break through. Your baby may bite your breast because she is biting everything and anything in an attempt to relieve the ache in her gums. Mothers may be given the go-ahead by their baby's doctor to give acetaminophen drops (Infants' Tylenol) or ibuprofen drops (Infants' Motrin, Infants' Advil) for teething pain. Some mothers use these medications an hour or so before nursing, but this may still not prevent biting. For more suggestions to help ease your baby's teething pain, see page 357, Coping with Teething.

Occasionally a baby's bite can cause a wound on the nipple. In the case of a painful wound, it may be necessary to temporarily express milk by using hand expression or pumping. Nipple wounds (like all human bites) can easily become infected. If a bite wound is not healing after a couple of days, it may contain bacteria, so you should seek help from your doctor and be treated with an antibiotic. Wounded nipples that are not healing may also lead to mastitis. Mastitis comes with fever and flu-like symptoms and can lessen milk production on that breast, which in some cases can become permanent.

Coping Measures for Biting

1. Avoid letting the baby snack at the breast during this period of biting. If the baby has nursed well within the past hour or so, delay the next feeding.

2. Shortly before your baby is due for a feeding, offer her a cold, damp washcloth or a chilled water-filled teething ring.

3. While you're nursing, watch for a change in your baby's nursing pattern. As soon as she stops taking long, even sucks and begins short, choppy ones, end the feeding—with your finger if necessary. If you notice a playful look on her face, end the feeding. Instead of paying attention to the TV, talking on the phone, or engaging in other activities, pay attention to your baby and stay vigilant during nursings so that you can tell when the baby is starting to lose interest and you can end the feeding.

4. If you resume nursing and the baby tries to bite again, she is obviously not hungry anymore. End the feeding.

Night Waking

Whether or not you've identified a reason for frequent night waking, you may be spending a considerable amount of energy trying to end it. Manipulating daytime naps, feeding solids late in the evening, giving medicine when the baby isn't sick or in pain, trying to keep the baby from falling asleep at the breast, consulting health-care providers, and trying different tactics in the middle of the night rarely work.

This is not to say that you shouldn't have your baby examined if you suspect a physical discomfort. She could be hurting from an ear infection (especially if she has had a runny nose in the past couple of weeks) or from teeth working their way in. Some babies who are distracted during daytime nursings may wake often at night out of hunger.

If your baby seems to be waking from teething pain, you can try giving her acetaminophen drops (Infants' Tylenol) or ibuprofen drops (Infants' Motrin, Infants' Advil). If the medication wears off before it's time to give another dose, you can "piggyback" the two pain relievers—that is, give the other in the meantime. But call your doctor's office for advice first.

Offering pacifiers, bottles, or other comfort objects in the night is not likely to get you a full night's sleep. Most parents who try these things must get up at night to find them when their babies wake up crying. Besides, unless a bottle is filled with water, a baby risks developing tooth decay when she falls asleep at night drinking from one.

There are simple ways you can help your baby sleep for longer periods at night. First, leave the baby alone if she doesn't need you immediately. Babies may make a lot of noises as they sleep, and not all of them signal a need to be fed. Listen before responding, and learn to distinguish which sounds are feeding requests and which are not. Soothing music can help a baby relax and drift off to sleep, and to fall back to

Childhood dental health becomes an important concern once a baby's teeth erupt. Clean the new teeth once or twice a day with a tiny amount of fluoride toothpaste and a soft cloth or very soft toothbrush. Although research indicates that breast milk has a protective effect against dental caries, some of that protection seems to be lost once a baby begins eating solids, and the presence of other carbohydrates along with breast milk in the diet can lead to caries. The American Academy of Pediatric Dentists recommends having a child's teeth first checked for decay at about the age of twelve months.

sleep when she wakes in the night. White noise (sounds of different frequencies combined together) is another tool that might lull the baby to sleep. You can buy a white-noise machine.

One way some parents succeed at making a baby sleep through the night is by letting her "cry it out" for a few nights or more. Several books tout this technique, perhaps the best known among them being Richard Ferber's *Solve Your Child's Sleep Problems*. The idea is to refuse to pick up your baby when she wakes during the night, and to let her cry herself back to sleep, until she finally learns that her crying is fruitless and stops crying in the night. Many parents report that this method has worked for them.

To other parents, though, the cry-it-out method seems too drastic, and some mental-health experts warn against it. No studies have shown that it is safe, these experts point out, and it certainly seems inconsistent with infants' emotional needs.

If you decide to try the cry-it-out method, or "controlled crying," choose a three- to four-day period in advance. When your baby wakes crying, go to her every 5 minutes. Lay her down, say "It's night-night time," and leave. Most babies cry for up to an hour or more the first night, and for a shorter time the next two or three nights. If this technique solves your night-waking problem, you can still continue nursing during the day.

A kinder way of training babies to sleep through the night is advocated by Elizabeth Pantley, a mother of four and the co-author of *The No-Cry Sleep Solution*. The no-cry method involves long naps early in the day, before-bed routines, and early bedtimes. Nighttime wakings are handled this way: As soon as the baby cries, you nurse her back to sleep. Over time, you gradually shorten the baby's time at the breast, with the aim of ending the nursing as soon as she stops actively sucking, before she is fully asleep (you must stay awake yourself, of course, to manage this). When the baby can fall back to sleep without extended sucking, you comfort her when she wakes just by patting her on the back and repeating a soothing word. Eventually, the baby should be able to go back to sleep on her own with just a word. If the baby shares your bed, you may want to help her stay asleep by holding her hand against your breast. Pantley's book includes sleep charts for tracking the baby's progress.

After developing her method with her own children, Pantley tested it on 200 other mother-baby pairs. More than half of the mothers had their babies sleeping through the night within three weeks, according to Pantley, and 92 percent succeeded within two months.

If Pantley's and Ferber's methods fail to work for you, consider the way nursing mothers all over the world have made night waking less disruptive: sleep with your baby. Despite what people say, your baby won't be smothered by the covers, by you, or by your mate. The baby won't keep you awake; babies with easy access to the breast rarely cry at night. After a few nights you'll adjust to the new sleeping companion, and her presence will not disrupt your sleep as much as would waking to her cries, getting out of bed, tending to her, and coming back to bed again. Neither you nor your baby will need to waken completely to nurse.

If having a baby in your bed sounds like a damper on sexual activity, couples who have adopted this approach seldom complain about a lack of sex. Parents do mention how much they enjoy watching their baby sleep, cuddling her warm little body, and waking up with her in the morning.

Families have come up with many inventive ways to make the "family bed" more comfortable, safe, and convenient. You might buy a larger mattress, build a platform for mattresses placed side by side, or simply put your mattress on the floor. Get a waterproof mattress pad so your mattress stays dry; so you stay dry, double-diaper the baby or use disposables at bedtime. This will eliminate most nighttime diaper changes; when you must get up, a low-wattage night-light will make things easier.

If you have doubts about sleeping with your baby, you might still try it for a couple of weeks before dismissing the idea. You can find more detailed advice on bed sharing in Dr. James McKenna's *Sleeping with Your Baby: A Parent's Guide to Cosleeping* (see page 423, References & Reading).

If you're still feeling worn out after you've found some way to get more sleep at night, you might examine your diet. Some lactating women may be vulnerable to fatigue because of vitamin B deficiencies. Although in such a case, the baby will generally grow well and get the nutrients she needs from her mother's milk, her mother may suffer from low energy levels. Be sure you are eating plenty of whole grains, which are rich in B vitamins.

You might also consider supplementing your diet with brewer's yeast, a potent source of B vitamins that is considered more effective and faster acting than B-complex supplements. Available in health-food stores, brewer's yeast can be taken as a tablet or as a powder. Starting with the daily dose recommended on the label, you can slowly increase the amount to two to four times the daily recommendation (increasing the amount too quickly could cause diarrhea in you and your baby).

Nursing Strike

Although nursing strikes can occur at any time, they usually happen in the second half of the baby's first year. A nursing strike is distinguished from weaning by its suddenness. Some babies wean themselves between eight and twelve months of age, but they usually do so gradually.

Reasons for nursing strikes vary greatly. They may include teething, a cold, an ear infection, a painful herpes sore in the mouth, or a change in the taste of the milk. They sometimes happen after a prolonged separation between a baby and his mother, or after a baby has bitten his mother and been frightened by her response. Sometimes, when a baby has become used to a bottle and its rapid flow of milk, his refusal to nurse is a response to his mother's dwindling milk supply. Some authorities believe a nursing strike may precede mastery of a major motor skill, such as crawling, standing, or walking.

Although some mothers decide to turn a nursing strike into final weaning, in most cases the baby can be coaxed to resume nursing. Strikes typically last a few days, but they may go on for as long as two weeks.

Treatment Measures for Nursing Strikes

1. Try a change in position, or nurse in a quiet, darkened room.
2. So long as the baby refuses to nurse, pump or manually express your milk frequently throughout the day. Offer the milk in a cup rather than a bottle.
3. Try to determine the cause for the nursing strike. Consider having the baby examined to rule out an ear infection or other physical problem. Check your milk supply, especially if the baby has

been nursing infrequently or has become increasingly dependent on a bottle: Do your breasts feel empty most of the time? Is the milk slow to letdown? Is the baby swallowing less?

4. Maintain frequent and close skin-to-skin contact with the baby without nursing. Offer the breast whenever the baby is sleepy.

Weaning the Older Baby

Weaning the older baby need not be hard, especially if she is crawling and busily exploring or has lost interest in some of her nursings. Ideally, weaning at any age should occur gradually, over several weeks at least. A good place to begin is with the nursing that the baby seems least interested in, most likely one during the day. Key to your success is providing an appealing substitute for the breast. This means offering not only something else to eat or drink, but also yourself. Nursing provides a mother's love and attention as well as food. You'll need to do a lot of cuddling and rocking and activities like reading a book or playing on the floor together.

You must choose whether to wean to a cup or a bottle. Although the older baby is developmentally ready for a cup, if she has trouble swallowing from one, the bottle may be best. However, giving the baby a bottle can lead to other difficulties, such as becoming overdependent on the bottle, losing interest in solid foods, and tooth decay. And if you wean the baby to a bottle, you will probably need to wean her *from* it later on.

Unless the baby is well established on table foods and eating three meals a day, give formula before offering solid foods.

Although weaning may progress quickly for some babies, concluding in a month or two, other babies take longer, especially those who are especially fond of nursing or are reluctant to give up certain feedings. The first nursing in the morning and those before naptime and bedtime are often most loved by the older baby. It may take longer to eliminate these completely. For helpful advice, read *The Nursing Mother's Guide to Weaning* (see page 423, References & Reading).

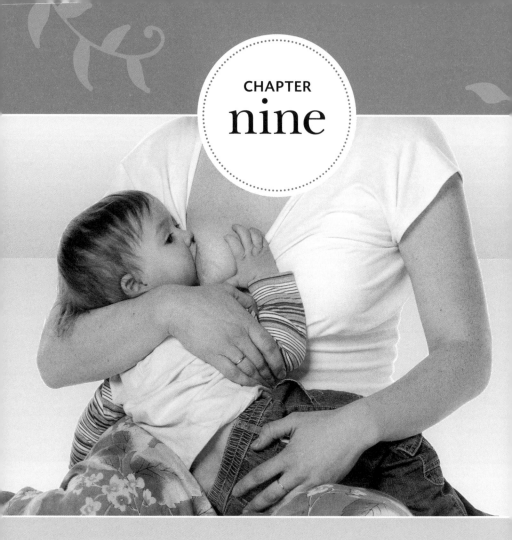

CHAPTER

nine

NURSING YOUR TODDLER

- Nursing during Pregnancy
- Tandem Nursing
- Your Toddler's Diet
- Weaning Your Toddler

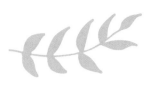

THE TODDLER IS TRYING TO ACCOMPLISH the major task of establishing himself as an individual. Although he is no longer a baby, he is still very dependent. One minute he is exploring and getting into everything, and the next he is turning to his mother for comfort and reassurance.

Many toddlers tend to nurse briefly. Some nurse just a few times a day, but many want the breast often. Or a toddler may nurse just a few times one day, and many times the next.

Even if a toddler nurses infrequently, nursing is important to him. The antibodies in breast milk are still present and protective. The toddler wants the breast for quick snacks, help in falling off to sleep, and intermittent comfort and emotional refueling. Sometimes nursing is one of the toddler's few connections to a busy mother. You may discover that nursing into toddlerhood is not only a convenient way of mothering, it is also one of the few times during the day that your child holds still long enough for cuddling and affection.

Some nursing toddlers still wake at night for feedings. See page 340, Night Waking, for suggestions and coping strategies. If you are sleeping with your baby, you might find additional help from the suggestions of Dr. Jay Gordon at www.drjaygordon.com/attachment/sleeppattern.html.

The young toddler may be quite insistent when he wants to nurse, regardless of the time or place. As he gets a bit older, he will become more willing to wait a little while.

Although children in many parts of the world are breastfed until they are two, three, or four years of age, nursing a walking, talking toddler is considered somewhat deviant in parts of Western society. Many toddlers are dependent on a bottle, pacifier, thumb, or blanket, and this is quite accepted, but a mother who is nursing a toddler may have to deal with veiled or point-blank suggestions that her child is too old for it. The concerns about nursing beyond infancy often reflect the fear that a child will become spoiled or overdependent. In fact, when a toddler's need for security is met, he becomes more self-assured and independent.

Mothers who are nursing toddlers usually enjoy socializing with others who are doing the same. La Leche League not only voices support for women who breastfeed beyond the first year but also offers meetings for those who are nursing one-, two-, three-, or even four-year-olds (see Appendix A, page 386, for more information on La Leche). Norma Jane Bumgarner's book *Mothering Your Nursing Toddler* is an excellent resource for those nursing beyond infancy (see page 423, References & Reading).

Nursing during Pregnancy

Although many people frown on breastfeeding during pregnancy, there is no reason you cannot continue nursing your child, if you're comfortable doing so, when you find out another is on the way. Fears that nursing will harm a fetus have no basis, even for mothers who are too queasy to eat much. No studies have shown that nursing during pregnancy leads to miscarriage or poor growth. When to stop nursing is up to you—but it's best to be sure your child is regularly eating solid foods and drinking from a cup before you give up nursing completely.

Even with frequent nursing, pregnancy often causes a decrease in milk supply, particularly at mid-pregnancy. The milk becomes quite salty as the supply diminishes, and at about the start of the third trimester, colostrum replaces milk in preparation for the newborn. If your baby is not yet a year old when you notice your milk supply declining, you may need to supplement your milk with formula. After the first year, though, you can substitute whole dairy milk, served in a cup (see page 380, Your Toddler's Diet).

It is thought that about half of nursing babies and toddlers wean during their mothers' pregnancies, some on their own and the rest with encouragement from their mothers. The other half do not seem to mind the changes in the milk and show no signs of wanting to give up nursing. This can be problematic, because many women who nurse while pregnant experience tender breasts and sore nipples. Caused by the hormonal changes of pregnancy, this soreness usually goes away as the pregnancy progresses, but in the meantime the pain may be so great that you feel you can't go on breastfeeding. In this case, see page 381, Weaning Your Toddler.

Some mothers feel agitated while nursing during pregnancy. This is apparently a physiological response.

Many nursing women also feel especially tired after becoming pregnant again. This is a normal response to pregnancy. Plenty of rest helps combat fatigue, especially in the first trimester. Nursing your baby or toddler may actually help you deal with fatigue, since breastfeeding is a relaxing way to mother a baby who is tired, hurt, or demanding of your time.

Some pregnant mothers may notice uterine contractions while nursing. No studies have shown that such contractions lead to premature labor, but if you have had a previous premature labor, you should discuss this possibility with your doctor.

Tandem Nursing

Mothers who have nursed throughout all or most of their pregnancies may find themselves nursing an older baby or toddler along with the new baby. This may be overwhelming for some, particularly if the older child is nursing frequently. But many have found it to be a generally positive experience.

Because the breasts receive more stimulation with two babies than with only one, the milk is usually plentiful. As a rule, the younger baby should be nursed first, but the supply is likely to be so abundant that the timing of feedings may not be essential. In fact, mothers nursing two often end up with an oversupply of milk.

It's hard to know how your nursing toddler will react to the baby's arrival. Some toddlers want to nurse more often after than during pregnancy, and others cut back or wean entirely. Some siblings sweetly bond while nursing together, but often toddlers become possessive of their mothers' breasts. Nursing or not, older children may struggle with having to share Mom with a new baby. You may need to set limits if your toddler acts out because of jealousy.

Should you decide to wean the older sibling while nursing the new baby, ideally you should do so gradually. It may be tricky to keep the older child's mind off nursing while breastfeeding the baby in front of him. Reducing the number and length of nursings and providing distractions can be helpful in gradual weaning. See opposite, Weaning Your Toddler.

Bumgarner's *Mothering Your Nursing Toddler* includes a detailed section on tandem nursing. A book wholly devoted to this topic is Hilary Flower's *Adventures in Tandem Nursing: Breastfeeding during Pregnancy and Beyond* (see page 423, References & Reading).

Your Toddler's Diet

Toddlers are notoriously sporadic eaters. Their appetites decrease during this time—first because their growth slows greatly from that of the first year, and second because they are often too busy to eat. The toddler grows more in length than in weight. Weight gain typically slows to no more than a pound every two months. (In Appendix C, page 399, you'll find the World Health Organization's new growth charts, which show the normal weight of breastfed babies and children all over the world.)

The toddler's feeding skills vary considerably. Sometimes she may feed herself, and other times she may want to be fed. Parents who worry about how little their child eats may be tempted to persuade, trick, or even force her to eat more. This turns meals into battles and may be the start of long-term eating problems. As Ellyn Satter author of *Child of Mine; Feeding with Love and Good Sense* (2000), says, "You are responsible for *what* your child is offered to eat, *where* and *when* it is presented. She is responsible for *how much* of it she eats."

The suggested minimum servings of foods for the toddler are similar to those for the older baby. A handy rule of thumb is this: Give 1 tablespoon per year of age or one-quarter of the adult serving, whichever is easiest to figure for the particular food. You would therefore offer your toddler 2 tablespoons of peas or one-quarter of an apple. The suggested daily minimum servings for each food group are as follows:

- Fruits and vegetables: 4 servings
- Grains (bread, cereal, noodles, rice): 4 servings

- High-protein foods: 2 servings
- Whole milk: 2 to 3 cups

Offering a meal or nutritious snack every three to four hours is a good approach with a toddler. Don't always offer milk just because she likes it; if she drinks more than three cups a day, it may replace other nutritious foods in her diet. Expect that your toddler may enjoy a certain food one day and refuse it the next. Make sure she comes to the table for meals and is offered whatever foods the family is eating. Do not play into her food whims by running out to the kitchen to fix something else for her when she refuses to eat.

Weaning Your Toddler

Ideally, complete weaning occurs when both the child and the mother are ready for it. Many times, though, a mother begins to think about bringing breastfeeding to a close while her toddler is still happily nursing. She may feel that full weaning will make things easier—that it will put an end to night waking, make the baby more independent, or improve her own energy level. Some mothers have a self-imposed deadline for ending breastfeeding and begin to feel pressured once it draws near. Others simply become fearful that their children will nurse forever if allowed. Most often, a mother considers full weaning when other people suggest that the baby should no longer need to nurse.

All mothers have mixed feelings about nursing at times. Keep in mind that ending breastfeeding will not help your child sleep through the night, improve your relationship with your partner, make you less tired or less bored, or make your child less dependent on you. Toddlers, especially, often demand to nurse more when their mothers become busier and when they receive little mothering except at the breast. At those times that young children need more attention, ironically, mothers often most feel that they need some kind of a break. Stopping breastfeeding during one of these times could be terribly upsetting for a child and for the rest of the family as well. Should the arbitrary date you had in mind for full weaning arrive, there is no need to follow through if you and your child are still enjoying nursing.

Knowing all this, you may still have trouble dealing with the disapproval of friends and family members. Families in particular can wield tremendous influence over a nursing relationship. You may be able to deal with criticism from others by either ignoring it or confronting it. Or you may choose to withdraw from those who are critical and find new friends who believe in nursing older babies; a mother-to-mother support group, such as the Nursing Mothers Counsel or La Leche League (see Appendix A, page 386), is one place to do this. Finally, you might simply keep your nursing secret from those who don't approve. This may be easy if you're nursing only at night and in the early morning.

When a baby is still nursing often and enthusiastically at the end of his first year, he will probably want to continue nursing throughout the second year and beyond. Some experts say that a child rarely initiates weaning before the age of four. For this reason friends may tell you to wean by your baby's first birthday if you have definite feelings against nursing a three-year-old. You may fear that if you wait, you will have a major struggle convincing your child to stop nursing in the months to follow. That toddlers seldom initiate weaning, however, doesn't mean that they always fight it. Should you find yourself still happily nursing at your baby's first birthday, be assured that there will probably be several opportune times to wean and numerous techniques to accomplish weaning after a year of age and before the age of four.

You might rightly stop breastfeeding if you have definite feelings against nursing a toddler or nursing while pregnant. Full weaning—or just limiting the number of daily feedings—may also be best if you are starting to resent nursing.

The decision to give up breastfeeding should be made carefully. Timing is important once you've decided to wean. Keep in mind that weaning is a process rather than an event. Weaning initiated by the mother should ideally occur gradually and empathetically over several weeks, at least. And there are better times than others to initiate the process. If the child is particularly clingy and needy, if he has recently had a stressful experience such as moving or starting childcare, or if you are actively trying to get him to sleep through the night, now is not the time to wean.

In general, mother-led weaning involves substituting for nursing something that the child enjoys as much. In this way weaning does not become a series of deprivations or rejections. If the pace of weaning is too rapid, most children will react with obvious unhappiness or increased dependency on a pacifier, a thumb, or a bottle. Occasionally, full weaning must be postponed for a few weeks because the child is simply unable to cope without nursing.

Unfortunately, no one technique works for every mother and toddler. The best recommendations involve finding substitutions and distractions that may satisfy the child while at the same time ensuring that his needs for food, love, and attention are met. No plan is likely to succeed, however, unless a mother is sure of her own desire to wean. Her attitude is most important to her success.

Before you begin, pay close attention to the child's nursing routine, and yours. Keeping a record for a few days, like the one below, may give you some valuable insights for developing an effective plan.

TIME	PLACE	INTEREST LEVEL	REASON FOR NURSING
1:15 P.M.	living room	moderate	attention (I was talking on the phone)
5:30 P.M.	kitchen	moderate	hunger
8:00 P.M.	living room	high	sleepiness

Take note of when and where you nurse, the child's level of interest in nursing, and what you think prompted his demand for the breast. From the toddler's point of view, nursing may be just the thing whenever he is bored, frustrated, or tired, or he wants your attention or comfort—as well as when he is hungry.

From your observations, you should be able to identify which nursings are least crucial to your toddler and get some clues as to what type of substitutions will most likely satisfy him. Some nursings may be easily replaced with a nutritious snack or something to drink. Substitutions for toddlers may include any number of activities—playing with a special toy, reading a book, taking a walk, or visiting with another toddler.

Warm-weather months may be an easier time to encourage weaning, as most toddlers enjoy exploring out of doors.

Although you may be able to substitute certain predictable daily nursings with other activities, if your toddler nurses sporadically all day, you may sometimes need to coax him to postpone nursings. Delaying daytime nursings works well for some toddlers, as long as some distraction is provided. This can be an effective way to further weaning.

Some of your nursings are probably associated with routines the two of you have established, and with recurrent situations in which your toddler wants to nurse to get your attention. Identify these instances so you can change the pattern. If you nurse in bed early in the morning, get up instead. Get dressed, and offer your child a breakfast of table food. If you have a favorite place to relax and nurse, stay away from it. If your toddler demands to nurse every time you talk on the phone, keep conversations short. If you sit in front of the television and nurse, do something else or he will want to continue with the usual pattern. Think creatively of ways your child can learn new routines.

You can also take advantage of your child's ability to understand language. Talk to him about nursing—especially if you are trying to postpone feedings. He may accept your wish to "save up the milk till naptime and night-night." Older toddlers may be able to agree to future weaning upon an upcoming birthday or other milestone, such as the start of preschool.

The bedtime nursing may continue as the child's favorite. Some mothers find this is a special time for themselves as well and continue with it for weeks or months after other feedings have been abandoned. If you want to wean your toddler completely, your partner or another family member may be able to help the child establish a non-nursing bedtime routine.

More suggestions for easing weaning can be found under Weaning the Older Baby, page 375, and in *The Nursing Mother's Guide to Weaning* (see page 423, References & Reading).

Once nursings become infrequent, your breasts may look smaller and feel less firm. Still, you may be able to express milk for several months after nursing has stopped. Your breasts will probably regain their former size and shape within six months of weaning.

Whether you initiate weaning or whether it is a mutual undertaking, you are bound to feel a little sad as the final days of nursing arrive, marking the end of the precious time you and your child spent together nursing. I hope you will also feel proud of yourself, for the wonderful start in life that you have given your child.

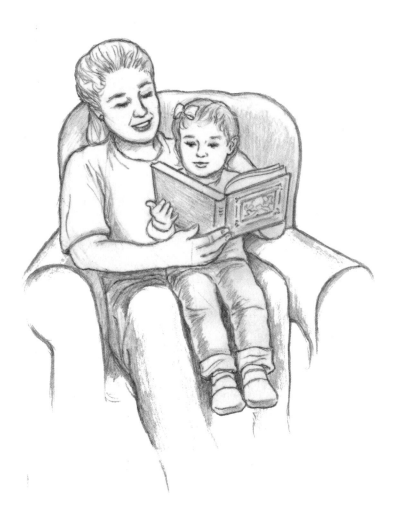

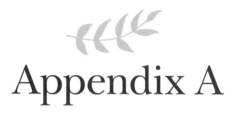

Appendix A
Resources for Nursing Mothers

....

BREASTFEEDING SUPPORT AND EDUCATION

The following organizations offer new mothers breastfeeding support and resources.

Boston Association for Childbirth Education and Nursing Mothers' Council
(617) 244-5102; www.bace-nmc.org
Local mothers can call or visit the website to find breastfeeding counselors in the area.

La Leche League International
1-800-LaLeche (1-800-525-3243); www.llli.org
This is an administrative contact number only. They do not provide breastfeeding assistance. Instead, they refer callers to local Leaders. Call or check the website for a referral to a local La Leche League group or La Leche League leader.

Nursing Mothers Counsel
San Francisco Bay Area Chapter: (650) 327-6455; www.nursingmothers.org
Santa Cruz Chapter: (831) 688-3954; www.nursingmothers.org
Counselors are available to take calls seven days a week. Free breastfeeding classes and home visits are available to mothers who live in the area. The San Francisco Bay Area Chapter rents and sells breast pumps and also has grant pumps available at reduced rates for those in need. Local chapters are also available. Check the website for more information.

LACTATION PROFESSIONAL REFERRAL SERVICES

International Lactation Consultant Association
(888) 452-2478 (United States and Canada); www.ilca.org
Call weekdays between 9:00 a.m. and 5:00 p.m. ET. To find a local breastfeeding resource, click on "find a lactation consultant" on the website.

DRUG AND MEDICATION SAFETY INFORMATION

You may find answers to your questions about medications and breastfeeding in Appendix D.

Infant Risk Center at Texas Tech University
(806) 352-2519; www.infantrisk.com
The Infant Risk Center, developed by Dr. Thomas Hale, is available to nursing mothers who have concerns about the safety and risks of taking medications—both prescriptions, over-the-counter, and recreational—and drugs of abuse. All calls are responded to within a day or two.

LactMed
https://www.ncbi.nlm.nih.gov/books/NBK501922
Dr. Anderson is also the author of LactMed, the government-run drugs and lactation database. The database contains information on most every medication.

GENERAL OVERALL HELPFUL WEBSITES

Baby Center
www.babycenter.com
This site offers thousands of original, medically reviewed articles on preconception, pregnancy, babies, and toddlers, plus live chats with experts, bulletin boards, and newsletters.

Breastfeeding After Breast and Nipple Surgeries
www.bfar.org
This site offers information for women who are breastfeeding after breast and nipple surgeries.

Kelly Mom
www.kellymom.com
This is a popular site for information for breastfeeding mothers. Kelly is an expert on evidence-based breastfeeding information and writes about numerous feeding issues.

Mothers Overcoming Breastfeeding Issues (MOBI)
www.mobimotherhood.org
MOBI is a nonprofit organization committed to supporting mothers who have experienced many of the difficulties that have interfered with their breastfeeding relationship. Founded by mothers who are grieving their own unsuccessful breastfeeding relationships, MOBI's goals are to promote the support of mothers with breastfeeding issues, with online support groups with education and research.

Resources for Nursing Families
www.lowmilksupply.org
This site offers information not only for mothers experiencing low milk supply but also about the milk supply process in general.

Special Supplemental Nutrition Program for Women, Infants, and Children (WIC)
www.fns.usda.gov/wic
WIC is a federally funded program that provides nutritional information, counseling, and food to low- and moderate-income pregnant and nursing mothers and their young children. Some WIC programs also offer breast pumps to nursing mothers. Eligibility for WIC services is determined by family income. To locate a WIC office near your home, contact your county or city health department or visit the website.

PUMP RENTALS

Ameda, Inc.
(866) 992-6332; www.ameda.com
Call or check the website to locate an Ameda station, where you can rent the full-size Platinum pump, the lightweight Lact-E pump, or the Elite pump.

Medela, Inc.
(800) 435-8316 ((800) TELL-YOU); www.medela.com
Call to be referred to a local rental station.

NURSING BRAS AND BUSTIERS

While nursing bras are not necessary for mothers who are nursing their infants, they can make things feedings easier to manage. It is usually a good idea to visit a store to try on bras ahead of time before giving birth. Even though nursing bras may be available at retail stores, keep in mind that the selection of styles and sizes may be too limited for you depending on your breast size. Large breasted women may not find an extensive array of styles in smaller shops. When trying on bras while you are still pregnant, know that your breasts will usually become larger once your milk comes in and your rib cage will shrink a bit. Getting a good fit is essential for comfort, as well as for avoiding plugged milk ducts. If you are considering purchasing underwire bras, be sure that the wires do not press on the area of breast tissue just below your arm pit. Working with an experienced bra fitter can be very helpful in selecting the best style and size for you.

Bravado! Designs: (800) 590-7802, www.bravadodesigns.com

This is a favorite line of nursing bras that is available in stores in both Canada and the U.S. as well as online. Some styles come in extra-large sizes. The company also sells a pumping bra (the "Bravado Clip and Pump").

LactaMed Simplicity Hands Free Pumping Bra: www.lactamed.com

This pumping aid is not actually a bra, but more of a configuration of straps that secures pump flanges in place for pumping. The idea behind this product is that it allows for "hands-on" pumping, or the ability to massage the breasts to assist in emptying the breast quickly and more completely. The straps come in pink, black, teal, and yellow.

Rumina: (425) 466-4409, www.ruminaformoms.com

Rumina is a company for nursing mothers that sells soft and inexpensive tanks and bras for both nursing and hands-free pumping. Bras range in size from small to extra-large and a sizing guide is on the website.

Simple Wishes: (888) 324-9474, www.simplewishes.com

Simple Wishes makes a "bustier" that allows for hands-free pumping. The flanges fit securely into small openings at the nipples, making it possible to move about freely while pumping. The bustier can be adjusted to fit a changing body, it covers more of the trunk than a bra, and it exposes little skin. Simple Wishes also offers the B3 All-in-One Bra, which can be used as both a regular nursing bra and a pumping bra. Call or visit the website to locate a retailer near you, or order online. Mothers can find these pumping bras less expensively at Target and through Lansinoh.

PUMPING ACCESSORIES

Pumpin' Pal
(877) 466-8283; www.pumpinpal.com

The angled, elliptical Pumpin' Pal Super Shields can be inserted into various other pump flanges for more comfortable pumping. The shields come in three sizes, determined by the mother's cup and nipple sizes. Visit the website or call to place an order, speak with a salesperson, or find a local retailer.

BeauGen Cushions
(845) 670-5034; www.BeauGen.com

BeauGen breast pump cushions are designed for more comfortable nursing. Mothers with uncomfortable pumping despite having the correct size flanges may benefit from these soft and stretchy cushions. The majority of mothers who rated the product highly say it helps with having very elastic nipples and inadequate milk flow. They're expensive, so take advantage of BeauGen's subscription option if you need to order more than once.

AIDS FOR SORE AND INJURED NIPPLES

Medela SoftShells and TheraShells
www.medela.com

The Medela SoftShells for Sore Nipples and the TheraShells are vented to keep nipples protected. The SoftShells have a flexible backing and the TheraShells have a stiff plastic backing. Purchase from retailers like Target and Walmart, or by telephone from Medela.

NIPPLE CREAMS

Lansinoh's Modified Lanolin
(800) 292-4794; www.lansinoh.com

Lansinoh's modified lanolin costs $10 for a 1.4-ounce tube. HPA "Minis" come in a three-pack of 0.25 ounce each for about $15. The cream is carried by many drugstores and discount stores; call or visit the website to find a local source.

Manuka Honey
Medical-grade Manuka honey is well-known for its healing and antibacterial properties. A ½-ounce tube can be purchased from a large health food store or ordered from Amazon or other online stores for about $12. Getting this honey with a UMF (Unique Manuka Factor) of 16 or higher is recommended for stronger healing ability. One recommended product is known as "MediHoney" gel, and it can be purchased at Walmart and large drugstore chains, as well as in some grocery markets that specialize in health foods. MediHoney is irradiated and does not have any live botulism spores that are dangerous to infants.

Motherlove Nipple Cream
(888) 209-8321; www.motherlove.com

Motherlove nipple cream contains organically grown healing herbs, marshmallow root, calendula, olive oil, shea butter, and beeswax. A 1-ounce jar costs $10. Visit Motherlove's website to order or locate a local distributor. There is also a "Store Locator" to help find somewhere local that you can find Motherlove products including the nipple cream.

INVERTED NIPPLE SUPPLIES

Breast Shells
Breast shells are marketed both to correct inverted nipples during pregnancy and/or to protect injured nipples from friction against clothing. Few women find the flexible Medela SoftShells for Inverted Nipples ($18.49 per pair) effective in treating inverted nipples. Supple Cups are more effective in treating inverted nipples during pregnancy; see below. The SoftShells for Sore Nipples ($18.95 per pair) and the TheraShells ($15.99 per pair) are vented to keep nipples protected. The SoftShells have a flexible backing and the TheraShells have a stiff plastic backing. Purchase from retailers like Target and Walmart, or by telephone from Medela

Supple Cups
www.supplecups.com

These are small silicone cups that are squeezed and centered over a flat or inverted nipples. They are worn for increasing amounts of time and help bring nipples outward for an easier latch by the baby. Interested mothers should visit the website for help in ordering the correct size and information on using the cups.

"DRIP" MILK COLLECTORS

There are some products that can be worn on one side while the baby nurses from the other for the purpose of collecting "drip" milk. There are three as of this writing.

Milkies Milk Saver
www.mymilkies.com

This product is designed to be worn on the opposite side when a mother is nursing on the other. This cup is centered over the nipple and can collect just a bit more than two ounces. Milkies can be purchased at Target for about $28 each or found online for less.

Milk-Saver On-the-Go
www.mymilkies.com

This product from the same company, includes two cups that fit flatter within a bra and collects just one ounce of milk per cup. The price of these two cups is about $19.95.

Lacti-Cups
www.lacti-cups.com

These are similar to Milkies with some notable differences. Two cups are included in each box and each cup can hold two and a half ounces of milk. Drip milk can be worn in the cups for up to four hours (but only two if saving milk for a premature or sick newborn). The price is about $27 online. Call to order.

Silicone Squeeze Breast Pumps

These pumps, such as the "Haaka" can be used as a milk collector when worn on one side and usually while a mother is nursing on the other. See Haaka pump in Chapter Five under "Silicone squeeze pumps" on page 312.

SILICONE NURSING PADS

Simply Lily
www.lilypadz.com

An alternative to conventional cloth or disposable pads, LilyPadz ($19.95 per pair or $37.95 for two pairs) don't absorb milk but instead apply a gentle pressure on the nipple to keep milk from leaking. The pads adhere gently to the skin, so they can be worn without a bra. Call or visit the website to order a pair or to locate a retailer near you.

NIPPLE SHIELDS

Silicone nipple shields are used by some mothers when their newborns are unable to latch into the breast. Shields come in various styles and a few companies make them. Know that some styles do not allow for much milk transfer to the baby. The following companies make the best shields but still, some babies will still not get enough milk. Ideally, it is best if a lactation professional can see you and your baby, and fit you with a pair that are both comfortable and ensure that your baby is getting enough milk. Lactation consultants may suggest that you pump after each feeding to ensure that your breasts are well-drained. Most newborns can be weaned off of shields when their ability at the breast improves.

Lansinoh
www.lansinoh.com

Lansinoh also makes shields in 20 mm and 24 mm sizes. A pair of nipple shields cost between $8-$13 for a pair.

Medela, Inc.
www.medela.com

Medela makes two different styles—one that is completely round and another that has an outer area that has been cut out that are known as "contact" shields. The shields come in three sizes: 16 mm, 20 mm, and 24 mm.

BABY SCALES

Medela, Inc.

www.medela.com

Highly accurate electronic scales are available from local pump rental stations. You may be able to locate a rental station by calling Medela.

Tanita Digital Baby Scale (model 1584)

This scale can be purchased from Amazon. It is fairly accurate. Less expensive scales are typically inaccurate.

NURSING SUPPLEMENTATION DEVICES

A nursing supplementation device provides supplementary milk or formula while a baby is breastfeeding. Such a device is most commonly used when a baby is adopted or a mother wishes to resume lactating after a period of not nursing. A supplementer may also help when a mother wishes to both build up and supplement a low milk supply, or when a baby has a weak or ineffective suck.

A supplementer consists of a container to hold breast milk or formula and a thin, flexible tube that is placed on the breast, ending at the nipple. The baby must latch on to the nipple and the soft tube at the same time. As the baby sucks, he receives the supplement along with whatever milk his mother is producing. These devices should be used with the guidance of a lactation professional experienced with them, who may also sell nursing supplementers. Medela and Lact-Aid can refer you to any local source or sell them directly. Check out their websites.

Medela, Inc.

www.medela.com

Medela's Supplemental Nursing System is made of hard plastic is available from the manufacturer and various stores, clinics, and online sources for $67 plus shipping.

Lact-Aid International

www.lact-aid.com

The Lact-Aid Nursing Trainer System is available from the manufacturer and from some lactation professionals for $57.95 for the standard kit and $69.95 for the deluxe kit. Disposable bags are filled with milk and soft tubing brings the milk to the nursing infant. Visit the website for additional information.

HERBAL REMEDIES FOR LOW MILK SUPPLY

Fenugreek

Fenugreek is available in capsule form in most health-food stores and some drugstores. A bottle of 100 capsules sells for $10 to $12. The typical lactation dose is three capsules three times daily (disregard the dosing recommendations on the label to treat other ailments).

Motherlove Capsules and Extract: More Milk Plus, More Milk Special Blend

www.motherlove.com

More Milk Plus (capsules and extract) both contain fenugreek seed, blessed thistle, nettle leaf, and fennel seed and are designed to increase milk production quickly. More Milk Special Blend capsules and extract, which contain goat's rue, as well as the herbs in More Milk Plus, are designed to stimulate the development of breast tissue and increase milk supplies in mothers who have had breast surgery, who have polycystic ovary syndrome (PCOS), who have insufficient glandular tissue, or who are adopting.

Capsules let you avoid the licorice-like flavor but are more expensive; extract may be absorbed faster. In either formulation, capsules cost $24 for 60 or $42 for 120. The extracts cost $20 for 2 ounces, $34 for 4 ounces, and $50 for 8 ounces. The usual dose for capsules is one capsule four times daily. The dose for the extracts depends on the woman's weight.

Motherlove products are available in some health food stores, baby supply stores, and lactation practices. You can contact Motherlove to find a local distributor by using the "store locator" on the bottom of the web pages or order direct from Motherlove by phone or through the website.

Malunggay

www.golacta.com

Malunggay is another popular herbal remedy containing the dried leaves of the Malunggay tree. One study showed that mothers who delivered premature infants and used a pump to bring in full milk production produced 200 percent more milk than mothers who did not use it in the early days after giving birth. The powdered leaves are also high in vitamin A, vitamin C, calcium, potassium, iron, and protein. The recommended dosage varies from product to product. The two popular companies that have a Malunggay product are Motherlove Herbals and Sugarpod Naturals. Sugarpod's product is Go-Lacta.

The typical dose of Go-Lacta is one to three capsules, two to three times a day. One bottle of 60 capsules costs $20; if you order from Go-Lacta's website, you can get free shipping when buying two or more bottles. The powder form is also available for $24.95. Mothers who have had previous supply issues can start taking Go-Lacta three weeks before their due date.

Domperidone (Motilium)

InHouse Pharmacy: (800) 868-9064, www.inhousepharmacy.vu; CanUSAMeds: (877) 469-9619; www.canusameds.com

Domperidone, also known by the brand name Motilium, is usually sold for treating disorders of the gastrointestinal tract. This drug has also been found to stimulate milk production, more safely so than another medication, Reglan. Side effects in the mother (headache, abdominal cramps, dry mouth) are uncommon with Domperidone, and very little of the medication reaches the baby. The use of Domperidone is approved for nursing mothers by the American Academy of Pediatrics. Unfortunately, Domperidone is not manufactured in the United States, although there are a couple of ways mothers can get this medication. The typical dose for Domperidone is 10-20 mg, four times a day to increase a breastmilk supply.

Mothers and get Domperidone without a prescription from any pharmacy in Mexico. This may work for you if you, or friends and family live nearby or visit there.

As of this writing, the most reliable source for Domperidone, without a prescription, is InHouse Pharmacy in New Zealand. Unfortunately, there are restrictions on their international shipment locations.

InHouse Pharmacy carries several brands of 10-milligram Domperidone tablets, each with different package sizes and different prices. The least expensive is Vomistop, at about $70 for a minimum order of 500 tablets and is the most popular choice. It is best to check prices on the website and prices as subject to change. Shipping to the United States is free and takes seven to fourteen days.

Another pharmacy, CanUSAmeds, will send Domperidone to mothers in the U.S. and Canada but only with a prescription. The price for 500 10-milligram pills is $134.98. The shipping takes anywhere from seven to twelve business days. Shipping cost is $13. CanUSAmeds does not accept credit cards, only personal (or "e checks").

NURSING PILLOWS

Zenoff Products

(415) 785-3890; www.mybrestfriend.com

The wearable My Brest Friend Nursing Pillows, each with a cushioned back support, make positioning the baby easier and sitting to nurse more comfortable. The pillow for a single baby in a variety of prints costs about $35.95; the deluxe model offers a baby-plush soft fabric and costs about $39.95. The model for twins costs about $59.95. Call or check the website to order or to find a dealer near you.

NURSING STOOLS

Zenoff Products

(415) 785-3890; www.mybrestfriend.com

Nursing stools help maintain a comfortable position for breastfeeding by lifting the lap and alleviating stress on the back, shoulders, and neck. These adjustable stools are available from the manufacturer and various stores, clinics, and online sources for $29.95.

SPECIALNEEDS FEEDER

Formerly called the Haberman Feeder, this device is designed for babies with cleft palates or other oral problems that make it difficult to maintain suction. A special valve and adjustable silicone nipple make it easy for a baby to withdraw milk through this feeder, which is available through Medela and online sources for about $30 for the 80-ml bottle.

Dr. Brown's

www.drbrownsbaby.com

Dr Brown's Specialty Feeding System is relatively new and unique. It was created in 2015 to help infants that are unable to feed easily at the breast or with a typical bottle. Other infants, including those with congenital issues heart or neurological problems, may also feed with less stress on this system. The development of this unique bottle system originated by requests from medical professionals to combine the Dr. Brown's Natural Flow bottle system and a one-way valve from a competitor cleft palate bottle system. This system can be purchased online through Walmart and Amazon for about $16 to $20 for a two-pack.

Medela, Inc.

www.medela.com

BREAST MILK STORAGE BAGS

Lansinoh Milk Storage Bags

www.lansinoh.com

These bags are used by many milk banks for their durability. You can get these either with or without adapters for pumping directly into the bag. A pack of 50 bags for about $11 dollars can be found on Amazon.

Medela, Inc.

www.medela.com

Medela Pump & Save Bags can be used with most Medela pumps except. The bags are available through Medela, discount and online stores for about $15 for a package of 100.

PUMP-SANITIZING MICROWAVE BAGS

Medela Quick Clean Micro-Steam Bags
www.medela.com
Medela Quick Clean Micro-Steam Bags allow you to disinfect pump parts in a microwave in about 3 minutes. Each bag can be used as many as 20 times. The bags are available from Medela and online stores for about $6 for a package of five.

PUMP WIRES

Medela Quick Clean Breast Pump and Accessory Wipes
www.medela.com
These wipes allow for convenient portable cleaning, with no need for soap and water after each pump session. These hygienic wipes are proven safe for cleaning pumps and accessories as well as highchairs, tables, cribs, and countertops. A pack of 24 wipes costs $9 and a pack of 40 wipes costs $19.99.

INFANT PROBIOTICS

Gerber Soothe Colic Drops
www.gerber.com
A study of breastfed infants showed that giving a baby just five drops a day of probiotics decreased colic symptoms by the end of one month. These drops are now being sold by Gerber as Gerber Soothe Colic Drops. A 0.17-ounce bottle (enough for 25 days) costs $24-$28 and can be purchased from Amazon and at some pharmacies. Another version containing Vitamin D is "Gerber Soothe Vitamin D and Probiotic drops is also available with L. reuteri.

Evivo
www.evivo.com
Another new probiotic preparation for infants suffering with colic symptoms is Evivo, a preparation which contains activated b. infantis. This bacterial strain is known to restore the infant gut microbiome after the use of antibiotics and/or c-sections have interrupted the transfer of "healthy bacteria" to the newborn infant during childbirth. Intended for infants who suffer with colic symptoms, this rather expensive product is mixed with breast milk and given orally once a day for as long as the baby is being breastfed. Evivo powder is kept either refrigerated or frozen before being mixed with breast milk and given to the baby. A one-month supply of Evivo is about $80/month. See more about ordering on the website.

"NEXT TO MOM" BABY BEDS

Arm's Reach Bedside Co-Sleeper
www.armsreach.com
Arm's Reach Bedside Co-Sleeper is a baby bed that connects to an adult-size bed to allow a mother and her baby to sleep safely and comfortably next to each other. Various models are available, priced from $164 to $250. Each can be converted into a bassinet, a playpen, a changing table, or even a love seat. For beds higher than 24 inches, a leg extension kit is available separately. Visit the website to find a local retailer.

Halo BassiNests
www.halosleep.com
This oval shaped bassinet with mesh walls swivels to bring the baby closer to mom in the night. Models range from $229 to $279. The sleeper can be used for babies up to about five months of age and up to 30 pounds. Visit the website for more.

MILK BANKS IN THE UNITED STATES AND CANADA

The Human Milk Banking Association of North America

www.hmbana.org

This nonprofit milk banking association screens its donors and pasteurizes the donated milk for vulnerable newborns and infants whose mothers are unable to provide enough milk. Women who wish to donate milk must be healthy nonsmokers who take no medications (with some exceptions). Most milk banks require a minimum number of ounces from each donor.

Donors freeze their milk before sending it to the milk bank. The milk banks send a large cooler and pay to have it shipped back to them at no cost to the mothers. There the milk is thawed, pooled with that of other donors, heat-treated to kill any bacteria or viruses, and refrozen (it retains its immunological properties through this processing). The milk is dispensed only after a cultured sample shows no bacterial growth. Then it is shipped frozen by overnight express to hospitals and individual recipients.

Because of all the work that goes into processing it, donated milk is expensive, and its supply is limited. Parents who want to buy donated milk must have a physician's prescription. Common conditions for which physicians prescribe donated milk include prematurity, allergies, formula intolerance, immunological deficiencies, infectious diseases, and inborn errors of metabolism. Doctors may also prescribe donated milk for short periods to provide superior nutrition for a baby recovering from surgery or to get an adopted baby off to a good start.

As of this writing the Human Milk Banking Association of North America has certified more than thirty banks in the United States and Canada, and others are in the process of becoming certified. **Visit the website and click "Find a Milk Bank" to find out if a milk bank is available in your area. Or, call (817) 810-9984.**

Appendix B

Determining Babies' Milk Needs
during the First Six Weeks

TEN-PERCENT WEIGHT LOSS

A newborn should lose less than 10 percent of her birth weight before she begins to gain weight. Find your baby's birth weight in the left column of the table. Look at the figure across from your baby's birth weight in the right column. If your baby weighs this amount or less, you'll want to compare her milk needs (see the following sections of this appendix) with your milk production, and take steps to increase her milk intake

Birth Weight (in pounds-ounces)	10% Less	Birth Weight (in pounds-ounces)	10% Less	Birth Weight (in pounds-ounces)	10% Less
4-8	4-2	7-0	6-5	9-8	8-9
4-9	4-2.5	7-1	6-6	9-9	8-10
4-10	4-3	7-2	6-7	9-10	8-10.5
4-11	4-3.5	7-3	6-7.5	9-11	8-11.5
4-12	4-4	7-4	6-8	9-12	8-12
4-13	4-5	7-5	6-9	9-13	8-13
4-14	4-6	7-6	6-10	9-14	8-14
4-15	4-7	7-7	6-11	9-15	8-15
5-0	4-8	7-8	6-12	10-0	9-0
5-1	4-9	7-9	6-13	10-1	9-1
5-2	4-10	7-10	6-14	10-2	9-2
5-3	4-11	7-11	6-15	10-3	9-3
5-4	4-12	7-12	7-0	10-4	9-4
5-5	4-12.5	7-13	7-0.5	10-5	9-4.5
5-6	4-13	7-14	7-1	10-6	9-5
5-7	4-14	7-15	7-2	10-7	9-6
5-8	4-15	8-0	7-3	10-8	9-7
5-9	5-0	8-1	7-4	10-9	9-8
5-10	5-1	8-2	7-5	10-10	9-9
5-11	5-2	8-3	7-6	10-11	9-10
5-12	5-3	8-4	7-7	10-12	9-11
5-13	5-4	8-5	7-8	10-13	9-12
5-14	5-5	8-6	7-9	10-14	9-13
5-15	5-5.5	8-7	7-9.5	10-15	9-13.5
6-0	5-6	8-8	7-10	11-0	9-14.5
6-1	5-7	8-9	7-11	11-1	9-15
6-2	5-8	8-10	7-12	11-2	10-0
6-3	5-9	8-11	7-13	11-3	10-1
6-4	5-10	8-12	7-14	11-4	10-2
6-5	5-11	8-13	7-15	11-5	10-3
6-6	5-12	8-14	8-0	11-6	10-4
6-7	5-13	8-15	8-1	11-7	10-5
6-8	5-14	9-0	8-2	11-8	10-5.5
6-9	5-14.5	9-1	8-2.5	11-9	10-6.5
6-10	5-15	9-2	8-3	11-10	10-7.5
6-11	6-0	9-3	8-4	11-11	10-8
6-12	6-1	9-4	8-5	11-12	10-9
6-13	6-2	9-5	8-6	11-13	10-10
6-14	6-3	9-6	8-7	11-14	10-11
6-15	6-4	9-7	8-8	11-15	10-12

BABIES' MILK NEEDS DURING THE FIRST FIVE DAYS

Find your baby's age in the left column. At right is the amount of milk he needs at each of eight daily feedings.

Baby's Age, in Hours	Milk Needed per Feeding in Milliliters	in Ounces
24–48	15	½
48–72	20	⅔
72–96	30	1
96–120	45	1½

BABIES' MILK NEEDS FROM FIVE DAYS TO SIX WEEKS OF AGE

Follow these steps to determine how much milk your baby needs.

Step 1. Weigh the baby naked, on an accurate scale, at least one hour after a feeding. Find the baby's weight in kilograms in the chart below. If the baby weighs 7 pounds, 5 ounces, for example, look down the column headed "7" and across the row headed "5." The baby's weight in kilograms is 3.317.

Ounces	4	5	6	7	Pounds 8	9	10	11	12	13	14
0	1.814	2.268	2.722	3.175	3.629	4.082	4.536	4.990	5.443	5.897	6.350
1	1.843	2.296	2.750	3.203	3.657	4.111	4.564	5.018	5.471	5.925	6.379
2	1.871	2.325	2.778	3.232	3.685	4.139	4.593	5.046	5.500	5.953	6.407
3	1.899	2.353	2.807	3.260	3.714	4.167	4.621	5.075	5.528	5.982	6.435
4	1.928	2.381	2.835	3.289	3.742	4.196	4.649	5.103	5.557	6.010	6.464
5	1.956	2.410	2.863	3.317	3.770	4.224	4.678	5.131	5.585	6.038	6.492
6	1.984	2.438	2.892	3.345	3.799	4.252	4.706	5.160	5.613	6.067	6.520
7	2.013	2.466	2.920	3.374	3.827	4.281	4.734	5.188	5.642	6.095	6.549
8	2.041	2.495	2.948	3.402	3.856	4.309	4.763	5.216	5.670	6.123	6.577
9	2.070	2.523	2.977	3.430	3.884	4.337	4.791	5.245	5.698	6.152	6.605
10	2.098	2.551	3.005	3.459	3.912	4.366	4.819	5.273	5.727	6.180	6.634
11	2.126	2.580	3.033	3.487	3.941	4.394	4.848	5.301	5.755	6.209	6.662
12	2.155	2.608	3.062	3.515	3.969	4.423	4.876	5.330	5.783	6.237	6.690
13	2.183	2.637	3.090	3.544	3.997	4.451	4.904	5.358	5.812	6.265	6.719
14	2.211	2.665	3.118	3.572	4.026	4.479	4.933	5.386	5.840	6.294	6.747
15	2.240	2.693	3.147	3.600	4.054	4.508	4.961	5.415	5.868	6.322	6.776

Step 2. To determine the approximate amount of milk a baby needs in a 24-hour period, multiply the baby's weight in kilograms by 6, and round the result to the nearest whole number.

Example: 3.317 kilograms × 6 = 19.902 ounces

If the baby weighs 3.317 kilograms, she needs approximately 20 ounces of milk per day.

Step 3. Calculate how much milk the baby needs at each feeding. Divide the amount of milk the baby needs daily by the number of times she nurses in each 24-hour period.

Example: 20 ounces ÷ 8 = 2½ ounces

If the baby needs 20 ounces of milk per day and nurses eight times per day, she needs 2½ ounces of milk at each feeding.

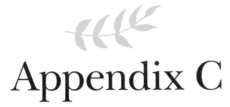

Appendix C

The World Health Organization
Growth Standards

The World Health Organization (WHO) Growth Reference Study was undertaken between 1997 and 2003 to generate new growth curves for assessing the growth and development of infants and young children around the world. Growth data was collected from about 8,500 children from widely different ethnic backgrounds and geographical settings (Brazil, Ghana, India, Norway, Oman, and the United States). The new growth charts provide a single international standard that best represents the normal physiological growth of children from birth to five years of age and establishes the breastfed infant as the model for normal growth. The charts differ from those used by most U.S. health-care providers, which are based mostly on the growth of formula-fed children. In the near future, I hope, the WHO charts will replace the ones currently in use in doctors' offices.

The original WHO weight charts are in kilograms only, but the versions on pages 400 and 401 also show a baby's weight in pounds.

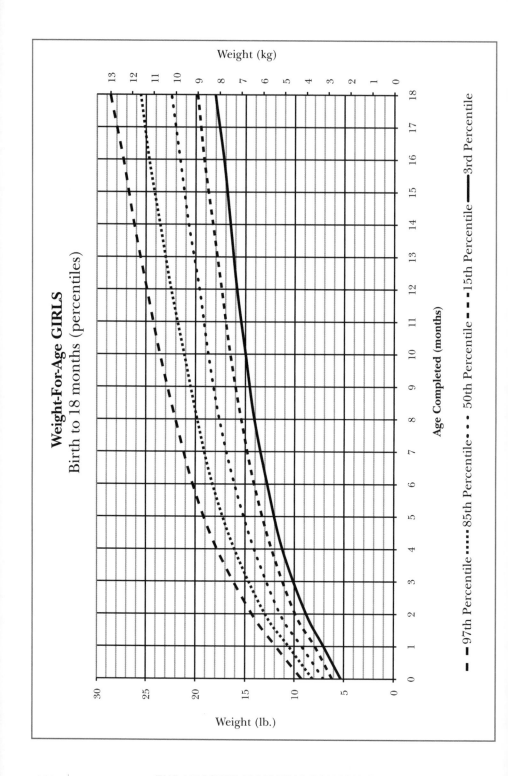

Weight-For-Age GIRLS
Birth to 18 months (percentiles)

Weight (kg)

Weight (lb.)

Age Completed (months)

■ ■ 97th Percentile ■■■■■ 85th Percentile ● ● 50th Percentile ■ ■ ■ 15th Percentile —— 3rd Percentile

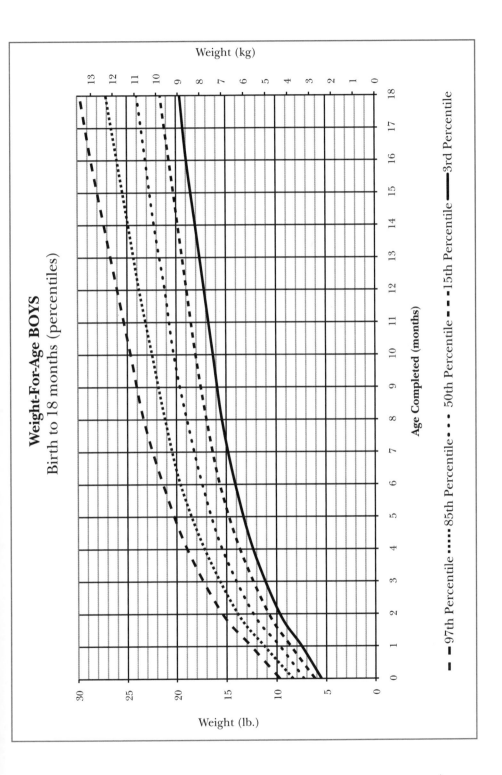

Weight-For-Age BOYS
Birth to 18 months (percentiles)

Weight (kg)

Weight (lb.)

Age Completed (months)

- -97th Percentile ·····85th Percentile· · · 50th Percentile - - -15th Percentile ——3rd Percentile

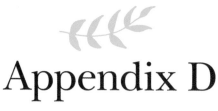

Appendix D
The Safety of Drugs during Breastfeeding

....

By Philip O. Anderson, Pharm.D., F.A.S.H.P., F.C.S.H.P.

If you are considering taking a medication while nursing, you are likely wondering what effects it may have on your baby and on milk production. Clear guidelines are sometimes hard to come by in this situation. This appendix will explain what you should consider before taking a particular drug, and how, if you take it, you can minimize its effects on your child.

THE PASSAGE OF DRUGS INTO MILK

Almost any drug you take will reach your milk in some quantity. Although you would never want to expose your baby to a foreign chemical unnecessarily, the amount of a drug that appears in milk is usually not great enough to harm a nursing child. One group of researchers found that 87 percent of drugs are transmitted in amounts of 10 percent or less of the mother's dose. About half of these are in amounts less than 1 percent of the mother's dose. Only about 3 percent of drugs reach the infant in amounts similar to the mother's dose. If you were taking a medication during pregnancy, the amount your infant is exposed to in breast milk is considerably less than during pregnancy. Several considerations are important when deciding whether to take a particular drug:

Your baby's age and maturity. Just as your baby becomes better able to move about as he grows older, his ability to detoxify and eliminate foreign chemicals and drugs improves with time. Premature infants have little ability to metabolize drugs; when a preemie needs treatment for a medical condition, drugs are given in much smaller doses than they would be for a full-term newborn or an older infant. The amount of medication in a mother's milk that is safe for a one-month-old might be risky for a premature infant. Likewise, a baby who is several months old has a much greater capability of handling drugs in breast milk than a one-month-old. And when an infant begins to eat solid food, he consumes less breast milk and, therefore, less of any drug it may contain. Most unwanted drug effects in breastfed infants occur in infants under two months old.

The persistence of the drug in the body. Some drugs are eliminated from the body after only a few hours, whereas others remain for a long time and accumulate. Accumulation potential is measured by the "half-life" of the drug; it takes four to five half-lives for a drug to be eliminated from the body. Drugs with long half-lives are more likely to persist in milk than are those with short half-lives. Drugs with long half-lives are also more likely to accumulate in the baby and affect her. A drug might have a longer half-life in a newborn than in a two-month-old for reasons discussed above.

Your needs. Maybe you have a serious medical condition that threatens your health and your ability to care for your child, and you must take medication for it. Or maybe you're suffering from only a minor discomfort, and can get by without a medication. Whatever your condition, you must evaluate its seriousness and the consequences of not taking a particular drug. Then weigh these consequences against the benefits of breastfeeding, as you see them. You may decide to pump your milk and discard it while you're taking the medication or, if necessary, give up nursing altogether rather than expose your baby to a potentially hazardous drug. Only infrequently does a mother's medication make it necessary for the mother to completely stop nursing, though. Researchers in Canada found that many mothers who were prescribed an antibiotic for an infection failed to take the medication for fear of harming their nursing infants, even after being told that the drug was safe to use during nursing. Such action could easily make the infection worse and require a more potent antibiotic.

The duration of treatment. If you have a chronic health problem, such as high blood pressure, you may be taking a drug daily over a long period. But perhaps you need medication for only a few days, as is usual with many antibiotics, or even just once, as with an anesthetic for a dental procedure or a diagnostic agent for an X-ray. If only brief drug therapy is needed, you can usually avoid exposing your infant to harmful amounts of the drug with minimal disruption to your normal pattern of breastfeeding.

The history of the drug. If a drug has been used for many years—especially if it has been given frequently to infants or to nursing mothers—the risks it poses to the breastfed baby are quite predictable. This is not so, however, for drugs that are new on the market, for most herbal remedies, and for drugs that have never been used in children or infants. With no safety record to go on, health-care providers may vary in their assessments of the risks your baby faces from small amounts of the drug in your milk. Drugs given to you as samples by your physician are usually very new and are unlikely to have information about use during breastfeeding. Ask your physician if he can prescribe an older medication that will be just as effective as the free sample of the new drug—the peace of mind is usually worth the cost of paying for the prescription.

Coordinating feedings and dosage. If a drug is quickly eliminated because of a short half-life, you may be able to time the doses in a way that will minimize the amount of drug in your milk at feedings. You might take a dose just after nursing, so the amount of drug in the milk is highest between feedings. If you are on a once-a-day medication, you might take it after the last feeding of the evening. By morning the amount of drug in your milk may be down to an acceptably low level. These strategies work best with older infants who are nursing at infrequent intervals.

Part of the reason you can limit your baby's drug exposure this way is that drugs pass in both directions between your bloodstream and breast milk. As the drug levels in your bloodstream decrease, the drug in your milk will pass back into your bloodstream. When breastfeeding must be withheld because of drug therapy that may harm an infant, expressing and discarding milk ("pumping and dumping") is sometimes advocated in the mistaken belief that the drug will be eliminated from the milk sooner. Because of the reverse passage of drugs from milk to the bloodstream and because only a very small fraction of the drug in your body is in your milk, pumping and dumping has very little effect on the eventual amount of drug your baby gets from your milk. Pumping the breasts can be useful, though, to maintain your milk supply and decreasing any pain from engorgement when you've temporarily stopped breastfeeding.

Route of administration. The way that you take a medication partially determines how much of the drug will get into your bloodstream and to your baby. Drugs you're given by injection go directly into your bloodstream and can reach the milk, but some injected drugs cannot be absorbed into the infant's bloodstream from her gastrointestinal tract. Medications you take by mouth usually appear in your bloodstream, except for some that are meant to work locally in the stomach or intestines. Small amounts of drugs can be absorbed from drops and ointments placed in the eye. Vaginal and rectal products can also be absorbed into the bloodstream. Drugs taken by inhaler generally reach the bloodstream in much smaller amounts than the same drug taken orally.

Since creams and ointments applied to the skin usually do not allow very much drug to enter into your bloodstream, they are generally safe to use while nursing. Be careful, though, not to get a medicated cream on your baby's skin or allow him to get any into his mouth. If you are applying medication to your nipples, wipe them gently before nursing and reapply the medication after nursing. It is better to use water-washable creams on the breast than greasy petrolatum (Vaseline)-based ointments, because the baby can ingest and absorb some of the petroleum-based oils found in petrolatum.

THE EFFECTS OF DRUGS ON LACTATION

Not only may the drugs you take affect your baby directly, but some may influence your milk production. This can happen in a number of ways, since several hormones work together to control lactation. Some drugs are used deliberately to stimulate or stop milk flow; however, a few medications intended for another purpose can affect lactation. Those that can decrease lactation are identified in this appendix.

SIDE EFFECTS IN THE BABY

Only infrequently must nursing be discontinued completely because of potential infant drug toxicity. Concern usually arises when the baby is a newborn or preemie or when the mother must take one of the most toxic drugs or a combination of potentially toxic drugs. But even drugs that are usually safe for nursing babies can occasionally cause mild but unpredictable allergic reactions, such as skin rashes. Minor side effects such as fussiness, drowsiness, and diarrhea occur sometimes but usually do not require medical attention. More serious side effects are rare.

You may also get different advice about medications from different physicians—your obstetrician and the baby's pediatrician, for example. Unnecessary alarm and confusion are often caused by statements concerning nursing made by a drug's manufacturer in the Physician's Desk Reference (PDR) or package insert. Many mothers stop nursing after receiving such confusing or inaccurate advice. It is important to consult a health professional with specific expertise in advising nursing mothers about medication use if you have questions about your drug. One such source is MotherToBaby, a free service that can be reached at toll free at 866-626-6847 or at https://mothertobaby.org/.

COMMON DRUGS AND THEIR SAFETY

If side effects or possible allergies become a problem for your baby while you're taking a drug, do not hesitate to seek help.

In the following list, common drugs are grouped into categories and subcategories according to their uses. Their potential effects on the breastfeeding infant are noted and, where applicable, effects on lactation also. Drug names that begin with a lower-case letter are generic names; those that begin with a capital letter are brand names with the corresponding generic name given after it. The names of combination products are followed by lists of the ingredients they contain; see the separate entry for each ingredient. Not all brands are listed, so if you can't find the name of a particular product in this list, look under the generic name of its ingredient or ingredients. A more complete listing of brand names is in the "Index to Common Drugs" at the end of this appendix. If you can't find the drug you're looking for here or need more detailed information, you might find it on the U.S. National Library of Medicine's Drugs and Lactation (LactMed) website, at https://www.ncbi.nlm.nih.gov/books/NBK501922/?term=lactmed. This website has been recommended by the American Academy of Pediatrics as a source of information on medication use during breastfeeding. Although the information on this site is mostly aimed at health professionals, the summaries are easy to understand. You might print out the detailed information for a particular drug so you can discuss it with your health-care provider.

Acne products. Even though the manufacturer cautions against it, tretinoin can be used during nursing if it is applied only to the face, because very little is absorbed into the bloodstream. Avoid touching the infant's skin with treated areas of your own skin, when you're nursing and when you're not. Other topical products, such as benzoyl peroxide, clindamycin, and erythromycin, can also be used. Isotretinoin taken by mouth should not be used while nursing. Daily use of tetracycline for acne for more than 2 weeks is not desirable while nursing. Doxycycline is the preferred tetracycline during breastfeeding.

Anesthetics. General anesthetics. Nitrous oxide is sometimes used for dental procedures and short outpatient procedures; it is rapidly eliminated from the milk. Injectable anesthetics such as midazolam and propofol, which are used for many short outpatient surgical procedures, have little or no effect on breastfed infants. Gaseous general anesthetics such as desflurane, enflurane, isoflurane, and sevoflurane, which are used in hospitals for major operations, have not been studied in nursing mothers and their babies, but they are eliminated rapidly. Generally, by the time a mother feels sufficiently recovered from anesthesia to breastfeed, you can resume nursing.

Local anesthetics. These drugs are given by injection for dental or other short procedures. Although many people refer to these drugs as "Novocaine" (the trade name for procaine), this old drug is no longer available. Information on the effects of local anesthetics during nursing is available for only three drugs, ropivacaine, lidocaine, and bupivacaine, all of which can be used while nursing. Although other local anesthetics are unlikely to affect a breastfed baby, breastfeeding may be withheld as a precaution for four hours after one of these other drugs is administered.

Antibiotics and other antimicrobials. Most drugs that are taken for infections reach the milk in only small quantities—quantities that would be too small to treat the same infections in your infant. Occasionally, though, these small drug amounts can disrupt the normal balance of microorganisms (the microbiome) in a baby's mouth and intestines. This may result in diarrhea or diaper rash, caused by an overgrowth of yeast or other organisms in the bowel or, less often, thrush, an overgrowth of yeast in the mouth. The likelihood of infant diarrhea or thrush occurring depends on the drug you are taking, especially if you need more than one course of therapy for a persistent or recurrent infection. Although these conditions generally are not serious and can be readily treated, it is important to watch for their signs while you are taking an antibacterial drug.

Aminoglycosides. These drugs (gentamicin, tobramycin, amikacin) are given primarily in the hospital, by injection. Amounts that appear in milk are very small and pose no danger to the breastfed infant because they are not absorbed by the baby.

Antitubercular drugs. Combinations of medications such as isoniazid, rifampin, and pyrazinamide are used to treat tuberculosis. Isoniazid is also used alone, to prevent tuberculosis in those exposed to the disease. In general, treating the nursing mother with these drugs is safer than exposing the infant to untreated tuberculosis, although isoniazid and pyrazinamide pose a slight theoretical risk of damage to the baby's liver. Although rare, watch the infant for signs of jaundice (yellowing of the skin and eyes) and contact your physician if this occurs.

Cephalosporins. These drugs are similar to penicillins, and the same precautions apply. Occasionally allergies develop to these drugs, so watch for signs of skin rash. Cephalexin is a cephalosporin commonly prescribed safely to nursing mothers.

Clindamycin. Clindamycin is best avoided if possible, but a few days of therapy is acceptable, as long as the baby is closely monitored for diarrhea and bloody stools. Clindamycin presents little risk to the infant if it is given vaginally rather than orally or intravenously. See also "Acne Products."

Linezolid. Information is limited on this antibiotic for resistant Staph. infections, but the dose in milk is much less than the dose given directly to newborn infants.

Macrolides. Erythromycin is a generally safe drug that is often given directly to infants. The closely related drugs azithromycin and clarithromycin appear to be equally safe. See also "Acne Products."

Metronidazole and tinidazole. Breastfeeding should be stopped temporarily during use of these medications, but can be resumed 24 hours after the last dose of metronidazole and three days after a dose of tinidazole. For postoperative (including C-section) infections, a cephalosporin or clindamycin should be considered as an alternative.

Nitrofurantoin. This drug appears in small amounts in breast milk. These amounts are generally not harmful to infants over one month of age, but the drug should be avoided with babies under 1 month of age, especially preemies.

Penicillins. These are very safe drugs that are often given directly to infants as treatment for infections. Occasionally allergies develop to penicillins, so the baby should be watched for skin rashes. If you see signs of rash, diarrhea, or thrush, call your health-care provider.

Quinolones. Ciprofloxacin, levofloxacin, moxifloxacin, and several others have not been well studied in nursing infants, although recent experience indicates that they are probably not particularly harmful during nursing.

Sulfonamides (sulfas). Septra and Bactrim are common drugs that contain trimethoprim and the sulfonamide, sulfamethoxazole. Large doses of sulfonamides given directly to newborn infants can increase the risk of jaundice (yellowing of the skin and eyes). Other medications are usually preferred if the baby is premature or less than 1-2 months of age. These drugs are acceptable while nursing older infants.

Tetracyclines. These are generally not given to children or pregnant women because they can cause permanent staining of the infant's teeth. The amounts that appear in milk, however, are very small and are partially inactivated by the calcium in milk. In fact, tooth staining caused by a tetracycline in breast milk has never been reported. Doxycycline is now considered safe to give directly to infants and children, so it is a good choice in this class of antibiotics. Other tetracyclines can be used by the nursing mother for up to two weeks, but they should be used only if no other drug will work. One tetracycline, minocycline, can cause the milk to turn black. See also "Acne Products."

Vancomycin. Vancomycin and the related drug daptomycin are excreted into milk in only small amounts and are not absorbed into the baby's bloodstream. They are acceptable during nursing.

Antifungals

Ciclopirox. This drug has not been studied during breastfeeding. Because only a small amount is absorbed after application to the skin, it is considered a low risk to the nursing infant. Avoid use on the nipples where the infant might directly ingest it.

Clotrimazole. Clotrimazole (dissolved from a lozenge) and miconazole have been safely used in the mouths of infants with thrush, often successfully after nystatin has failed, and these antifungals are also safe to use for a mother's vaginal infections. Numerous related drugs, such as butoconazole, econazole, oxiconazole, and terconazole, are also available for vaginal use. Since little is known about their absorption into the bloodstream of a nursing infant, it is preferable to use clotrimazole or miconazole when a vaginal antifungal is needed.

Fluconazole. This is a potent, low-risk antifungal that is taken orally. A single dose for vaginal infections can be used while nursing. Fluconazole can also be used simultaneously in the mother and infant to treat breast infections and thrush when other drugs have failed. At least two weeks of therapy is required in this situation.

Ibrexafungerp. This drug has no information on use during breastfeeding. Although it is not prohibited in nursing mothers, ibrexafungerp should be used with caution during breastfeeding, especially while nursing a newborn or preterm infant.

Ketoconazole. You should not take ketoconazole orally or apply the cream to your nipples because it can be absorbed into the baby's bloodstream and may be toxic. Application of the cream elsewhere on your body or use of the shampoo is not harmful to the baby.

*Naftifine.*This drug has not been studied during breastfeeding. Because only a small amount is absorbed after application to the skin, it is considered a low risk to the nursing infant.

Polyenes. Since amphotericin B and nystatin aren't absorbed into the baby's bloodstream, you can safely use them in your infant's mouth or on your nipples to treat thrush. You can also safely take them orally or receive amphotericin B by injection.

Antiparasitics. Albendazole is used for various worm (parasite) infestations. Excretion into breastmilk is minimal and it is considered acceptable to use during breastfeeding.

Insecticides. These are used to treat scabies, a skin condition caused by mites, and pediculosis, or infestation with lice. An old medication, lindane, is a very fat-soluble insecticide that can persist in milk for a long time. Although no harm has been reported in breastfed infants due to lindane, it does persist in the infant's body, so this drug is best avoided. Safer alternatives include pyrethrins (RID, for example) or permethrin (Nix) for lice, and a higher potency permethrin (Elimite) for scabies.

Ivermectin. Ivermectin is poorly excreted into breastmilk after oral administration. It would not be expected to cause any adverse effects in breastfed infants. No data are available on excretion after use on the skin, but amounts in breastmilk should be very low. Avoid application to the breast area where the infant might directly ingest the drug.

Mebendazole. This is used for various worm (parasite) infestations. Since it is poorly absorbed from the intestinal tract, it is unlikely to cause adverse effects in breastfed infants. Contrary to one old report, it does not inhibit lactation.

Antivirals

Acyclovir. This antiviral drug is used to treat newborns and is well tolerated by the nursing infant.

Amantadine and rimantadine. These antiviral agents for influenza may decrease lactation and cause side effects in the breastfed baby. They should therefore be avoided while nursing.

Famciclovir. This drug and its derivative, penciclovir, which is available as a topical cream, have not been studied in infants or during nursing. It is best to avoid famciclovir, but application of penciclovir away from the breast is acceptable.

Monoclonal antibodies for COVID-19. This can be given during breastfeeding. Very little of the monoclonal antibodies enter the milk and much less is absorbed by the infant. It is not known how much protection against COVID-19 these antibodies provide to the infant when given to a nursing mother.

Oseltamivir. This antiviral drug for influenza enters milk in very low levels and is acceptable to use during breastfeeding. The similar drug zanamivir has not been studied, but since it is inhaled and little drug reaches the mother's bloodstream, its use is also acceptable.

Valacyclovir. This breaks down in the mother's body to acyclovir, so it can also be used during nursing.

Blood formation and coagulation drugs

Clopidogrel. Clopidogrel, prasugrel, and ticagrelor act in a different way to decrease blood platelet function. None have been studied during nursing, and so they should be avoided during breastfeeding.

Dabigtran. Several new oral anticoagulants are available. Dabigatran and rivaroxaban seem like they would not affect the breastfed infant because only very small amounts are found in milk. Apixaban appears in milk in rather high amounts and should be avoided during breastfeeding.

Epoetin alfa. This is an injection that stimulates the production of red blood cells. Although small amounts enter breast milk, the drug is not absorbed from the infant's intestinal tract and so has no adverse effects on the infant. Darbepoetin is a long-acting form of epoetin alfa and is also acceptable to use during breastfeeding.

Filgrastim. Filgrastim and sargramostim are similar to epoetin alfa but stimulate production of white rather than red blood cells. These drugs are also not absorbed from breast milk. These drugs are acceptable to use during breastfeeding.

Heparins. Heparin, enoxaparin, and dalteparin, are given by injection and can be used during lactation because they do not pass well into milk, nor does the infant absorb them from milk.

Tranexamic acid. Used to help decrease bleeding and is used in women with postpartum hemorrhage, studies have found no increased risk of adverse effects in breastfed infants whose mothers receive the drug after delivery.

Warfarin. This drug is poorly excreted into milk. It can be used during breastfeeding.

Antiepileptic drugs. Antiepileptics (anticonvulsants) are used to treat epilepsy, mood disorders, and nerve pain. Because these medications are used continuously and are often long acting, they should be taken with caution during breastfeeding. Your baby may show no effects other than subtle behavioral changes, so be vigilant. Infants of mothers taking anticonvulsants tend to have more difficulty nursing and to wean earlier than other babies. You may need to have your infant's blood drawn to determine if the drug is affecting him. Infants of mothers taking other medications along with an anticonvulsant are more likely to have problems with drowsiness, feeding difficulties, and growth. Recent studies on some of these drugs indicate no harmful effects on the infant's development. Additionally, if you are taking one of these drugs, it is important to take folic acid (vitamin B9), because it has been shown to improve mental function in exposed infants. It should be started before pregnancy and continued throughout breastfeeding.

Carbamazepine. This drug is known to pass into milk in moderately large amounts. Breastfeeding with carbamazepine taken alone does not appear to adversely affect infant growth or development. Although most breastfed infants of women taking the drug show no effects from it, three infants have had liver problems. Watch for jaundice (yellowing of the skin and eyes) while using carbamazepine. Also make sure that your infant is nursing and growing well.

Clobazam. Maternal clobazam resulted in low levels in milk in a few mothers. Monitor the infant for drowsiness, adequate weight gain, and developmental milestones.

Clonazepam. Use of clonazepam during nursing can cause drowsiness and sluggishness in breastfed infants. Other drugs are preferred, if possible.

Eslicarbazepine. No information is available on eslicarbazepine, but it is a derivative of carbamazepine, so its effects are expected to be similar.

Gabapentin. Only small amounts of gabapentin are found in breast milk. Monitor the infant for drowsiness, adequate weight gain, and developmental milestones.

Lacosamide. This drug has not been well studied in breastfeeding, but it did not adversely affect development in a few infants who were breastfed for 7-9 months.

Lamotrigine. Numerous infants have been safely breastfed during maternal therapy, but infants have measurable blood levels of the drug. Breastfeeding with lamotrigine taken alone does not appear to adversely affect infant growth or development. Rarely, lamotrigine can cause very severe skin reactions, so use caution until more information is available; if your infant develops a rash, stop breastfeeding immediately and check with your health-care provider.

Levetiracetam. Limited information is available on this drug, but only small amounts appear in milk.

Oxcarbazepine. A few infants have been breastfed while their mothers used oxcarbazepine. All of the infants have done well, but watch your infant carefully until more information is available.

Phenobarbital. This drug has been given directly to infants for many years, usually with no severe adverse effects. You can use it during breastfeeding, although it may make the baby drowsy and less interested in nursing, especially newborns. The baby's behavior, weight gain, and blood levels should be monitored if there is concern. Women taking phenobarbital sometimes have to stop nursing because of its sedating effects on their infants.

Phenytoin. This drug has been used for many years by breastfeeding women. Very low amounts enter milk, and there have been no consistent reports of problems in breastfed infants from the drug in breastmilk. Breastfeeding with phenytoin taken alone does not appear to adversely affect infant growth or development.

Pregabalin. Limited information indicates that the amounts of this drug in milk are low.

Primidone. This drug is similar to phenobarbital; the same precautions apply.

Tiagabine. Information on tiagabine is very limited. Use this medication with caution, and observe your infant carefully for drowsiness and feeding difficulties, especially in the newborn period.

Topiramate. A few infants have been breastfed while their mothers used this drug, and no adverse effects have been reported. Most of the infants had no detectable topiramate in the bloodstream. One infant had diarrhea from topiramate in breast milk.

Valproic acid and divalproex. Both of these drugs are converted to valproate in the body. Only very small amounts of valproate enter milk, and many nursing mothers have used it safely. Rarely, the drug may cause liver damage or interference with blood platelets. The infant should be watched for unusual bruising and signs of jaundice (yellowing of the skin and eyes). Breastfeeding with valproate taken alone does not appear to adversely affect infant growth or development.

Vigabatrin. Limited information indicates that the amounts of this drug in milk are low.

Zonisamide. Information on the safety of this drug during breastfeeding comes from only a few mother-infant pairs. Rather large amounts are found in breast milk, and some breastfed infants have detectable zonisamide in their blood. No adverse effects have been reported, but use zonisamide with caution until more information is available, especially in newborns.

Diabetes and weight-loss products

Artificial sweeteners. Excretion of all sweeteners into breastmilk appears to be below conventional toxic limits. A concern is that if sweeteners increase the sweetness of milk, they might predispose infants to later increased sugar intake and obesity. It is probably prudent to limit artificial sweetener consumption while breastfeeding, given the lack of information regarding short- and long-term consequences of exposure during infancy. Aspartame may be the preferred high-intensity artificial sweeteners for nursing mothers because it does not reach the mother's bloodstream or appear in milk. High-fructose corn syrup (HFCS), which is found in many non-diet sodas, causes unnatural elevations in milk fructose concentrations. Although the full health implications for infants are not confirmed, maternal HFCS intake may increase the growth rate of breastfed infants, possibly leading to obesity. Maternal HFCS intake should be limited during breastfeeding.

Insulin. A normal component of human milk, insulin is not absorbed by the infant, but may have beneficial local activity in the intestinal tract. Breastfeeding improves postpartum glucose tolerance in mothers with gestational diabetes and reduces the insulin requirement of patients with type 1 diabetes. The cause is the use of glucose to make milk. Insulin dosage requirements may be different after birth than before pregnancy, but this is variable. Close monitoring of blood glucose is necessary during breastfeeding.

Metformin. Levels of metformin in milk are low and apparently do not affect breastfed infants. Metformin should be used with caution while nursing newborn and premature infants, because not as much information is available in these infants.

Dipeptidyl peptidase-4 inhibitors. This includes alogliptin, linagliptin, saxagliptin, and sitagliptin. No information is available on their excretion into milk or use in lactation. These drugs can be used during breastfeeding, but careful monitoring of the infant is required. Saxagliptin and linagliptin might be preferred during breastfeeding because they may have less impact on the infant.

Glucagon-like peptide-1 receptor antagonists. These include dulaglutide, exenatide, liraglutide, lixisenatide, and semaglutide. Current labeling recommends against nursing with all of these drugs, because there are no reports of their use in mothers who are breastfeeding infants.

Sodium–glucose cotransporter 2 inhibitors. These drugs increase glucose excretion in the urine, include canagliflozin, dapagliflozin, empagliflozin, and ertugliflozin. These drugs have no human lactation information and are not recommended because of the theoretical risk of injury to the developing kidney.

Sulfonylureas. These have fallen out of favor in the treatment of type-2 diabetes because they can cause hypoglycemia and weight gain. The advantage for nursing mothers is that information exists on the excretion into breast milk for two of the currently used second-generation agents, glyburide and glipizide, which are undetectable in milk. Checking the breastfed infant's blood glucose is advisable during maternal therapy with sulfonylureas.

Thiazolidinediones. These include pioglitazone and rosiglitazone. Although no information is available, it is unlikely that either would be transmitted into milk in significant amounts. Pioglitazone is preferred because it is not contraindicated in breastfeeding according to the drug's labeling.

Acarbose and miglitol. These two drugs prevent glucose absorption from the gastrointestinal tract. Because they are poorly absorbed by the mother, it is unlikely that these drugs would affect the infant through breast milk, although no reports of their use by nursing mothers have been published.

Repaglinide and nateglinide. These are "not recommended" during breastfeeding, according to their labeling. These drugs can cause hypoglycemia and have no information in breastfeeding, they are probably not good choices in nursing mothers until more data become available.

Pramlintide. Pramlintide is given by subcutaneous injection. If any reaches the milk, it is most likely digested by the nursing infant, rather than absorbed. It can cause hypoglycemia, so monitoring of the infant's serum glucose is recommended.

Weight-loss products. Rapid, excessive weight loss during lactation should be avoided, because many fat-soluble environmental contaminants (such as some insecticides and fire-retardants) are stored in body fat. When body fat is lost rapidly, contaminants might be released into the bloodstream and appear in the fat of breast milk in larger than usual amounts. In addition, some weight-loss agents can affect infants or the milk supply. Many weight-loss products contain vitamins that may also be in multivitamin products prescribed by your physician. If you take both products, your vitamin intake may be excessive.

Arthritis, pain, and migraine medications

Acetaminophen. This drug is often used in infants and is safe to use during breastfeeding.

Antirheumatic drugs. Several drugs are used for severe rheumatoid arthritis. Hydroxychloroquine has been well studied and is acceptable during breastfeeding. Azathioprine and cyclosporine are also considered acceptable to use during breastfeeding. Penicillamine has been used safely in the mothers of many breastfed infants. Low (25 mg or less) weekly doses of methotrexate may be acceptable during breastfeeding as well, although some believe it should be avoided (see also "Immunosuppressants and Immunomodulators"). Leflunomide, mycophenolate and sirolimus have not been studied in nursing infants and are currently considered incompatible with breastfeeding.Many new drugs used for rheumatoid arthritis and inflammatory bowel disease are monoclonal antibodies, which pass poorly into breastmilk and are not absorbed by the infant. Their generic names usually end in "-mab". These drugs are generally considered acceptable to use during breastfeeding, including adalimumab, certolizumab pegol, infliximab, rituximab and tocilizumab. Several similar drugs have not yet been studied during breastfeeding. Etanercept is similar to these drugs and is also considered to be acceptable during nursing.

Aspirin. When large doses are taken daily, as for arthritis, problems can sometimes occur. Generally, it is best to avoid aspirin; ibuprofen is a better choice. If you take an occasional aspirin, do not breastfeed for at least one hour after the dose.

Ergotamine. This is a component of several products, such as Cafergot, used in the treatment of migraine headaches. Some ergot alkaloids might cause vomiting in breastfed infants whose mothers have taken the drugs. Although ergotamine itself has not been studied in nursing mothers, avoiding it while breastfeeding is a good idea. Ergotamine might also suppress lactation.

Muscle relaxants. Most of these drugs have not been studied during nursing. Muscle relaxants taken by mouth, such as carisoprodol, chlorzoxazone, diazepam, and methocarbamol, are sedatives and can be expected to cause drowsiness in breastfed infants, especially if they are taken with other drugs that cause drowsiness. In general, it is best to avoid these drugs while breastfeeding, if possible. Cyclobenzaprine doesn't reach high levels in milk, and one mother breastfed her infant without any infant side effects. Taking ibuprofen (Motrin, Advil) or acetaminophen (Tylenol) along with mild to moderate exercise will usually ease muscle spasms and pain as well as muscle relaxants.

Opioids. Drowsiness due to opioids in milk occurs more commonly in infants than formerly thought—about 20 percent of breastfed babies whose mothers have taken an opioid are affected. The degree of drowsiness varies with the dosage, and babies under one month old are particularly at risk. Limiting the dosage to one tablet (such as 30 mg of codeine, 5 mg of hydrocodone or oxycodone every four hours for three or four days is advisable; acetaminophen (Tylenol) or ibuprofen (Motrin, Advil) can be taken in addition. Larger amounts of opioids have caused sedation and decreased breathing in some infants as well as interfered with nursing. Single injections of an opioid during nursing usually cause no problems, but intravenous narcotics given during labor can sometimes interfere with the establishment of lactation. Meperidine (Demerol) is the worst in this regard; morphine causes fewer problems and fentanyl the least. Epidural administration causes fewer nursing problems than intravenous use. Only a small amount of tramadol appears in milk, and infants are not adversely affected by this amount, so tramadol can be used during breastfeeding. Methadone, when used for maintenance in opioid use disorder during pregnancy, appears not to adversely affect breastfed infants. The methadone in breast milk reduces the abstinence symptoms of newborn infants. Beginning methadone after delivery while breastfeeding is not safe for the baby. Buprenorphine for opioid use disorder in one mother caused severe symptoms in her breastfed infant. It should be used with caution by nursing mothers.

Nonsteroidal anti-inflammatory drugs (NSAIDs). Ibuprofen, diclofenac, and flurbiprofen appear in only minute amounts in milk; they seem safe to use while nursing an infant of any age. If your infant is over one month old, you can also use fenoprofen, ketoprofen, ketorolac, naproxen, tolmetin, celecoxib, indomethacin, and long-acting drugs such as diflunisal, meloxicam, piroxicam, and sulindac. The more toxic drug mefenamic acid should be avoided during breastfeeding. Ibuprofen is the best choice among the NSAIDs.

Triptans. Very little sumatriptan appears in milk, even when it is given by injection, and the small amount that reaches the infant is poorly absorbed. Eletriptan also passes poorly into breast milk. These two drugs are preferred. Rizatriptan, zolmitriptan and almotriptan also appear to be acceptable to use because the amounts in milk are small. Naratriptan is acceptable while nursing an older infant, but not a newborn. No information is available on frovatriptan, so the other triptans are preferred.

Cancer chemotherapy. Because the older drugs in this class are among the most toxic used in medicine, very few women have breastfed while taking them. Little is known about the passage of these drugs into milk, but even small amounts, should they reach the baby, could cause harm. Because these drugs are used for only very serious conditions, it is usually more important for the mother to take the drug than it is for her to nurse her baby. Generally, therefore, breastfeeding should be avoided, although occasionally short-acting chemotherapy drugs that are given intermittently may allow a woman to resume nursing after stopping temporarily, for example, stopping for one week out of four. Some of the newer targeted biotechnology drugs, such as monoclonal antibodies with generic names ending in "-mab," are likely safer during breastfeeding than the older drugs, but they have not been studied thoroughly enough to recommend them during breastfeeding at this time. The new kinase inhibitors are recognizable by their generic names, which generally end in "-nib." Very little information is available with these drugs during breastfeeding. Because of their potential toxicity to the infant, breastfeeding is generally avoided when they are used. The oldest drug in this category, imatinib, has some information indicating that it might be acceptable during breastfeeding, but it is usually not allowed.

Cough, cold, allergy, and asthma medications. The various drugs used for these respiratory conditions are often taken together in combination products, which should generally be avoided during breastfeeding. Usually only one or two symptoms are troublesome, and a single-ingredient product can treat them effectively. For example, hay fever and other allergies can be treated with an antihistamine alone, and a cough can be treated with a cough syrup that has only one or two active ingredients. Oral sustained-release products should be avoided. Common sore throat lozenges (such as Sucrets, Chloraseptic, and Hall's) are safe to use. Drugs taken as nasal sprays or by inhaler reach the milk in lesser quantities than those taken orally and pose little risk of harm to the nursing infant.

Antihistamines. These are used in many products for allergy, colds, coughs, and inducing sleep, although their use for colds is not justified. These drugs can reach the infant through breast milk in amounts large enough to cause drowsiness or fussiness. High doses of antihistamines, particularly when in combination with a decongestant, may decrease the milk supply. Use no more than necessary to control symptoms; often a single dose at bedtime is enough. If you are planning to use an oral product, choose one with 2 mg or less of chlorpheniramine or brompheniramine per dose, 25 mg or less of diphenhydramine per dose, or 5 mg or less of cetirizine per dose, or 2.5 mg or less of levocetirizine and avoid sustained-release products. Loratadine, desloratadine, and fexofenadine in milk are well tolerated by infants and are preferable to the sedating antihistamines. Most nonprescription medications for motion sickness, such as dimenhydrinate and meclizine, are also antihistamines. One or two doses of these medications should have no effect on the infant other than temporary drowsiness. They are preferred over scopolamine in the patch form, which is more likely to decrease the milk supply.

Asthma inhalers and nasal inhalers. These may contain a bronchodilator (such as albuterol, salmeterol, or ipratropium) or a corticosteroid (such as beclomethasone, fluticasone, flunisolide, or triamcinolone). All of these reach the mother's bloodstream in very low levels, and levels in milk are even lower. Try to avoid swallowing excess medication after using an inhaler, because swallowed medication may enter the blood from the intestinal tract and reach the milk. Rinse your mouth and throat and spit out the excess medication.

Cough medicines. The two most common drugs are guaifenesin and dextromethorphan, both of which are acceptable to use during breastfeeding.

Decongestants. Nasal sprays (such as Afrin) are preferable to oral drugs, especially if your baby is a newborn. A saltwater spray or rinse is safe to use during nursing. Oral decongestants can cause agitation or fussiness in an infant. Most important, they can decrease the milk supply and might eventually cause the milk to dry up. If you are planning to use an oral product, choose one with 30 mg or less of pseudoephedrine or phenylephrine per dose. Avoid sustained-release (long-acting) and combination products.

Theophylline. Aminophylline and other theophylline products have been well studied in breast milk. Occasionally they can cause jitteriness or fussiness in infants, usually newborns. In general, though, they are acceptable to use.

Ergot alkaloids.

Bromocriptine. This has been used after birth to suppress lactation, but it is no longer approved for this use because it can be severely toxic to mothers. In mothers with increased prolactin levels, an appropriate dose of bromocriptine might still allow breastfeeding.

Cabergoline. This potent, long-acting drug can stop lactation after a single dose. You shouldn't use it if you intend to nurse your baby.

Ergonovine and methylergonovine. These drugs are sometimes given to mothers right after delivery to diminish uterine bleeding. Methylergonovine is preferred, because ergonovine can suppress lactation. With the usual doses and the normal length of treatment, these drugs cause no problems in the breastfed newborn. Large amounts, however, might cause nausea, vomiting, and diarrhea in the baby. These effects may occasionally occur when the drugs are used beyond the immediate postpartum period.

Gastrointestinal drugs. Many of the drugs in this class act only in the stomach and intestine and are not absorbed into the bloodstream; they cannot, therefore, appear in milk. Other gastrointestinal drugs are absorbed and can affect the infant through breast milk. If a choice exists, choose a drug that is not absorbed.

Antacids. These drugs are poorly absorbed and are safe to use during breastfeeding.

Antidiarrheals. Loperamide and diphenoxylate have not been well studied, but one or two small daily doses should pose little risk to the nursing infant. Larger amounts might affect the infant. Bismuth subsalicylate is best avoided because of the large amount of absorbable salicylate it contains. Salicylate in large amounts can be toxic to the baby.

Antinauseants. Many drugs used for nausea and vomiting are phenothiazine derivatives (see "Psychotherapeutic Agents"), such as prochlorperazine and promethazine, taken in low doses. Another commonly used drug is trimethobenzamide. These drugs may cause transient drowsiness or, rarely, abnormal movements in infants, but can be used for a short time. Newer antinauseants such as dolasetron, ondansetron, and granisetron are used for more severe nausea due to cancer chemotherapy, general anesthesia or after cesarean section. Although these drugs have not been studied well in breastfeeding women, they are not absorbed well into the baby's bloodstream if they do get into the mother's milk, so the risk they pose to the baby seems minimal. No adverse infant effects have been reported after ondansetron use in nursing mothers and the drug has been used safely when given directly to infants.

Domperidone. This drug is used to stimulate intestinal movement. Like metoclopramide, it has been used to increase milk production. It appears to be less likely to cause serious side effects in the mother and infant than metoclopramide. However, domperidone is not licensed for sale in the United States, so drug acquisition and quality can be a problem. Domperidone should not be used in women with a personal or family history of heart arrhythmias or in women who take certain drugs, such as erythromycin, fluconazole and others.

Histamine H-2 antagonists. During breastfeeding, famotidine and nizatidine are the preferred drugs in this class, especially if the baby is young, because they reach the mother's milk in the lowest amounts. Cimetidine is the least desirable of this group and should be avoided.

Laxatives. Many of the more potent laxatives are absorbed into the bloodstream and have caused increased frequency of stools in breastfed infants. Cascara should be avoided while nursing, because it can affect the breastfed infant if taken in high doses. Senna can be used occasionally in small amounts. Bulk-forming laxatives such as bran and other fibers such as psyllium (Metamucil) and calcium polycarbophil (FiberCon) are not absorbed into the bloodstream and are therefore safe to use. Likewise, stool-softening agents such as docusate are not absorbed. Bisacodyl is a stronger laxative that is also not absorbed into the bloodstream. Saline cathartics such as Phospho-Soda and milk of magnesia are poorly absorbed and do not affect the composition of milk. Glycerin suppositories are also safe to use.

Mesalamine derivatives. Diarrhea and bloody stools have occurred rarely in infants of mothers using mesalamine, olsalazine, or sulfasalazine. These drugs may be used during nursing, but the baby should be observed for diarrhea.

Metoclopramide. This medication is used mainly to stimulate intestinal movement and nausea. It has also been used to increase the milk supply in women who are producing insufficient quantities of milk, such as mothers of premature or sick infants, and in adoptive mothers. Metoclopramide does not appear to harm the infant if it is used for two weeks or less. Because this drug may cause or worsen depression, it should not be used by women with a history of depression, and it should not be used for long periods of time or repeatedly because of the risk of causing depression or movement disorders.

Proton pump inhibitors. Omeprazole and pantoprazole are the only drugs of this type that have been studied during nursing. Information is limited, but levels in milk appear to be very low, and no harm has occurred in breastfed infants. Omeprazole is also used in infants. Esomeprazole is a form of omeprazole and should be equally safe. Other drugs in this class (dexlansoprazole, lansoprazole and rabeprazole) have not been studied during breastfeeding, so for now omeprazole is preferred.

Sucralfate. This drug acts locally in the mother's intestinal tract and poses no harm to the breastfed infant.

Heart and blood pressure drugs. These drugs are not often used in women of breastfeeding age, and information about them is therefore limited. Very little is known about newer agents.

ACE inhibitors. Benazepril, captopril, enalapril, and quinapril can be used while nursing. No other drugs in this class have been studied during breastfeeding.

Amiodarone. This drug has caused low thyroid levels and delayed growth in a breastfed infant, so some experts recommend avoiding nursing while taking this drug. However, a few other infants have been breastfed without harm. Using this medication while nursing requires close monitoring of the infant, including tests of thyroid function.

Angiotensin-II blockers. There is almost no information on the use of drugs in this class (such as eprosartan, losartan, irbesartan, olmesartan, telmisartan, and valsartan) during nursing or in infants. One mother It is best to avoid them until more is known. Candesartan levels in milk were very low in three mothers and not found in their infants' bloodstreams, so it is probably acceptable to use.

Beta blockers. The oldest drug in the group, propranolol, is also the best studied and safest. Metoprolol and labetalol can be used, too, because these drugs reach the milk in insignificant amounts. The long-acting beta blockers, such as acebutolol, atenolol, nadolol, sotalol, and timolol, reach the milk in higher quantities and are also more likely to accumulate in the infant's bloodstream. These should be avoided while breastfeeding a newborn.

Calcium channel blockers. Nifedipine has been well studied and is safe to use; it is sometimes used to treat painful nipple vasospasm (Raynaud's syndrome) that occurs occasionally during nursing. Information on diltiazem and verapamil is limited, but amounts in milk do not appear to be large enough to affect nursing infants.

Clonidine. Clonidine and the related drug guanfacine may decrease milk production. Clonidine reaches the milk in high levels, and breastfed infants have blood concentrations of the drug approaching those of their mothers. Other blood-pressure drugs are preferable, but if these drugs can't be avoided, they should be used with caution during breastfeeding.

Digoxin. This drug is excreted into milk in only small amounts. It can be used safely during lactation.

Diuretics. Large doses of diuretics, especially the most potent ones and those that are long acting, can decrease milk production. Their passage into milk has not been well studied, but the amounts that reach infants are likely to be small. These small amounts might in rare instances cause rashes or other allergic reactions. Chlorthalidone is a very long-acting diuretic should not be used during breastfeeding because it suppresses lactation. It might also accumulate in the infant's body. Furosemide has been used to suppress lactation. It should be used only with caution during breastfeeding, in small doses. Hydrochlorothiazide given once daily in doses of 25 mg or less, this drug appears safe. Small doses of torsemide did not suppress lactation in one study when mothers continued to breastfeed. Larger doses given several times daily have been used to suppress lactation. Long-acting thiazides should be avoided during breastfeeding. Spironolactone appears in insignificant amounts in milk.

Flecainide. Flecainide appears to be acceptable to use during breastfeeding because milk levels are fairly low.

Hydralazine. Amounts of this drug excreted into milk are small. Hydralazine can be used during lactation.

Methyldopa. Amounts of this drug excreted into milk are small, and methyldopa has been used safely during nursing for many years.

Mexiletine. Mexiletine is not expected to cause any adverse effects in breastfed infants, because amounts in milk are low.

Procainamide. Amounts that reach the milk are small. This drug appears acceptable to use while nursing.

Propafenone. Levels of this drug in milk are very low and should not cause a problem for the nursing infant.

Reserpine. Because this drug can cause nasal stuffiness in infants, it should be avoided during lactation.

Herbals. There is a mistaken tendency to think that because herbal drugs are "natural" they are never toxic. This is not true. Each herbal product must be evaluated individually on its own merits and risks. Unfortunately, almost none of these products have been studied during lactation, and very few have been studied in infants. Because these drugs are poorly regulated in the U.S., the quality and amounts of ingredients and even the ingredients themselves can vary widely from batch to batch and from one manufacturer to another. Additionally, because plant products may contain dozens of chemicals that can cause allergies, they may be more likely than conventional medications to cause problems like asthma and skin rashes in your infant or lead to plant allergies later in his life. For all these reasons, it is somewhat of a gamble to use herbal products during nursing. Information on some of the most commonly used herbals is listed below.

Barley. Barley has a component that might increase milk supply, which is how beer might stimulate lactation. It is safe to eat during breastfeeding, as in soup, but the alcohol in beer can affect the infant.

Blessed thistle. This is sometimes used to stimulate lactation, but there are no scientific studies that confirm its effectiveness. In fact, there have been no studies of the herb's effects during lactation. Blessed thistle appears to be fairly safe, but allergies have been reported, especially in those allergic to ragweed.

Chamomile. Various preparations have been used to treat mastitis and cracked, bleeding nipples and to increase lactation. No scientific data support these uses, but chamomile seems to be generally safe during breastfeeding. Allergic skin reactions occur occasionally in the mother.

Chasteberry. Some weak evidence shows that chasteberry might be useful for breast pain (mastalgia). It is well tolerated, but it might inhibit lactation.

Echinacea. There have been no studies of this herb during lactation. Although it is often used to prevent colds, scientific studies have shown it to be of little benefit. Some of its chemical components have been found in breast milk.

Elderberry. Most often used for influenza and immune stimulation, there is no information on the appearance of elderberry in breast milk or on the safety of elderberry in nursing mothers or infants.

Evening primrose oil. This oil contains various fatty acids and vitamin E. Some weak evidence shows that it might be useful for cyclic breast pain (mastalgia). It is well tolerated can be used while breastfeeding.

Fennel. Fennel is included in some proprietary mixtures that are promoted to increase the milk supply. Only a minimal amount of data support this use.

Fenugreek. Most commonly used as a spice, fenugreek seeds are often used to stimulate lactation and increase milk supply. Although there have been no high-quality scientific studies to substantiate this use, fenugreek is considered a safe food substance in small amounts; it is used as a flavoring in artificial maple syrup. It can lower blood sugar, and can interfere with warfarin, so diabetic women and those on warfarin should not use it without consulting a physician. Allergic reactions have also been reported.

Feverfew. Feverfew has no specific uses for breastfeeding. It is most often used to prevent migraine. No data exist on the excretion of feverfew into breastmilk or on the safety and efficacy of feverfew in nursing mothers or their infants.

Fish oil. A source of omega-3-fatty acids such as DHA and EPA, fish oil appears to have some benefit in mothers with severe postpartum depression. Although not harmful to breastfed infants, evidence for beneficial effects in the infants is weak.

Ginkgo biloba. No studies on the use of ginkgo during lactation are available. Maternal side effects are generally mild, but allergic skin reactions have occurred, and these could occur in the nursing infant as well as in the mother. People who take ginkgo sometimes experience headaches and gastrointestinal problems.

Goat's rue. This has a long history of use to increase milk supply, but very minimal scientific data exist on the safety and efficacy of goat's rue in nursing mothers or infants. In general, goat's rue is well tolerated, but it might lower blood sugar, so caution should be used in women with diabetes.

Ma huang. Also called ephedra, this common herbal ingredient in diet products contains an amphetamine-like stimulant that can suppress lactation and may affect a nursing infant. These diet products, many of which contain other stimulants as well, should definitely be avoided during lactation. See also "Weight-Loss Products."

Milk thistle. Milk thistle is said to increase milk supply, but very little evidence supports this use. However, very little is excreted into milk, so it is unlikely to harm the infant.

Moringa. The leaves of this tree, called malunggay in the Philippines, have been used to increase milk supply. Some studies indicate that it might have some activity as a galactogogue in mothers of preterm infants.

Peppermint. This plant contains menthol and supposedly increases milk supply, but no scientifically valid information supports this use.

Raspberry. The leaf supposedly increases milk supply; however, no scientifically valid clinical trials support this use.

Sage. Sage has been used to decrease lactation and to aid with weaning or an overabundant milk supply; however, no scientific studies substantiate this use or the safety of sage in nursing mothers or infants.

Saint John's wort. Colic, drowsiness, and lethargy have occurred in breastfed infants whose mothers were taking St. John's wort, and compounds from the plant are found in the bloodstream of breastfed infants. In fair-skinned persons, the drug may cause allergic skin reactions with light exposure. The drug is not very effective for depression, and the wisdom of self-medication for a serious condition such as depression is doubtful. St. John's wort should be avoided during lactation.

Stinging nettle. This has been used to treat anemia and as a galactogogue; however, no scientifically valid clinical trials support the safety and efficacy in nursing mothers or infants for any use.

Turmeric. Turmeric has been used in some countries to increase lactation and decrease breast pain, but good studies are lacking. It can cause nausea and diarrhea, and allergic reactions have been reported. It may increase the risk of bleeding in patients taking anticoagulants. No information is available on its effects on breastfed infants.

Valerian. Valerian is most commonly used to treat anxiety and sleep disturbances, and occasionally for self-treatment of postpartum blues or depression. No data exist on the safety and efficacy of valerian in nursing mothers or infants, but some of its components are potentially toxic. It is probably best avoided during nursing.

Wild asparagus. Called shatavari in India, wild asparagus has a long history of use as a galactogogue in India. The safety of wild asparagus has not been rigorously studied, but two small studies found no adverse effects in mothers or their nursing infants.

Thyroid drugs

Thyroid products are used to replace the thyroid hormone that is lacking or low in the mother's bloodstream. When a woman takes proper doses, her thyroid levels become approximately normal. Thyroid replacement, therefore, poses no risks to the breastfed infant. Large daily doses of thyroid hormone (more than about 100 micrograms daily of levothyroxine) might affect the infant. Breastfeeding during treatment with the antithyroid drugs, propylthiouracil (PTU) and methimazole, is acceptable. However, methimazole is now preferred because of rare toxic reactions to PTU. Monitoring of the infant's blood for adequate thyroid function may be necessary. Radioactive iodine-131should never be used in nursing mothers and if it is, breastfeeding of this infant should be discontinued permanently.

Female hormonal drugs

Clomiphene. This synthetic hormone-like drug affects the activity of estrogen in the body and stimulates ovulation. There is no information on the drug during nursing; however, it can suppress lactation. Because it could have serious adverse consequences on the sexual maturation of your infant, and because it could remain in your body and milk for weeks after you take it, you should discontinue nursing if you take it.

Contraceptives. Hormonal contraceptives can be divided into two categories: combination and progestin-only. The combination products contain estrogen, decrease lactation, and can cause premature weaning, although long-term effects on growth and development in infants have not been found. Included among the combination contraceptives are the vaginal ring (NuvaRing), the contraceptive patch (Ortho Evra), and one injectable product (Lunelle). These contraceptives are not preferred, especially immediately after birth, because they might interfere with the establishment of lactation or affect the newborn. It is best not to use a combination contraceptive during breastfeeding unless you intend to stop nursing soon.

If you plan to use hormonal contraception, a progestin-only oral product such as norethindrone or levonorgestrel, or a progestin given by injection (Depo-Provera, Implanon, Nexplanon), is preferable. Some intrauterine devices (IUDs) release small amounts of progesterone or progestin (for example, Progestasert and Mirena) and are considered as safe as other progestin-only contraceptives. Nonhormonal intrauterine devices, including copper-containing devices (Copper-T), can be used during lactation without concern of adverse effects on the infant or lactation. Progestin-only contraceptive injections or implants are sometimes given within a few days after birth. Usually, this does not affect nursing.

The short duration of exposure to morning-after contraceptives, such as levonorgestrel (Plan B), should not adversely affect the nursing infant and at worse should have only a minimal, temporary effect on lactation.

Estrogens. Estrogens have been used after birth to suppress lactation, but they are no longer used this way because they are dangerous for the mother. Estrogen products such as Premarin and Estrace, taken orally or vaginally, probably interfere with nursing.

Corticosteroids. Drugs in this category include cortisone, methylprednisolone, prednisone, and triamcinolone. Usual low doses of these drugs that are used for long-term immunosuppression in lupus, after organ transplantation or other chronic conditions are not a concern for the breastfed infant. Mothers who require one or more large intravenous doses for disease flares can minimize the exposure of the infant by avoiding nursing for two to four hours after the dose.

Dexamethasone and betamethasone are long-acting agents that have not been studied during nursing. It is best to avoid these two drugs.

Immunosuppressants and immunomodulators

Azathioprine. Numerous mothers have safely breastfed their infants while taking azathioprine following organ transplantation. See also antirheumatic drugs.

Cyclosporine. Some mothers have breastfed while taking this medication without harm to the baby, but the nursing infant should be carefully monitored, possibly with blood testing. See also antirheumatic drugs.

Glatiramer. Limited information exists on the use of this drug during breastfeeding. Because it is unlikely to be absorbed by the infant from breast milk, harmful effects are unlikely in the infant.

Interferons. Several interferon drugs are available. These drugs are unlikely to pass into milk and affect an infant, as was found to be the case in studies of three breastfeeding women who were taking interferon alfa. Also, these drugs are active only when given by injection, so any interferon that would enter breast milk would have little or no effect on the infant. Some information on breastfeeding and interferon beta found no harm to breastfed infants and most experts feel that this drug can be used during breastfeeding.

Methotrexate. Methotrexate should not be used during breastfeeding in the doses required for cancer chemotherapy, but this drug might be acceptable in the low doses used for arthritis. See "Arthritis, Pain, and Migraine Medications."

Mycophenolate mofetil. This has not been adequately studied during breastfeeding, so it is generally considered to be undesirable to nurse while taking it.

Tacrolimus. Experience with tacrolimus during nursing has found no harm to breastfed infants and amounts in milk are small. It is acceptable to use during nursing. Tacrolimus can be used on the skin during breastfeeding as long as it is not applied to the breast or other areas where the infant would come into direct contact with it.

Everolimus and sirolimus. These drugs have very little information during breastfeeding. Although no adverse reactions have been reported in breastfed infants, better-studied drugs are preferred when possible.

Iodine and iodide. Use of povidone iodine, especially as a douche, but even on the skin, can result in high iodine blood levels in the mother. Iodine becomes concentrated in milk and then in the infant's thyroid gland, possibly causing abnormal thyroid function; iodide rashes have also occurred in breastfed infants. Iodides should not be used during lactation. See also "Radio-Opaque Agents."

Lipid-lowering drugs. None of the cholesterol-lowering drugs have been studied during nursing. Because cholesterol is essential for the proper development of the infant's brain and nervous system, drugs that can enter the milk should generally not be taken during nursing.

Statins. Statis are the most potent and commonly used drugs and include atorvastatin, fluvastatin, lovastatin, pitavastatin, pravastatin, rosuvastatin, and simvastatin. They have not been studied well, but pravastatin and rosuvastatin have a small amount of information indicating that the amount is milk is low and atorvastatin was used safely in a small number of infants.

Fibrates. These are other lipid-lowering drugs that can enter the milk and include fenofibrate and gemfibrozil. Fibrates should be avoided during nursing.

Ezetimibe. This has not been studied during breastfeeding and should also be avoided.

Resins. Cholestyramine, colestipol, and colesevelam are resins that work only in the mother's intestinal tract and are not absorbed. They can be used during nursing.

Niacin. Niacin in high doses has not been studied in nursing mothers. It is unclear whether high-dose niacin can affect the nursing infant.

Nonmedical drugs. Since drugs used for nontherapeutic purposes are not essential to the well-being of the mother, and their effects on a breastfed infant are often unknown, their use is generally discouraged. Additionally, even small amounts can cause positive drug tests in your infant's urine, which with some drugs could lead to legal problems.

Alcohol. Alcohol readily passes into the milk. Large amounts of alcoholic beverages consumed over a short time can make a baby drunk and can inhibit the let-down reflex. Even small amounts of alcohol taken right before nursing can cause disruption in nursing behavior and the mother-infant interaction. Right after you drink an alcoholic beverage, your infant may suck more but consume up to 25 percent less milk (the baby may make up for this later in the day if you take no more alcohol). Heavy daily drinking can lead to hormonal imbalances in a breastfed infant, and even small to moderate amounts of alcohol taken daily or nearly every day while nursing appear to cause delayed muscular development and coordination in infants, although the severity of this problem depends on the amount of alcohol used. An occasional alcoholic beverage does not pose a danger to the infant, but you should wait at least two hours per drink before nursing. This period of time allows alcohol to leave the breast milk. Because breastfeeding is more frequent in the first month after birth and your infant is more susceptible, it is probably a good idea to avoid alcohol during this important time.

Amphetamines. Amphetamine and methamphetamine ("crystal," "crystal meth") have not been formally studied during nursing. However, they are potent stimulants. Breastfeeding mothers who take these drugs might have fussy infants who cry a lot, cannot be comforted easily, and do not sleep well. Amphetamines probably also inhibit the mother's milk production. These drugs should not be used during nursing; if they are, the mother should temporarily stop nursing for 24 to 48 hours after taking them recreationally. Lower doses of amphetamine or methylphenidate prescribed to treat medical conditions appear not to affect breastfed infants.

Caffeine. Low to moderate intake of beverages containing caffeine (such as 2 cups of coffee or 3 to 4 cups of tea per day) is unlikely to cause problems in the infant, since the amount of caffeine that reaches the milk is usually small. But very high caffeine intake (more than ten cups of coffee or cola per day, for example) can make the baby jittery and agitated.

Cocaine. Cocaine is extremely toxic to infants because they metabolize it very slowly. Great agitation and continuous crying are often noted in breastfed infants of cocaine users, and cocaine applied to the nipples to treat soreness can cause convulsions in the infant. Cocaine should be avoided during nursing. If a mother does use it, she should stop breastfeeding for at least 24 hours afterward.

Hallucinogens. Information is lacking on the effects of these drugs (such as LSD, psilocybin and ecstasy) during breastfeeding; however, levels in milk should be low by the time the mother has stopped feeling the effects of the drug.

Cannabis. There are few reports of the effects of cannabis in breastfed babies. After a single use, the psychoactive component, tetrahydrocannabinol (THC), levels in milk are apparently low, but the active component of the drug can build up in the body with daily or near-daily use. Early studies on THC in milk have been inconsistent, but THC persists in milk for at least 6 days and perhaps up to 6 weeks with heavy use. Note, too, that an infant in the same room with a smoker will breathe in significant quantities of marijuana, probably more than through breast milk. Breastfed infants whose mothers use cannabis heavily have sometimes shown delayed muscular development and coordination. THC and its metabolites are detectable in the urine of breastfed infants whose mothers use cannabis products. Much more study is needed to clarify the effects of cannabis products on infants whose mothers use them while pregnant and nursing, especially with today's high potency products. The best advice is to avoid cannabis while nursing. See "Tobacco" below for ways to minimize infant exposure.

Cannabidiol (CBD oil). Even less information is available on cannabidiol (CBD oil), which may have some medical uses. However, use on the skin is not likely to affect the infant unless she is able to touch or lick the product from the mother's skin. Many CBD products are contaminated with THC and other chemicals from cannabis.

Phencyclidine (PCP). Large amounts of this drug have been measured in the breast milk of users. PCP must be entirely avoided during breastfeeding. It might take several days for PCP to clear from breast milk.

Tobacco. Nicotine from smoking tobacco appears in breast milk. Other toxic substances in smoke reach the milk as well. Smoking interferes with lactation, which causes smokers to start supplementing and stop nursing sooner than nonsmokers. Infants of smokers are more likely than other babies to have colic symptoms and respiratory infections. Additionally, although breastfeeding reduces the risk of sudden infant death syndrome (SIDS), smoking negates this advantage. If you can't stop smoking while you are nursing, you should (1) decrease your smoking as much as possible, (2) avoid nursing just after smoking, (3) avoid smoking in the same room with your baby, and (4) cover your regular clothing while you smoke and remove the covering before holding your infant. Although amounts of nicotine in breast milk during the use of a nicotine patch appear to be about the same as those in the milk of smokers, using a nicotine patch or nicotine chewing gum during breastfeeding is preferable to smoking.

Psychotherapeutic agents. For many of these drugs, little is known about excretion into milk or effects on breastfed infants. Undertake nursing with caution if you are using one of these medications. Combinations of two or more of these drugs are more likely to adversely affect the infant than a single drug.

Major tranquilizers. These drugs include the phenothiazines, such as chlorpromazine, thioridazine, trifluoperazine, perphenazine, and fluphenazine; the closely related thioxanthenes, such as thiothixene; the butyrophenones, such as haloperidol; and the newer "atypical" drugs such as clozapine, olanzapine, paliperidone, quetiapine, risperidone, and ziprasidone. Small amounts of these drugs appear in breast milk, and occasionally they have caused drowsiness in breastfed infants. Long-term effects on the infant are not well known. One study found no altered development in infants exposed to one of these drugs through breast milk; however, use of two or more of the drugs together could adversely affect the infant's development. It is acceptable to breastfeed with most of these drugs, but nursing is not recommended during clozapine therapy, which can cause harmful side effects in the infant.

Antidepressants. Postpartum depression occurs in about one of eight women. Untreated depression can have serious and long-lasting effects on infant growth and development, so treatment is essential. None of the medications used in treating depression are known to decrease milk production. If you took one of the following drugs during pregnancy, it is best to continue on the same medication during breastfeeding, because amounts in milk are much less than those passed across the placenta.

Tricyclic antidepressants. Drugs such as amitriptyline, imipramine, nortriptyline, and desipramine are found in milk in small amounts and do not seem to affect the growth and development of the breastfed infant. Drowsiness can result with some of the more sedating drugs, such as doxepin, which should be avoided. Nortriptyline appears to be the safest and best studied of all the tricyclic antidepressants. It is found in only small amounts in milk, and little or none reaches the infant's bloodstream. If possible, take tricyclic antidepressants in the evening, after the final nursing session of the day, to minimize the dose that the breastfed infant receives.

SSRI antidepressants. Fluoxetine appears in milk in higher amounts than most other antidepressants; it is very long acting; and side effects in the infant (colic, fussiness, and drowsiness) have been reported during its use, although infants older than one month can probably tolerate it better than younger babies. If fluoxetine is being continued from pregnancy or is needed for another reason, the benefits of using this medication while breastfeeding usually outweigh the risks to the infant, but watch the infant carefully for side effects. Citalopram is also found in relatively large amounts in milk, and it may cause drowsiness in the infant, especially when the baby is a newborn. Escitalopram is a form of citalopram that is taken in a lower dose;

however, it, too has caused infant side effects occasionally. Fluvoxamine, paroxetine, and sertraline are found in lower amounts in milk and are shorter acting than fluoxetine. Sertraline and paroxetine are the best studied and do not seem to affect nursing infants in the short or long run. They are good choices when an antidepressant is needed during nursing, with sertraline recommended most frequently.

Brexanolone. Brexanolone is a hormonal antidepressant that is given intravenously over 60 hours. The amounts in milk are low and the drug is not absorbed well by the baby, so if brexanolone is required, it is not a reason to discontinue breastfeeding. However, excessive drowsiness or sudden loss of consciousness can occur during brexanolone infusion, so it is suggested that nursing mothers provide a separate caregiver for any child who is present during the infusion.

Bupropion. Bupropion has been studied in a small number of mother-infant pairs and appears not to adversely affect nursing infants.

Nefazodone. This drug has also not been well studied, but it has caused drowsiness and poor feeding in one newborn infant, so it is best avoided if you are nursing a newborn.

Venlafaxine. Venlafaxine is found in relatively high amounts in milk and in the nursing infant's bloodstream. Experience with it during breastfeeding is limited, but side effects in infants have not been seen. If possible, avoid venlafaxine if you are nursing a newborn. Desvenlafaxine produces lower levels in milk than venlafaxine and may be preferable.

Vortioxetine. This appears in milk in low amounts that are unlikely to affect a nursing infant, but it has not been studied extensively.

Other antidepressants. Limited data indicate that duloxetine, mirtazapine, and trazodone are probably also acceptable to take during breastfeeding, but watch for excessive drowsiness if you are nursing a newborn. Amoxapine, maprotiline, and vilazodone have been less well studied, so no judgment can be made on their safety.

Monoamine oxidase inhibitors. Drugs such as phenelzine and tranylcypromine, are very potent drugs and should not be used while breastfeeding. If they are essential, breastfeeding should probably be stopped.

Lithium. This drug reaches breast milk in rather high levels. Lithium can accumulate in the infant's bloodstream and cause side effects in a premature or newborn infant who becomes dehydrated due to diarrhea or a viral illness. A healthy infant can be breastfed during lithium therapy, but only with careful monitoring—including, in some cases, blood tests for lithium. If your infant becomes ill for any reason during lithium therapy, contact your health-care provider.

Sedatives and sleep medications. Several types of drugs are included in this category. Although all of them can make an infant drowsy, some are more likely to do so than others. The drugs also differ in how long they persist in the body, which affects their tendency to accumulate in the infant.

Barbiturates. Drugs in this class include amobarbital, butalbital, pentobarbital, phenobarbital, secobarbital, and others. All of them, especially phenobarbital, may occasionally cause drowsiness in breastfed infants, but none are particularly hazardous to the baby otherwise, unless she becomes so drowsy that she nurses less.

Benzodiazepines. These are the most frequently used sedative drugs. They include alprazolam, chlordiazepoxide, diazepam, flurazepam, lorazepam, oxazepam, triazolam, and others. Although these drugs are safe in adults, newborn infants do not readily metabolize them; the long-acting drugs in this group accumulate in the infant's body. These include clorazepate, chlordiazepoxide and diazepam. They may make the baby drowsy and, in some cases, may interfere with the binding of bilirubin in the bloodstream. These problems are accentuated in premature and newborn babies. Short-acting benzodiazepines, such as lorazepam, oxazepam and triazolam, reach breast milk in lesser amounts, and are therefore unlikely to cause drowsiness. Some sleeping medications similar to the benzodiazepines are eszopiclone, zaleplon and zolpidem.

These are relatively short acting and appear in milk in very small amounts, so they can be used while nursing.

Buspirone. Occasional use of buspirone during nursing appears to be acceptable, but long-term daily use should be avoided because the amount of information available is inadequate.

Over-the-counter sleep medications. These usually contain diphenhydramine; the general precautions for the sedating antihistamines apply. (See "Cough, Cold, Allergy, and Asthma Medications.")

Radiologic agents. A number of compounds are used in the X-ray diagnosis of various conditions. These compounds fall into three categories: MRI contrast agents, radio-opaque contrast agents, and radioactive agents. The radiologist administering these tests usually has guidelines on breastfeeding with the specific agents. X-rays themselves, of teeth, bones, or the chest, pose no hazard to the breastfed infant.

MRI contrast agents. These agents, gadobenate, gadobutrol, gadodiamide, gadofosveset gadopentetate, gadoterate, gadoteridol, gadoversetamide, and gadoxetate, contain gadolinium rather than iodine and are relatively safe and rapidly eliminated. There is no need to stop nursing for any length of time after receiving one of these agents.

Radio-opaque agents. Also called iodinated contrast agents or x-ray contrast media, these are generally compounds that contain iodine, but the iodine is tightly bound to the compound and does not enter breast milk in large amounts. None of these agents require cessation or withholding of breastfeeding.

Radioactive agents. Breastfeeding must be stopped for a time after some of these agents are administered. The period of time varies depending on the agent and the dose given; a few of these agents such as iodine-131 persist in breast milk for so long that complete weaning of the baby is necessary. After exposure to some of these agents your body could give off radiation, particularly at close range. This means that not only would you have to stop breastfeeding temporarily, but you might not be able to hold your baby for some time, since doing so would expose her to radioactivity. Technetium-containing agents, such as pertechnetate often require no waiting period or only a short waiting period. Be sure to tell the radiologist that you are breastfeeding before you receive any of these agents. You can ask to have your milk tested to see how much radioactivity is remaining and when it is safe to resume nursing.

For nursing mothers with overactive thyroid glands, the most commonly prescribed of these agents are iodine-123 (for diagnosis) and iodine-131 (for treatment). Iodine-123 is usually eliminated in two to three days. Discontinuation of nursing is definitely required after iodine-131. A future baby can be safely breastfed after receiving these agents. Technetium 99m pertechnetate is the preferred alternative for diagnostic use during breastfeeding.

Vaccines and skin tests. No routine vaccine or skin test (such as the one for tuberculosis, PPD), when given to a mother, is known to pose a hazard to her breastfed infant. Killed vaccines, including diphtheria, hepatitis A and B, injectable influenza, injectable polio, and tetanus vaccines, are inactive in breast milk. Although routine live vaccines are occasionally transmitted through breast milk, they do not endanger the baby. Live vaccines include inhaled influenza, measles, mumps, oral polio, rubella, oral typhoid, and varicella. With the exceptions of the smallpox and yellow fever vaccines, the U.S. Centers for Disease Control and Prevention (CDC) states that no vaccination should be withheld from a woman or delayed because she is breastfeeding.

Several types of vaccines for COVID-19 are available. The mRMA vaccines are safe and effective in nursing mothers. They result in high antibody levels in milk that help protect your infant from COVID-19. As of this writing, less breastfeeding information is available about the use of adenovirus vector vaccines; however, the Centers for Disease Control and Prevention states that nursing mothers can receive any of the vaccines available in the United States.

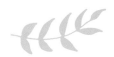

References & Reading

References

Breastfeeding without Birthing: A Breastfeeding Guide for Mothers

O Mireles: *Markers of lactation insufficiency: A study of 34 mothers, in*: K. Auerbach, Ed. Current Issues in Clinical Lactation 2000. Jones and Bartlett, Sudbury, MA. Pp. 25-35). see K Huggins, E Petok,

American Academy of Pediatrics. "Policy Statement: Breastfeeding and the Use of Human Milk." *Pediatrics* 115 (2005): 496–506.

————. "Prevention of Pediatric Overweight and Obesity." *Pediatrics* 112 (2003): 424–30.

————. "Report on the Assessment of Scientific Evidence Relating to Infant-Feeding Practices and Infant Health." *Pediatrics* 74 (1984): 191–97.

Anderson, A. M. "Disruption of Lactogenesis by Retained Placental Fragments." *Journal of Human Lactation* 17 (2001): 142–44.

Arenz, S., et al. "Breast-Feeding and Childhood Obesity: A Systematic Review." *International Journal of Obesity and Related Metabolic Disorders* 28 (2004): 1247–56.

Auerbach, Kathleen G. "Employed Breastfeeding Mothers: Problems They Encounter." *Birth* 11 (1984): 17–20.

Auerbach, Kathleen G., and Laurence Gartner. "Breastfeeding and Human Milk: Their Association with Jaundice in the Neonate." *Clinics in Perinatology* 14 (1987): 89–107.

Auerbach, Kathleen G., and E. Guss. "Maternal Employment and Breastfeeding: A Study of 567 Women's Experiences." *American Journal of Disease in Childhood* 138 (1984): 958–60.

Bachrach, V. R., et al. "Breastfeeding and the Risk of Hospitalization for Respiratory Disease in Infancy: A Meta-Analysis." *Archives of Pediatrics and Adolescent Medicine* 157 (2003): 237–43.

Ballard, Jeanne L., et al. "Ankyloglossia: Assessment, Incidence, and Effect of Frenuloplasty on the Breastfeeding Dyad." *Pediatrics* 110 (2002): 62–68.

Bauer, G., et al. "Breastfeeding and Cognitive Development of Three-Year-Old Children." *Psychology Report* 68 (1991): 1218.

Bener, A., et al. "Longer Breast-Feeding and Protection against Childhood Leukaemia and Lymphomas." *European Journal of Cancer* 37 (2001): 234–38.

Bier, J. A., et al. "Human Milk Improves Cognitive and Motor Development of Premature Infants during Infancy." *Journal of Human Lactation* 18 (2002): 361–67.

Bishara, R. "Volume of Foremilk, Hindmilk, and Total Milk Produced by Mothers of Very Preterm Infants Born at Less Than 28 Weeks of Gestation." *Journal of Human Lactation* 25 (2009): 272–79.

Bishop, N., M. McGraw, and N. Ward. "Aluminum in Infant Formulas." *Lancet* 1 (1989): 490.

Bowen, A. B., and C. R. Braden. "Invasive *Enterbacter sakazakii* Disease in Infants." *Emerging Infectious Diseases Journal* 12 (2006): 1185–89.

Brazelton, T. Berry. *Infants and Mothers: Differences in Development*, rev. ed. New York: Delta/Seymour Lawrence, 1983.

Brent, N., et al. "Sore Nipples in Breast-Feeding Women: A Clinical Trial of Wound Dressings versus Conventional Care." *Archives of Pediatric and Adolescent Medicine* 152 (1998): 1072–82.

Brewster, Dorothy Patricia. *You Can Breastfeed Your Baby . . . Even in Special Situations.* Emmaus, PA: Rodale Press, 1979.

Byers, T., et al. "Lactation and Breast Cancer: Evidence for a Negative Association in Pre-Menopausal Women." *American Journal of Epidemiology* 121 (1985): 664–74.

Bystrova, K., et al. "Skin to Skin Contact May Reduce Negative Consequences of 'the Stress of Being Born': A Study on Temperature in Newborn Infants, Subjected to Different Ward Routines in St. Petersburg." *Acta Pediatrica* 3 (2003): 320–26.

Christensson, K. "Temperature, Metabolic Adaptation, and Crying in Healthy, Full-Term Newborns Cared for Skin-to-Skin or in a Cot." *Acta Paediatrica Scandinavica* 81 (2009): 488–93.

Coles, J. "Qualitative Study of Breastfeeding After Childhood Sexual Assault." *Journal of Human Lactation* 25 (2009): 317–24.

Collaborative Group on Hormonal Factors in Breast Cancer. "Breast Cancer and Breastfeeding: Collaborative Reanalysis of Individual Data from 47 Epidemiological Studies in 30 Countries, Including 50,302 Women with Breast Cancer and 96,973 Women without the Disease." *Lancet* 360 (2002): 187–95.

Colson, S. D., et al. "Optimal Positions for the Release of Primitive Neonatal Reflexes Stimulating Breastfeeding." *Early Human Development* 84 (2008): 441–49.

Cotterman, K. J. "Reverse Pressure Softening: A Simple Tool to Prepare Areola for Easier Latching During Engorgement." *Journal of Human Lactation* 20 (2004): 227–37.

Courtney, K. "Maternal Anesthesia: What Are the Effects on Neonates?" *Nursing for Women's Health* 11 (2007): 499–502.

Cumming, R. G., and R. J. Klineberg. "Breastfeeding and Other Reproductive Factors and the Risk of Hip Fractures in Elderly Women." *International Journal of Epidemiology* 22 (1993): 684–69.

Davis, M. K., D. A. Savitz, and B. I. Graubard. "Infant Feeding and Childhood Cancer." *Lancet* 2 (1988): 365–68.

DeCarvalho, M., M. Hall, and D. Harvey. "Effects of Water Supplementation on Physiological Jaundice in Breast-fed Babies." *Archives of Disease in Childhood* 56 (1981): 568–69.

Dewey, K. G., et al. "Breast-Fed Infants Are Leaner than Formula-Fed Infants at 1 Year of Age: The DARLING Study." *American Journal of Clinical Nutrition* 57 (1993): 140–45.

————. "Maternal Weight-Loss Patterns during Prolonged Lactation." *American Journal of Clinical Nutrition* 58 (1993): 162–66.

Dowling, D. A., et al. "Cup-Feeding for Preterm Infants: Mechanics and Safety." *Journal of Human Lactation* 18 (2002): 13–20.

Eglash, A., et al. "History, Physical and Laboratory Findings, and Clinical Outcomes of Lactating Women Treated with Antibiotics for Chronic Breast and/or Nipple Pain." *Journal of Human Lactation* 22 (2006): 429–33.

Ehrenkranz, R., and B. Ackerman. "Metoclopramide Effect on Faltering Milk Production by Mothers of Premature Infants." *Pediatrics* 78 (1986): 614–20.

Elias, Marjorie F., et al. "Sleep/Wake Patterns of Breastfed Infants in the First Two Years of Life." *Pediatrics* 77 (1986): 322–29.

Estrella M. C., et al. "A Double-Blind, Randomized Controlled Trial on the Use of Malunggay (*Moringa oleifera*) for Augmentation of the Volume of Beastmilk among Non-Nursing Mothers of Preterm Infants." *Philippine Journal of Pediatrics* 49 (2000): 3–6.

Ferber, Richard. *Solve Your Child's Sleep Problems: The Complete Practical Guide for Parents.* New York: Simon and Schuster, 1985.

Fiocchi, A., et al. "Food Allergy and the Introduction of Solid Foods to Infants: A Consensus Document." *Annals of Allergy, Asthma, and Immunology* 1 (2006): 10–20.

Friedland, G., and R. Klein. "Transmission of the Human Immunodeficiency Virus." *New England Journal of Medicine* 317 (1987): 1125–35.

Gardiner, D. T., et al. "Breast-Feeding Increases Sleep Duration of New Parents." *Journal of Perinatal and Neonatal Nursing* 21 (2007): 200–206.

Gillman, M. W., et al. "Risk of Overweight among Adolescents Who Were Breastfed as Infants." *Journal of the American Medical Association* 285 (2001): 2461–67.

Gordan, C. M., et al. "Prevalence of Vitamin D Deficiency among Healthy Infants and Toddlers." *Archives of Paediatric Medicine* 162 (2008): 505–12.

Gupta, J. K., and V. C. Nikoderm. "Position for Women during Second Stage of Labor." *Cochrane Library* 3. Oxford: Update Software, 2003.

Gwinn, M. L., et al. "Pregnancy, Breastfeeding, and Oral Contraceptives and the Risk of Epithelial Ovarian Cancer." *Journal of Clinical Epidemiology* 43 (1990): 559–68.

Hahn-Zoric, M., et al. "Antibody Responses to Parenteral and Oral Vaccines Are Impaired by Conventional and Low Protein Formulas as Compared to Breastfeeding." *Acta Paediatrica Scandanavica* 79 (1990): 1137–42.

Hill, P. D., et al. "Comparison of Milk Output Between Mothers of Preterm and Term Infants: The First 6 Weeks After Birth." *Journal of Human Lactation* 21 (2005): 22–30.

————. "Initiation and Frequency of Pumping and Milk Production in Mothers of Non-Nursing Preterm Infants." *Journal of Human Lactation* 17 (2001): 9–13.

Horne, R. S., et al. "Comparison of Evoked Arousability in Breast and Formula Fed Infants." *Archives of Disease in Childhood* 89 (2004): 22–25.

Horwood, L. J., et al. "Breast Milk Feeding and Cognitive Ability at 7–8 Years." *Archives of Disease in Childhood–Fetal and Neonatal Edition* 84 (2001): 23–27.

Huggins, Kathleen, and Sharon Billon. "Twenty Cases of Persistent Sore Nipples: Collaboration Between Lactation Consultant and Dermatologist." *Journal of Human Lactation* 9 (1993): 155–60.

Huggins, Kathleen, et al. "Markers of Lactation Insufficiency: A Study of 34 Mothers." *Current Issues in Clinical Lactation* 1 (2000): 25–35.

Hurst, N. M., et al. "Mothers Performing In-Home Measurement of Milk Intake During Breastfeeding of Their Preterm Infants: Maternal Reactions and Feeding Outcomes." *Journal of Human Lactation* 20 (2004): 178–87.

Jain, L. "Morbidity and Mortality in Late-Preterm Infants: More Than Just Transient Tachypnea!" *Journal of Pediatrics* 151 (2007): 445–46.

Jensen, Rima. "Fenugreek: Overlooked but Not Forgotten." *UCLA Lactation Alumni Association Newsletter* 1 (1992): 2–3.

Jernstrom, H., et al. "Breast-Feeding and the Risk of Breast Cancer in BRCA1 and BRCA2 Mutation Carriers." *Journal of the National Cancer Institute* 96 (2004): 1094–98.

Kalies, H., et al. "The Effect of Breastfeeding on Weight Gain in Infants: Results of a Birth Cohort Study." *European Journal of Medical Research* 10 (2005): 36–42.

Karp, Harvey. "The 'Fourth Trimester': A Framework and Strategy for Understanding and Resolving Colic." *Contemporary Pediatrics* 21 (2004): 94–114.

Kavanaugh, Karen, et al. "Getting Enough: Mothers' Concerns about Breastfeeding a Preterm Infant after Discharge." *Journal of Obstetric, Gynecologic, and Neonatal Nursing* 24 (1995): 23–32.

Keating, J. P., G. J. Schears, and P. R. Dodge. "Oral Water Intoxication in Infants: An American Epidemic." *American Journal of Disease in Childhood* 145 (1991): 985–90.

Kennedy, K. I., et al. "Lactational Amenorrhea Method for Family Planning." *International Journal of Gynaecology and Obstetrics* 54 (1996): 55–57.

Klingelhafer, S. K. "Sexual Abuse and Breastfeeding." *Journal of Human Lactation* 23 (2007): 194–97.

Koetting, C. A., and G. M. Wardlaw. "Wrist, Spine, and Hip Bone Density in Women with Variable Histories of Lactation." *American Journal of Clinical Nutrition* 48 (1988): 1479–81.

Kotaska, A., et al. "Epidural Analgesia Associated with Low-Dose Oxytocin Augmentation Increases Cesarean Births: A Critical Look at the External Validity of Randomized Trials." *American Journal of Obstetrics and Gynecology* 194 (2006): 809–14.

Kramer, M. S., et al. "Breastfeeding and Child Cognitive Development: New Evidence from a Large Randomized Trial." *Archives of General Psychiatry* 65 (2008): 578–84.

Labbok, M. H., and G. E. Hendershot. "Does Breastfeeding Protect against Malocclusion? Analysis of the 1981 Child Health Supplement to the National Health Interview Survey." *American Journal of Preventative Medicine* 3 (1987): 227–32.

Lawrence, Ruth A., and Robert M. Lawrence. *Breastfeeding: A Guide for the Medical Profession.* St. Louis: Mosby, 2010.

————. *A Review of the Medical Benefits and Contraindications to Breastfeeding in the United States.* Arlington, VA: National Center for Education in Maternal and Child Health, 1997.

Layde, P. M., et al. "The Independent Associations of Parity, Age of First Full-Term Pregnancy, and Duration of Breastfeeding with the Risk of Breast Cancer." *Journal of Clinical Epidemiology* 42 (1989): 963–93.

Lee, S. Y., et al. "Effect of Lifetime Lactation on Breast Cancer Risk: A Korean Women's Cohort Study." *International Journal of Cancer* 105 (2003): 390–93.

Lieberman, E., and C. O'Donoghue. "Unintended Effects of Epidural Anesthesia: A Systematic Review." *American Journal of Obstetrics and Gynecology Supplement* 186 (2002): s31–68.

Lindenberg, C. S., et al. "The Effect of Early Post Partum Mother-Infant Contact and Breastfeeding Promotion on the Incidence and Continuation of Breastfeeding." *International Journal of Nursing Studies* 27 (1990): 179–86.

Livingstone, Verity, and L. Judy Stringer. "The Treatment of *Staphyloccus aureus* Infected Sore Nipples: A Randomized Comparative Study." *Journal of Human Lactation* 15, no. 3 (1999): 241–46.

Lopez, J. M., et al. "Bone Turnover and Density in Healthy Women during Breastfeeding and after Weaning." *Osteoporosis International* 6 (1996): 153–59.

Lucas, A., et al. "Breastmilk and Subsequent Intelligence Quotient in Children Born Preterm." *Lancet* 339 (1992): 261–64.

Main, E. K., et al. "Is There a Useful Cesarean Birth Measure? Assessment of the Nulliparous Term Singleton Vertex Cesarean Birth Rate as a Tool for Obstetric Quality Improvement." *American Journal of Obstetrics and Gynecology* 194 (2006): 1644–52.

Marasco, L., et al. "Polycystic Ovary Syndrome: A Connection to Insufficient Milk Supply?" *Journal of Human Lactation* 16 (2000): 143–48.

Mayer, E. J., et al. "Reduced Risk of IDDM among Breastfed Children." *Diabetes* 37 (1988): 1625–32.

McJunkin, J. E., W. G. Bithoney, and M. C. McCormick. "Errors in Formula Concentration in an Outpatient Population." *Journal of Pediatrics* 111 (1987): 848–50.

McTiernan, A., and D. B. Thomas. "Evidence for a Protective Effect of Lactation on Risk of Breast Cancer in Young Women." *American Journal of Epidemiology* 124 (1986): 353–58.

McVea, K. L., et al. "The Role of Breastfeeding in Sudden Infant Death Syndrome." *Journal of Human Lactation* 16 (2000): 13–20.

Meier, Paula. "A Program to Support Breastfeeding in the High-Risk Nursery." *Perinatology/ Neonatology* 4 (1980): 43–48.

————. *Professional Guide to Breastfeeding Premature Infants.* Columbus, OH: Abbott Laboratories, 1997.

Meier, Paula, and G. Anderson. "Responses of Small Preterm Infants to Bottle- and Breast-Feeding." *Maternal-Child Nursing* 12 (1987): 97–105.

Meier, Paula, et al. "Nipple Shields for Preterm Infants: Effect on Milk Transfer and Duration of Breastfeeding." *Journal of Human Lactation* 16 (2000): 106–14.

THE NURSING MOTHER'S COMPANION

Merchant, J. R., et al. "Respiratory Instability of Term and Near-Term Healthy Newborn Infants in Car Safety Seats." *Pediatrics* 108 (2001): 647–52.

Merrett, T. G., et al. "Infant Feeding and Allergy: Twelve-Month Prospective Study of 500 Babies Born in Allergic Families." *Annals of Allergy* 61 (1988): 13–20.

Mikiel-Kostyra, K., et al. "Effect of Skin to Skin Contact after Delivery on Duration of Breastfeeding: A Prospective Cohort Study." *Acta Paediatrica* 91 (2002): 1301–6.

Minutes of the Panel on Recommendations Relating to PBB and Nursing Mothers. Lansing: Michigan Department of Public Health, 1976.

Mitchell, E. A., et al. "Cot Death Supplement: Results from the First Year of the New Zealand Cot Death Study." *New Zealand Medical Journal* 104 (1991): 71–76.

Morino, C., and Susan M. Winn. "Raynaud's Phenomenon of the Nipples: An Elusive Diagnosis." *Journal of Human Lactation* 23 (2007): 191–93.

Morrow-Tlucak, M., R. H. Haude, and C. B. Ernhart. "Breastfeeding and Cognitive Development in the First Two Years of Life." *Social Science Medicine* 26 (1988): 635–39.

Morse, Janice M., and Margaret J. Harrison. "Social Coercion for Weaning." *Journal of Nurse Midwifery* 32 (1987): 205–10.

Mortensen, E. L., et al. "The Association between Duration of Breastfeeding and Adult Intelligence." *Journal of the American Medical Association* 287 (2002): 2365–71.

Morton, Jane, et al. "Combining Hand Techniques with Electric Pumping Increases Milk Production in Mothers of Preterm Infants." *Journal of Perinatology* 29 (2009): 757–64.

Moscone, S. R., and M. J. Moore. "Breastfeeding during Pregnancy." *Journal of Human Lactation* 9 (1993): 83–88.

Mosko, S., et al. "Infant Arousals during Mother-Infant Bed Sharing: Implications for Infant Sleep and Sudden Infant Death Syndrome Research." *Pediatrics* 100 (1997): 841–49.

Neifert, M. R., and J. M. Seacat. "Contemporary Breastfeeding Management Clinics." *Perinatology* 12 (1995): 319–42.

Newman, J., and T. Pitman. *Dr. Jack Newman's Guide to Breastfeeding.* Toronto: HarperCollins Canada, 2009.

Nommsen-Rivers, L. A., et al. "Newborn Wet and Soiled Diaper Counts and Timing of Onset of Lactation as Indicators of Breastfeeding Inadequacy." *Journal of Human Lactation* 24 (2008): 27–33.

Oddy, W. H., et al. "Breast Feeding and Respiratory Morbidity in Infancy: A Birth Cohort Study." *Archives of Disease in Childhood* 88 (2003): 224–28.

————. "Association between Breast Feeding and Asthma in 6-Year-Old Children: Findings of a Prospective Birth Cohort Study." *British Medical Journal* 319 (1999): 815–19.

Owen, C., et al. "Does Breastfeeding Influence Risk of Type 2 Diabetes in Later Life? A Quantitative Analysis of Published Evidence." *American Journal of Clinical Nutrition* 84 (2006): 1043–54.

————. "Infant Feeding and Blood Cholesterol: A Study in Adolescents and a Systematic Review." *Pediatrics* 110 (2002): 597–608.

Quigley, M. A., et al. "Breastfeeding and Hospitalization for Diarrheal and Respiratory Infection in the United Kingdom: Millennium Cohort Study." *Pediatrics* 119 (2007): e837–42.

Rayburn, W. F., and J. Zhang. "Rising Rates of Labor Induction: Present Concerns and Future Strategies." *Obstetrics and Gynecology* 100 (2002): 164–67.

Reynolds, A. "Breastfeeding and Brain Development." *Pediatric Clinics of North America* 48 (2001): 159–71.

Rickert, V. I., and C. Merle Johnson. "Reducing Nocturnal Awakening and Crying Episodes in Infants and Young Children: A Comparison between Scheduled Awakenings and Systematic Ignoring." *Pediatrics* 81 (1988): 203–12.

Righard, L., and M. O. Alade. "Effect of Delivery Room Routines on the Success of First Breastfeed." *Lancet* 336 (1990): 1105–7.

Rinker, B. D., et al. "The Effect of Breastfeeding upon Breast Aesthetics." *Aesthetic Surgery Journal* 28 (2008): 534–37.

Riordan, Jan, and Francine Nichols. "A Descriptive Study of Lactation Mastitis in Long-term Breastfeeding Women." *Journal of Human Lactation* 6 (1990): 53–58.

Riordan, Jan, and Karen Wambach. *Breastfeeding and Human Lactation.* St. Louis: Mosby, 2009.

Riordan, Jan, et al. "The Effect of Labor Pain Relief Medication on Neonatal Suckling and Breastfeeding Duration." *Journal of Human Lactation* 16 (2000): 7–12.

Roberts, J. E. "The 'Push' for Evidence: Management of the Second Stage." *Journal of Midwifery and Women's Health* 47 (2002): 2–15.

Roberts, J. E., et al. "The Effects of Maternal Position on Uterine Contractility and Efficiency." *Birth* 10 (1983): 243–49.

Romano, A., and J. Lothian. "Promoting, Protecting, and Supporting Normal Birth: A Look at the Evidence." *Journal of Obstetric, Gynecologic, and Neonatal Nursing* 37 (2008): 94–105.

Rosenblatt, K. A., D. B. Thomas, and WHO Collaborative Study of Neoplasia and Steroid Contraceptives. "Lactation and the Risk of Epithelial Ovarian Cancer." *International Journal of Epidemiology* 22 (1993): 192–97.

Sanchez-Ramos, L., et al. "Expectant Management versus Labor Induction for Suspected Fetal Macrosomia: A Systematic Review." *Obstetrics and Gynecology* 100 (2002): 997–1002.

Satter, Ellyn. *Child of Mine: Feeding with Love and Good Sense.* Palo Alto, CA: Bull Publishing, 2000.

Savino, F., et al. "*Lactobacillus reuteri* versus Simethicone in the Treatment of Infantile Colic: A Prospective Randomized Study." *Pediatrics* 119 (2007): e124–30.

Schach, B., and M. Haight. "Colic and Food Allergy in the Breastfed Infant: Is It Possible for an Exclusively Breastfed Infant to Suffer from Food Allergy?" *Journal of Human Lactation* 18 (2002): 50–52.

Simpkin, Penny, and M. O'Hara. Non-Pharmacologic Relief of Pain during Labor: Systematic Reviews of Five Methods. *American Journal of Obstetrics and Gynecology Supplement* 186 (2002): s131–59.

Souto, Gláucia C., et al. "The Impact of Breast Reduction Surgery on Breastfeeding Performance." *Journal of Human Lactation* 19 (2003): 43–49.

Tita, A. T., et al. "Timing of Elective Repeat Cesarean Delivery at Term and Neonatal Outcomes." *New England Journal of Medicine* 360 (2009): 111–20.

Tonkin, S., et al., "Apparently Life Threatening Events in Infant Car Safety Seats." *British Medical Journal* 333 (2006): 1205–6.

Torvaldsen, S., et al. "Intrapartum Epidural Analgesia and Breastfeeding: A Prospective Cohort Study." *International Breastfeeding Journal* 1 (2006): 24.

Vennemann, M. M., et al. "Does Breastfeeding Reduce the Risk of Sudden Infant Death Syndrome?" *Pediatrics* 123 (2009): e406–10.

Victora, C. G., et al. "Use of Pacifiers and Breastfeeding Duration." *Lancet* 341 (1993): 404–6.

Von Kries, R., et al. "Breast Feeding and Obesity: Cross-Sectional Study." *British Medical Journal* 319 (1999): 147–50.

Walker, Marsha. "A Fresh Look at the Risks of Artificial Infant Feeding." *Journal of Human Lactation* 9 (1993): 97–107.

Weintraub, R., G. Hams, M. Meerkin, and A. Rosenberg. "High Aluminum Content of Infant Milk Formulas." *Archives of Disease in Childhood* 61 (1986): 914–16.

Wickizer, Thomas M., Lawrence B. Brilliant, Richard Copeland, and Robert Tilden. "Polychlorinated Biphenyl Contamination of Nursing Mothers' Milk in Michigan." *American Journal of Public Health* 71 (1981): 132–37.

Wilson, A. C., et al. "Relation of Infant Diet to Childhood Health: Seven-Year Follow-up of Cohort of Children in Dundee Infant Feeding Study." *British Medical Journal* 316 (1998): 21–25.

Wilson-Clay, B. "Case Report of Methicillin-Resistant *Staphylococcus aureus* (MRSA) Mastitis with Abscess Formation in a Breastfeeding Woman." *Journal of Human Lactation* 24 (2008): 326–29.

Woolridge, M. W., and Chloe Fisher. "Colic, 'Overfeeding,' and Symptoms of Lactose Malabsorption in the Breast-fed Baby: A Possible Artifact of Feed Management?" *Lancet* 2 (1988): 3828.

Suggested Supplmental Reading

Balaskas, Janet. *Active Birth: The New Approach to Giving Birth Naturally*, rev. ed. Boston: Harvard Common Press, 1992.

Bumgarner, Norma Jane. *Mothering Your Nursing Toddler*. Shaumburg, IL: La Leche League International, 2000.

Flower, Hilary. *Adventures in Tandem Nursing: Breastfeeding during Pregnancy and Beyond*. Shaumburg, IL: La Leche League International, 2003.

Fraiberg, Selma H. *The Magic Years*. New York: Charles Scribner's Sons, 1996.

Gromada, Karen Kerkhoff. *Mothering Multiples*. Shaumburg, IL: La Leche League International, 2007.

Huggins, Kathleen. *The Expectant Parents' Companion: Simplifying What to Do, Buy, or Borrow for an Easy Life with Baby*. Boston: Harvard Common Press, 2006.

Huggins, Kathleen, and Jan Ellen Brown. *The Nursing Mother's Companion Breastfeeding Diary*. Boston: Harvard Common Press, 2010.

Huggins, Kathleen, and Jan Ellen Brown. *25 Things Every Nursing Mother Needs to Know*. Boston: Harvard Common Press, 2009.

Huggins, Kathleen, and Linda Ziedrich. *The Nursing Mother's Guide to Weaning*, rev. ed. Boston: Harvard Common Press, 2007.

Karp, Harvey. *The Happiest Baby on the Block*. New York: Bantam Books, 2003.

Kleiman, Karen R., and Valerie D. Raskin. *This Isn't What I Expected: Overcoming Postpartum Depression*. New York: Bantam Books, 2013.

Kropp, Tori. *The Joy of Pregnancy: The Complete, Candid, and Reassuring Companion for Parents-to-Be*. Boston: Harvard Common Press, 2008.

McKenna, James. *Sleeping with Your Baby: A Parent's Guide to Cosleeping*. Washington, DC: Platypus Media, 2007.

Pantley, Elizabeth, and William Sears. *The No-Cry Sleep Solution*. New York: Contemporary Books, 2002.

Pryor, Gale, and Kathleen Huggins. *Nursing Mother, Working Mother*, rev. ed. Boston: Harvard Common Press, 2007.

Rapley, Gill, and Murkett, Tracey. *Baby-Led Weaning: Helping Your Baby to Love Good Food, The Experiment*, 2019.

Robertson, Laurel, Carol Flinders, and Brian Ruppenthal. *The New Laurel's Kitchen*. Berkeley, CA: Ten Speed Press, 1986.

Sears, William, Martha Sears, Robert Sears, and James Sears. *The Baby Book: Everything You Need to Know about Your Baby from Birth to Age Two*, rev. ed. Boston: Little, Brown, 2013.

Simkin, Penny. *The Birth Partner: A Complete Guide to Childbirth for Dads, Doulas, and All Other Labor Companions*, 3rd ed. Boston: Harvard Common Press, 2007.

Simkin, Penny, Janet Whalley, and Ann Keppler. *Pregnancy, Childbirth, and the Newborn: The Complete Guide*. Minnetonka, MN: Meadowbrook, 2001.

Vartabedian, Bryan. *Colic Solved: The Essential Guide to Infant Reflux and the Care of Your Crying, Difficult-to-Soothe Baby*. New York: Ballantine Books, 2007.

Index

A

ABO incompatibility, 106
abscess, 204, 205, 206–207
accelerated Newman-Gold-
farb protocols, 142, 143
acetaminophen (Tylenol)
after birth, 50, 74
after cesarean birth,
60, 173
before nursing, 96
fever, alternatives for, 206
for engorged breasts, 79
for headache, 210
for sore nipples, 88
for teething pain, 340–341,
357, 369, 371
A+D ointment, 93
adopted babies. *See also*
babies
donated milk for, 141
Newman-Goldfarb proto-
cols, 142–144
nursing, 84, 140–141,
142–144
Adventures in Tandem Nursing
(Flowers), 380
Advil, Infants', 340, 357, 369,
371. *See also* ibuprofen
Affordable Care Act, 8,
38, 47, 101, 130, 242, 246,
283, 324
afterpains, 74
air travel with baby, 316–317,
325
alcohol, 128, 151–152,
180, 184
allergies (baby), 6, 183, 204,
216, 357. *See also* food
allergies
allergies (mother), 70, 92–93,
204, 210
All-Purpose Nipple Ointment
(APNO), 90–91, 93, 198
altitude, high, 250

aluminum in infant
formula, 6
amber necklaces, 341,
357–358
Ameda Elite pump, 278
Ameda Mya Joy pump, 290
Ameda One-Hand pump, 311
Ameda Platinum Breast
pump, 248, 257, 278
amniotic fluid, 25, 69
amphetamines, 151
anal fissure, 225
Anderson, Philip O., 13, 20
anemia (baby), 140, 358
anemia (mother)
breast infection and,
204, 206
iron for, 179, 346
post-gastric bypass surgery,
risks of, 140
anesthesia
during birth process, 23,
25–26, 65, 80
headache caused by, 209
nursing and, 189, 208, 318
safety of, 208, 318
tongue-tie revisions, 122
antacids, 229
antibacterials, 16–17, 88,
91, 198
antibiotic cream, 93, 200
antibiotics
for breast infections,
204–205, 346
bite wounds, 370
epidural fevers and, 26
impetigo, 200
Lyme disease and, 134
nipple injuries, 89–90, 370
mastitis, 204–206
oral, 90, 200
plugged ducts, 346
probiotics and, 233
thrush infection following
administration of, 92, 195

antibodies
ABO incompatibility
and, 106
birth preparation and, 23
breast milk as source of,
189, 328, 352, 365, 377
colostrum as source of,
156, 258
anticonvulsants, 148
antidepressants, 214–215
antifungals, 196, 197–198
antihistamines, 338
anti-inflammatory cream,
93, 198
anti-inflammatory drugs, 357
anxiety, 46, 72, 74, 151, 173,
174, 185, 210–215, 339, 353,
356–357
apnea, 40, 156, 223
APNO, 90, 91, 93, 198
appetite (baby), 182, 192, 219,
220, 337, 363, 380
appetite (mother)
depression-related, 102,
211, 213
hypothyroidism, 149
in mothers of multiple
babies, 165
postpartum, 72, 174,
176, 179
apples, 226, 360, 380
ARA (arachidonic acid), 4
ARDO Calypso Breast pump,
284, 304
Ardo Calypso Pro pump, 281
Ardo Carum pump, 279
areola
breast shells, 30
compression during nurs-
ing, 20, 52–53, 55, 57, 90,
96, 100
compression during pump-
ing, 256, 311
during engorgement, 71,
89, 101, 110
eczema and, 200

herpes lesions on, 148
incision on or near, 65, 84,
125, 129, 138–139, 208,
238, 255
insufficient glandular tissue
(IGT) and, 134
Montgomery's tubercles, 16
during pregnancy, 16
soap and shampoo, avoiding
on, 18, 69
softening, 78, 101, 110
thrush and, 195, 197
armchair for nursing, 39, 56
artificial nipples
baby familiar with, 51, 251
preference for, 63, 99,
109, 113
for premature babies, 161
and refusal to nurse, 114,
218, 350
sanitizing, 197
selection of, 271
slow-flow, 274, 330
Asian-descended babies, bilirubin levels of, 106
aspirin, 226
asthma, 4, 7, 223
Augmentin, 204
au pairs, 322
Avent bottle nipples, 272
Avent Comfort Manual Breast
pump, 311
Avent Double Electric Breast
pump, 296–297
Axid, 229
azithromycin, 204

B

babies. *See also* adopted babies;
premature babies
digestive system of, 50, 63,
155, 183, 192, 225, 229, 343
drugs prescribed for, 87
equipment for, 36–39
fever following epidural, 26
physical contact with, 4, 132,
156, 169, 327, 335, 375
prenatal development of, 23
temperament of, 221
urine, 39, 69, 73
wrapping snugly, 103,
124, 159
baby beds, 40–45, 108, 150,
372, 373
baby blues, 72
BabyBuddha, 301–302
Baby Ddrops, 187

baby doctor, selecting, 32–33
baby food, 183, 343
Baby-Friendly designation, 32
baby-led bottle feeding, 273–274
baby-led weaning, 360
Baby-Led Weaning (Rapley and
Murkett), 360
Baby Orajel, 357
baby scale, 128, 130, 145
bacteria
in breast infection, 92, 203
immune system and, 3–4
in infant formula, 5–6
MRSA, 204–205
in open wound (nipple), 89,
92, 370
probiotics, 230–231
in stored milk, 265–267
bacterial meningitis, 5
Bactroban (mupirocin), 200
Balm Barr, 92
band size, 34, 36
barium swallow, 231
Barton, Jessica, 274
baths, 24, 102, 172, 213
bed rails, 44
bedtime routines, 384
beer, 128, 151–152, 180, 237
Belly Bandit (band), 173
betamethasone ointment, 198
Bethanechol (Urecholine), 229
bilirubin
Asian-descended babies, 106
jaundice, 105–109
production of, 105
in stools, 50
water supplements and, 108
birth, natural, 23–27
birth control
milk production and, 143,
264, 336, 338, 348
options, 335–337
before resumption of
periods, 353
birth defects
nursing babies with, 167–169
pumping for babies with, 170,
245, 258–261
birthing centers, 32
birth weight
loss, 64–65, 67, 69, 79, 81–82,
125–126, 135, 255
low, 5, 51, 106, 133, 147, 163
regaining, 67, 108, 155, 181–
182, 191, 234
bisphenol-A (BPA), 6

biting during nursing
coping measures, 370
myth of, 8, 365
overview, 368–370
refusal to nurse after, 374
teeth eruption and, 340, 358
warning signs, 370
blanched nipples, 120, 198–200
blebs, 201, 203
blessed thistle
after breast surgery, 139
milk production and, 84–85,
135, 139
overview of, 84
pumping and, 265
relactation and, 144
as underfeeding treatment
measure, 237
bloating, 229
blood, deoxygenation of, 199
blood pressure
high, 25, 65, 80, 85
low, 25
blood sugar, 24, 28, 31, 51, 63,
146–147
blood type incompatibilities,
106
bone density, 178
bone meal, 178
bottle
acceptance of, 244, 251,
271–272
getting baby accustomed
to, 252
holding own, 10, 327
introduction of, 244, 251,
271–272
for milk storage, 267, 269
reluctance to take, 223,
272–273
selection of, 271
toddler use of, 377, 383
bottle feeding
alternatives to, 82, 113–114,
117, 128, 137, 169
baby-led, 271, 273–274
breastfeeding compared to, 7,
152, 159, 265–266
breastfeeding readiness after
period of, 141, 264
caregiver instructions concerning, 327–328, 330
cerebral palsy, babies
with, 170
circumstances requiring,
218, 238
cleft lip and palate, babies
with, 168

cup *vs.*, 99, 113, 117, 128, 273,
362–363, 374–375
of expressed milk, 240
hospital policies on,
30–32, 52
for latch-on difficulty, 101
milk intake requirements,
168–169, 327–328
for multiple babies, 165
night wakings and, 340
after nursing, 137, 145,
238, 272
nursing after, 238, 264
nursing supplement
through, 137
overfeeding, 263–264
paced, 271, 273–274
pitfalls of, 6–7, 51, 63,
371, 375
for premature babies,
159, 161
refusal to nurse and, 111,
113–114, 217–218, 223, 374
resources on, 129
scheduling of, 327–328
by sexual abuse survivors, 151
sleeping patterns and, 356
starting on, nursing after, 145
for sucking problems, 117–118
for supplements, 127,
128–129
bottle nipples. *See* artificial
nipples
botulism, 88, 91
bovine disease, 5
bowel movements
anal fissures, 225
colostrum and, 50, 64
diarrhea, 190–191
excessive, 125, 234
frequency and color of, 64,
69, 104–105, 108, 191,
338, 362
late onset milk production, 79
nursing and, 110
solid food effect on, 362
stimulating, 50
bradycardia, 156
brain development, 2, 155, 364
bras. *See also* nursing bras
breast shells, 30, 70
hands-free, 260
ill-fitting, 202, 204–205, 345
material for, 35
pregnancy and, 9, 16
selecting guidelines, 34–36
breads, whole-grain
benefits of, 213, 362
recommendations for, 362
at six months of age, 359

breast abscess, 204, 205,
206–207
breast biopsy, 138, 207, 208
breast cancer
benefits of breastfeeding
and, 11
lump as sign of, 201–202, 207
ruling out, 207
breast infections. *See also*
mastitis
causes of, 35, 89–90, 370
in diabetic mothers, 147
milk discarding with, 157
nursing during, 157
preventing, 89–90, 165, 181
signs and symptoms of, 147,
203, 207, 210, 216
treatment measures for,
345–346
breast lumps, 201–202, 207–208
breast milk. *See* milk
breast-milk jaundice, 106
breast pads
advance purchase of, 35–36
changing, frequency of, 89,
95, 197, 204, 345
dressings on, 89
holding in place, 34
for leaks, 71, 95, 329
obtaining, 35–36
breast pumps. *See also* clinical-
grade pumps; electric pumps;
expressing milk
double-electric, 283–284,
286–302
for "drip milk," 95
engorgement, use during, 71,
77, 79
exclusive use of, 261–264
flanges, 243, 256–257
functioning of, 242–243,
249–250
hand-operated, 250–251
insurance and, 8, 246–247,
285
late-onset production and,
81–83
loaner pumps, 280
manual pumps, 310–311
models, review of, 275–276
purchase, timing of, 38, 244
secondhand, 249
selecting, 242–244, 285
separation and, 60, 251,
317–318
silicone squeeze pumps,
312–313
single pumps, 309–310
sore nipples and, 86, 88–89
wearable, 250, 303–307

breast shells
areola softening with, 78
nipple shape improvement
with, 29–30, 36, 70, 101
precautions concerning, 70,
95, 209, 329
for sore nipples, 89
sterilizing, 197
breast surgery
breast augmentation, 65,
125, 135
breast reduction, 65, 125,
138, 139
herbal remedies after, 139
milk production, insufficient
following, 65, 125, 129,
238, 255
nursing after, 65, 125, 129,
138–139, 189, 318
pumping after, 139, 255
breathing
bra measurement and, 34
in car seat, 37, 72
difficulty, 217, 223
laryngomalacia, 165–166
heart defects and, 167
near-term babies, 153
noisy, 165–166
pattern establishment, 41
premature babies, 156
waterbeds, 44
brewer's yeast
colic symptoms caused
by, 226
for mothers of multiple
babies, 165
for mothers of older babies
(over six months), 352
for nursing mothers, 179
for vitamin B deficiency, 374
for working mothers, 331
Brewster, Dorothy, 148
bronchitis, 180, 223
B-streptococcal infection, 205
Bumgarner, Norma Jane,
378, 380
bupropion, 215
burping
after nursing at one
breast, 104
for babies with colic or reflux,
222–224, 232
during bottle-feeding, 274
fussiness and, 124
how to, 62
need for, indication of, 217
spitting up during, 222
"Business Case for Breastfeeding, The," 326
bust measurement, 34

C

caffeine
  avoiding or limiting during nursing, 179, 199
  benefits of, 210, 215
  depression and anxiety and, 213
  dysphoric milk ejection reflex (D-MER) and, 215
  headaches and, 210
  Raynaud's phenomenon and, 199
calcium
  absorption of, 186
  gastric bypass surgery and, 140
  intake guidelines, 165, 178
  during period, 265, 353
  Raynaud's phenomenon and, 199
  sources of, 158, 178
  soy milk fortified with, 364
calcium carbonate, 178
calcium supplements
  dairy product elimination, 228
  guidelines, 178
  for mothers of multiples, 165
  period resumption and, 265, 353
  for premature babies, 157–158
caloric intake (baby)
  "drip milk," 251
  hindmilk, 158, 167
  milk, 140, 158
  premature babies, 158, 162
  solid foods, 342, 349
caloric intake (mother)
  depression and anxiety and, 213
  diabetes and, 146–147
  "empty" calories, 178, 333
  fatigue and, 333
  gastric bypass surgery, 139–140
  multiple babies and, 165
  nursing, adjustment during, 175–176
  postpartum, monitoring, 177
  postpartum, requirements, 175–178
  premature delivery risk, 162
cancer
  breastfeeding as protection against (baby), 7
  breastfeeding linked to reduced risk of (mother), 11
  gut health and, 3
  lactoferrin and, 5

signs of, 201–202, 207–208
and sun exposure, 186
and vitamin D deficiency, 186
carbohydrates, 177, 213, 371
cardiac abnormalities, hindmilk and, 158, 167
milk pumping for babies with, 245
caregiver
  bottle offered by, 327–328, 330
  choosing, 321–324
  instructions for, 326–328
  nursing at home of, 328, 329
car seats, 36–38, 43, 72–73, 316
car travel with baby, 72–73, 232, 316
casein, 226
castor oil, 203
cavities, 188, 226
cephalexin (Keflex), 204
cephalosporins, 204
cereals
  ability to handle, 183
  in bottle, 340
  colic and, 232
  commercial infant cereals, 359
  cooked, 363
  depression and anxiety and, 213
  introduction, 183, 232, 359
  night walking and, 340
  reflux and, 232
  vegetarian diet and, 362
  as vitamin D source, 186
cereals, whole-grain, 213, 359, 362
cerebral palsy, 155, 169–170
cervical cap, 335–336
cesarean section
  antibiotics following, 92, 195
  depression and, 103
  induced labor followed by, 24
  for mothers with herpes, 148
  incidence of, 23–25, 148
  nursing following, 56, 59–60, 65, 80
  pain medication following, 74, 173
  placental fragments following, 81
  scheduling, 28
  "vaginal seeding" after, 4
cesarean support groups, 103
chair for nursing, 39, 54, 56, 148, 325

cheese
  allergy to, 226, 228
  calcium in, 178
  hard, 228, 361
  recommendations for, 364
  semi-hard, 361, 364
  as snack, 177, 331
chemical safety, 6, 20–21, 22
chest retraction, laryngomalacia and, 166
chewing, learning, 359, 360
chicken pox (varicella) in mothers, 134
child abuse, risk factors for, 231
childbirth classes, 27
childcare, 213, 320, 321–324
chocolate
  allergies, 92, 224–225
  consumption, maternal, 179
choking
  during bottle feeding, 273, 274
  cereal, precautions concerning, 232
  digestive disorder testing, 231
  laryngomalacia and, 166
  during nursing, avoiding, 217
  overabundant milk and, 208
  as reflux symptom, 223, 231–232
  self-fed vs. spoon-fed baby, 360
cholesterol
  benefit of breastfeeding and, 7, 11
  levels during pregnancy and lactation, 333–334
cimetidine (Tagamet), 229
citrus, 179, 225, 360, 363
clarithromycin, 204
cleft lip and palate, 66, 167–169, 254
clicking sound during sucking, 68, 112, 114–115, 120, 160
clindamycin, 204
clinical-grade pumps. See also breast pumps
  Affordable Care Act (ACA) and, 246–247
  breast abscess and, 207
  breast draining with, 114, 117–118
  cleft lip and palate, babies with, 168
  engorgement, use during, 79
  hypoplasia, use by mothers with, 135
  instructions for, 248–249

jaundice, absence due to, 109
for latch-on difficulty,
110, 114
for mastitis, 205–206
in maternity units, 258
milk production estimation
with, 126, 145, 235
milk production stimulation
with, 235, 260–262, 264
for missed feedings, 109,
317–318
models, review of, 276–283
for multiple babies, 163–164
for near-term babies, 154
Newman-Goldfarb protocol
role of, 142
nipple shape and, 99, 101
obtaining, 38, 246–247, 248
overview of, 245, 248–249
personal use pump compared
to, 249
for plugged ducts, 203
refusal to nurse, use
during, 218
sore nipples, use in event of,
86, 89
sucking problems, use in
event of, 116–118
cloth diapers, 36, 38
clotrimazole powder, 198
cloxacillin, 204
CMV (cytomegalovirus),
133, 249
cocaine, 151
cocoa butter, 70, 92
cod liver oil, 187
cold, avoiding, 199
cold packs, 78–79
colds
air travel and, 317
antibodies in milk, 189
medications for, 5, 189, 226
night wakings due to, 341
nursing difficulties and, 190,
201, 217
refusal to nurse due to, 374
solid food introduction
and, 342
cold sores, 133, 148
colic
caffeine as factor in, 179
causes of, 179, 224, 226, 228
cereal for, 232
coping measures, 232–233
definition and overview of,
222–224
formula-feeding and, 6
"gripe water" for, 230

hyperlactation syndrome as
cause of, 228–229
pumping in event of, 245
symptoms, 192, 223–224
treatments and tests for,
229–231
colostrum
adequate intake, signs of, 61,
64, 69
benefits of, 19, 49–50, 156
composition and overview of,
49–50
diabetes and, 147
expressing, 81–82, 98–99,
110, 113, 117, 147, 240–241
feeding, 82, 99, 110, 113, 117,
156–157
jaundice treatment with, 106
meconium and, 105–106
microbiome and, 4
milk mixed with, 70
milk replaced by, 51, 378
for premature babies,
155–157
production of, 17, 49–50, 62
pumping, 255, 258, 259, 277
spitting up, 68
swallowing, 61
comfort nursing, 129, 238
comfort objects, 371
comfort sucking, 150, 220
complicated birth, 23
compulsive behaviors, 211
concentration inability, 179, 211
confusion, 211
constipation
anal fissure caused by, 225
B_{12} deficiency, 140
breastfed babies free of,
6, 105
dehydration and, 175, 177,
331, 333
in formula-fed babies, 6
grunting and, 69, 105
low-carb diets and, 177
postpartum, 173
preventing, 175, 177, 331, 333
contraception, 142, 334,
335–337
contractions
epidural effect on, 25
induced, 24
postpartum, 50
premature births and,
162, 379
resting between, 27
cow's milk. See also dairy
products
allergy to, 216, 226, 361

alternatives to, 6
formulas based on, 226
human milk compared to,
2, 5
introduction to, 364
as supplement, 378
as vitamin D source, 186–187
cradle hold (cuddle hold)
pros and cons of, 53–54
side-lying position compared
to, 58
for twins, 163, 164
crossover hold
cradle hold compared to, 54
football hold compared to,
56–57
inverted or dimpled nipples
and, 98
overview of, 54–56
for premature babies,
159–160
sucking, aiding with, 117
tongue sucking problem,
treating with, 113
crying (baby)
at the breast, 109, 217
laryngomalacia, 166
lessening of, 219–221,
230, 233
nighttime handling of, 124,
150, 371–372
reasons for, 192–193, 219,
222–223
crying (mother), 74, 173, 211
cuddle hold. See cradle hold
(cuddle hold)
cups
drinking from, 252, 273
milk cups, 292, 297, 302–303,
305
sippy cup, 273, 363
supplements, feeding
with, 236
cyst, breast lump as, 207
cytomegalovirus (CMV), 5,
133, 249

D

dairy products. See also
cow's milk
galactosemia and, 152
introduction of, 361
maternal consumption of, 22,
226–227
for mothers of multiples, 165
recommendations for
baby, 228

day-care centers, 269, 322–323, 326, 330
dehydration, 79, 177, 185, 189–191, 201, 216
dental health, childhood, 123, 188, 363, 371
depression (postpartum). See postpartum depression
developmental problems, babies with, 169–170
DHA, 4, 5, 213
diabetes
  caloric intake (mother) and, 146–147
  colostrum and, 147
  gut bacteria and, 4
  jaundice in babies with, 106
  labor induction for, 25
  nursing and, 7, 11, 66, 80, 146–147
  PCOS and, 138
  thrush and, 92, 147, 194
  type 1, 7, 186
  type 2, 7
diaper rash
  oral medication administration followed by, 206
  treatment for, 92, 196, 221–222
  yeast as cause of, 92, 195–196, 221–222
diapers
  blood in, 97, 190, 224–225
  selecting, 38
  wetting, frequency of, 64, 69, 73, 191, 338
diarrhea
  B_{12} deficiency and, 140
  brewer's yeast and, 374
  food allergies as cause of, 361
  in formula-fed babies, 5–6, 190–191
  juice as cause of, 363
  maternal eating as factor in, 179, 189
  motility drugs and, 229
  narcotic withdrawal and, 74, 173
  nursing and, 5, 6, 179, 189
  stools, newborn, compared to, 104–105
diets and dieting (mother)
  babies, effect on, 179, 187, 189, 192, 216–217, 221, 224–228
  balanced diet, 165, 213
  brewer's yeast, 374
  dietary supplements, 97, 179, 199, 213, 226, 374
  fats in, 346

log of food and beverages, 227
mothers of older babies, 352
postpartum guidelines, 175
precautions concerning, 176, 177–178
premature delivery and, 162
toxic chemicals and, 22
vegetarian/vegan, 178
vitamin B deficiencies, 373
after weaning, 147
Domperidone (Motilium)
  milk production stimulation with, 87, 128, 135, 139, 157, 237
  Newman-Goldfarb protocol, 143
  obtaining, 87
  relactation with, 145
donated milk
  adopted babies and, 141
  casual sharing, 182
  milk banks, 183–184
double collection kits. See also breast pumps; clinical-grade pumps; electric pumps
  advantages of, 248, 262
  for babies with cleft lip and palate, 168
  during hospitalization, 189
  for late-preterm newborns, 154
  milk production estimation with, 126
  milk production stimulation with, 66, 144, 236, 248, 264
  for multiple babies, 163
  for near-term newborns, 154
  Newman-Goldfarb protocol role of, 142
  nursing, use after, 66, 144, 236, 255
  obtaining, 38, 81, 189
  overview of, 66–67, 248
  sore nipples and, 86, 88–89
  sucking problems and, 117
  underfeeding treatment role of, 126–127, 235
Down syndrome, 66, 169–170
Dr. Brown "CustomFlow" Double Electric Breast Pump, 299–300
duration
  for babies with heart defects, 167
  engorgement and, 77–78
  factors affecting, 67
  guidelines, 127
  for older babies, 352

time required for nursing, 52, 78, 233–234
  for toddlers, 380
  variations in, 181

E

ear infections. See also infections
  in babies with cleft lip and palate, 168
  in formula-fed babies, 5
  night waking due to, 341, 357, 371
  nursing patterns and, 190, 218
  pacifier use and, 51
  preventing, 168
  as reflux symptom, 223
  refusal to nurse due to, 218, 355, 374
  risk factors, 180
  solid food introduction, associated with, 342
electric pumps. See breast pumps; clinical-grade pumps; double-collection kits
Elvie Catch squeeze pump, 313
Elvie Curve squeeze pump, 313
Elvie pump, 306
Elvie Stride pump, 307
engorgement
  breast pain due to, 200
  causes of, 52, 70, 77
  decline in milk production, 77, 238
  herbs for, 85
  latch-on difficulty related to, 77
  nursing time and, 52
  overabundant milk and, 79
  preventing, 253, 324
  pumping and, 71, 77, 79
  sore nipples and, 89
  treatment measures for, 71
  weight loss (baby) and, 125, 129, 234
epidurals
  anesthesia for, 209
  breastfeeding affected by, 23
  delaying, 27
  milk production affected by, 65, 80
  patient-controlled, 26
  pros and cons of, 25–26
estrogen
  contraceptives with, 264, 334, 338, 348
  milk production affected by, 334, 336, 338, 348
  production of, 142

exercise
  antidepressant effect of, 213
  D-MER treatment with, 215
  in first two months after
    birth, 173, 174
  for tongue-tie revisions, 122
  for torticollis, 111
expressing milk. *See also* breast
  pumps
  air travel and, 317
  anesthesia and, 189
  areola, softening by, 71, 78
  for babies with birth
    defects, 167
  for babies with cleft lip and
    palate, 168
  for babies with hydrocephalus
    or spina bifida, 170
  bottles for, 169
  colostrum, 81–83, 98, 147
  engorgement treatment, 71,
    77, 79
  feeding, 99, 270–274
  feeding frequency, 337
  hand-expression, 240–242
  infectious conditions and,
    132, 134, 148, 205
  iodine, radioactive treatment
    and, 149
  for latch-on problems, 99, 113
  methods of, 240–251
  for near-term babies, 155, 269
  nipple wounds, 90, 370
  for non-nursing babies, 110,
    113, 258–261, 374
  for occasional separations,
    251, 317
  one-sided nursing, treating
    with, 350
  overabundance of milk
    and, 347
  overview of, 240
  for plugged ducts, 202
  refusal to nurse, treatment
    measures for, 110, 113,
    218, 234
  before returning to work, 252
  for sick babies, 155
  storage, 265–266, 268
  for sucking problems,
    115–118
  supplementers and, 137
  supply, maintaining by, 109,
    160, 163, 190, 318
  for underfeeding, 127–129,
    235–236
  weaning off of expressed
    milk, 83
  weight gain and, 348
  in workplace, 253–254, 324–
    326, 328–329

Evenflo Advanced Double
  Electric Pump, 295–296
Evenflo Advanced Single
  Electric Pump, 310

F

Fair Labor Standards Act, 324
Family Medical Leave Act
  (FMLA), 320
famotidine (Pepcid), 229
fat
  accumulated, milk produc-
    tion role of, 11
  colic and, 228, 244
  colostrum, 50
  "drip milk," 251, 312
  frozen milk and, 268, 270
  gastric bypass surgery
    and, 140
  hindmilk, 158
  losing excess, 176–177
  milk quality and, 22, 140, 252
  saturated, reducing, 346
  soapy smell from, 268
  sources of, 361, 364
  thrush mistaken for, 195
fatigue (mother)
  depression-related, 210–211
  dietary considerations, 177,
    333, 373
  hypothyroidism and, 149
  mastitis and, 204
  postpartum, 102, 174
  during pregnancy, 379
  weaning and, 365
fatigue (baby), 23
fenugreek
  after breast surgery, 139
  for hypoplasia, 135
  milk production stimulation
    with, 84–85, 138, 237, 265
  before period, 353
  for Polycystic Ovary Syn-
    drome, 138
  relactation and, 144
  as underfeeding treatment
    measure, 237
fever
  following epidural, 26
  infections and, 190, 203
  mastitis and, 204, 206, 370
  nursing frequency during,
    191
  placental fragments and, 81
  plugged milk ducts and, 207
  vomiting with, 216
First Years Quiet Expressions
  Double Breast Pump, 296

flange (breast pump)
  fit, 256–257, 258–259,
    262, 265
  need for, 116
  obtaining, 116
  placement of nipple in,
    248–249, 251
  selecting, 243, 256
  shields for, 345
food allergies. *See also* allergies
  (babies)
  blood relatives and, 361
  categories of, 224–226
  dairy products, 364
  development, causes of, 183
  eggs, 363
  family members with, 361
  fenugreek and, 84
  formula-feeding and, 6
  identifying, 361
  signs of, 361
  solid food introduction, 183,
    232, 342
football hold
  after cesarean section, 60
  benefits of, 54, 56
  cleft lip and palate, babies
    with, 168
  heart defects, babies with, 167
  for let-down problems, 217
  one-sided nursing, 111, 350
  overview of, 56–57
  for premature babies, 56,
    159, 160
  for problem nipples, 98
  refusal to nurse, 110, 217
  silicone pumps and, 312
  for sleepy babies, 104
  sucking, aiding with, 116–117
  tongue problems, 112–113
  for twins, 164
foremilk, 158, 167, 228, 244
formula
  adoptive mother use of, 141
  allergies and, 226
  body image and, 9
  bowel movements and, 69
  breastfeeding-as-contracep-
    tion and, 337
  "breastfeeding kits," 71
  breast milk compared to, 2,
    4–5, 10
  circumstances requiring, 13,
    67, 152
  colic and, 6, 231
  contaminants and toxins in,
    5, 6
  costs of, 10, 162, 168, 243, 248
  decreasing or eliminating, 83,
    375, 378
  emotional barriers and, 151

fussiness and, 124, 192, 218
growth pattern *vs.* nursing,
  338
hospital staff and, 31, 33, 51
hypoallergenic, 225, 364
lactose-free, 152
late-onset milk production
  and, 82–83
late-preterm newborns
  and, 155
medical reasons for, 152
for mother-baby separation,
  317, 330
for multiple babies, 162
near-term newborns and, 155
night wakings and, 340
overfeeding and, 263
phenylalanine-free, 152
pitfalls of, 183
for premature babies,
  155, 158
probiotics in, 6
and refusal of bottle, 272
and refusal to nurse, 63
relactation and, 145
risks of, 6–7
sexual abuse survivor use
  of, 151
as SIDS risk factor, 40
slow weight gain and, 349
sucking problems and, 115
supplementer systems
  and, 137
underfeeding and, 125, 127,
  129, 233, 234, 235, 236
as vitamin D source, 186–187
weaning baby off of, 83,
  375, 378
working mother use of,
  253, 254
Freemie Independence II pump,
  303–304
Freemie Liberty II pump,
  303–304
Freemie milk cups, 308
frenulum, short
  clipping, 121
  latch-on problems and,
    112, 119
  pumping for babies with, 254
  sucking problems and, 119
  underfeeding risks, 66
frequency
  after surgery (baby), 217
  appetite spurts and, 220
  for bed-sharing mothers, 40
  bottle-feeding schedule,
    327–328
  for breast infection, 205–206
  contraceptives and, 336–337

diabetic mothers, babies with,
  146–147
for diarrhea, 190–191
Down syndrome, babies with,
  169–170
eight months or older, 253
engorgement and, 70–71, 77
expressing milk, scheduling
  based on, 328
during fever, 190
first two months, 182, 185,
  191–193, 209
four to seven months, 253
guidelines, 60–61, 96, 181,
  183, 231
letdown reflex and, 96
for mastitis, 205
milk production delay and, 81
milk production reduced by
  insufficient, 134
milk supply increase based
  on, 192, 264
night waking, 124
normal, 125
nursing on demand, 123–124
plugged ducts, 201, 345
reflux and, 223, 231
for refusal to nurse, 109
six to twelve months, 354
sore nipples and, 88
stress during feedings, 167
sucking problems, 117
teething effect on, 357
toddlers, 377, 380
two to six months, 337–338
typical, 63–67
underfeeding and, 127, 236
for underweight babies,
  348–349
fussiness
  appetite spurts, 220
  bottle, offering during, 327
  bowel movements, 105
  colic, 231–232
  coping measures, 124
  diaper rash, 221
  dietary supplements and, 179
  fluoride and, 188
  frequent nursing and,
    192, 233
  fussy babies, seeking out
    mothers with, 219
  gripe water, 230
  hyperlactation syndrome, 228
  before mother's period, 353
  night-waking and, 123–124
  nutrition of mother and, 179,
    224–228
  during nursing, 63, 217–218,
    223

reasons for, 4, 179, 192, 220,
  221, 264
reflux and, 223, 231, 232
teething, 340, 357
temperament and, 221
yeast infections, 221

G

gastroesophageal reflux
  diagnosing, 216, 222
  overview of, 222–224
  spitting up, 216
  tests for, 231
  underfeeding, 234, 235–236
Ghaheri, Bobby, 122
glandular tissue, insufficient,
  80, 125, 129, 134–137, 238
Goldfarb, Lenore, 141
gripe water, 229–230
Gordon, Jay, 377

H

Haaka Ladybug squeeze
  pump, 313
Haberman Feeder, 168
hair loss, postpartum, 173–174
Hale, Thomas, 87
headaches
  acetaminophen (Tylenol)
    for, 210
  anesthesia and, 209–210
  aspirin and, 226
  caffeine and, 210
  Domperidone and, 87
  hormone drop and, 210
  ibuprofen for, 210
  lactation and, 210
  mastitis, 204
  nifedipine and, 199–200
  phenylpropanolamine
    and, 226
heartburn (baby), 222–224, 234
heart defects, nursing babies
  with, 167
heart disease, 3, 11
heart rate (baby), 25, 72,
  156, 159
hemorrhage, postpartum, 50, 81
hemorrhoids, 102, 172–173
hepatitis A, 5, 132
hepatitis B, 5, 132–133
hepatitis B-specific immunoglobulin (HBIG), 133

hepatitis B surface antigen (HBsAe), 132–133
hepatitis C, 133
herbs, milk production stimulation with
  adoptive mothers, 143
  blessed thistle, 84–85, 135, 139
  breast surgery and, 139
  vs. drugs, 83, 128, 145
  fennel, 84
  fenugreek, 84–85, 138, 237, 265
  hypoplastic breasts, 125, 129, 135, 238
  late onset and, 83
  Malunggay tree, 85
  moringa, 85
  nettle leaf, 84
  overview of, 84–85
  polycystic ovary syndrome (PCOS) and, 138
  before period, 353
  premature babies, 157
  pumping and, 265
  relactation and, 144–145
  selecting, 84–85
  sick babies, 157
  slow weight gain and, 348–349
  underfeeding treatment with, 127, 237
  wild asparagus root, 85
herpes, nursing mothers with, 133, 147–148, 374
hiccuping, 68–69, 110, 223
high-protein foods
  for babies, 363–364
  for mothers, 102, 165
  for toddlers, 381
hindmilk
  for babies with heart defects, 167
  colic treatment and prevention with, 228, 244
  one-breast nursing and, 181
  for premature babies, 158
  for sick babies, 158
HIV (human immunodeficiency virus), 22, 133, 249
home birth, 32
honey, 88, 91
hopelessness, feelings of, 211, 215
hormonal contraceptives, 336
hormones
  alcohol and, 151, 152, 180
  breastfeeding readiness, 19, 20, 142

drop, headaches caused by, 210
dysphoric milk ejection reflex (D-MER) and, 215
estrogen, 142
labor initiation and, 23
lactogen, 142
leptin, 6
microbiome and, 3
milk production stimulation and, 85, 87
oxytocin, 6, 7, 20, 210
placenta delivery and, 50, 80
postpartum shift, 73
progesterone, 142
prolactin, 19, 20, 85, 87, 152, 180, 254
vitamin D, 185, 186
hyperlactation syndrome, 224, 228
hypertension, 142, 200
hyperthyroidism, 149
hypoallergenic detergents, 93
hypoallergenic formula, 225, 364
hypoplasia/hypoplastic breasts
  appearance and identification of, 134–135
  milk production insufficient due to, 134, 135, 137
  overview of, 134–137
  pumping in cases of, 135
hypothyroidism, 84, 149
Hygeia EnDeare Pump, 280–281
Hygeia Evolve, 291

I

ibuprofen
  after birth, 50, 74
  after cesarean birth, 60, 173
  before nursing, 88, 96
  for engorged breasts, 79
  for fever, 206
  for headaches, 210
  for sore nipples, 88
  for teething, 340, 357, 369, 371
immune system
  solid food early introduction, impact on, 183
  microbiome and, 3, 4
  vitamin D role in, 186
  zinc role in, 359
immunities, milk role in, 4
impetigo, 92, 200
infant carriers, 148, 272, 316
infant car seats, 37–38, 316

infections. See also breast infections; ear infections; thrush; yeast infections
  cleft lip and palate, 168
  colostrum and, 19
  cytomegalovirus (CMV), 133
  diabetes and, 147
  Down syndrome, 170
  fever as sign of, 26, 190
  formula and, 5, 6
  heart defects as risk factor for, 167
  herpes, 133
  induction and, 25
  maternal antibodies and, 23
  microbiome and, 4
  pacifiers and, 51
  premature baby risk of, 28, 155
  second-hand smoke and, 180
  solid food, early introduction and, 342
  tattoos and, 22
  tuberculosis and, 132
  underwire bras and, 35
  vitamin D role in prevention of, 186–187
  vomiting as sign of, 216
  weaning and, 365
infectious diseases, 4, 141, 321
insurance carriers, for pumps, 8, 246–247, 285
insurance pumping
  clinical-grade pump, 245
  overview of, 254–255, 258
  reasons for, 240
intrauterine devices (IUDs), 335, 336
iron (baby)
  iron-deficiency anemia, 358
  lactoferrin and, 5
  overview of, 188
  premature babies, supplements for, 158, 188
  preparation for birth and, 23
  at six months, 359
  solid-food sources of, 358, 359, 361
iron (mother)
  after gastric bypass surgery, 140
  depleted, 343
  postpartum anemia treatment with, 179, 346
irritability (baby), 188, 192, 218, 219
irritability (mother), 73, 174, 179, 211, 216

J

jaundice
bilirubin and, 50, 105,
106–107
breastfeeding and, 103, 107
breast-milk jaundice, 106
colostrum and, 50
developmentally immature
newborns, 24
diabetic mothers, babies
with, 146
frequent feedings and, 103
glucose and, 63
incidence and severity,
105–106
late-preterm babies and, 153
milk production delay as
cause of, 23, 79
nursing babies with, 103, 107
overview of, 105–107
phototherapy for, 105, 107
physiologic jaundice, 105–106
risk factors for, 24, 63, 79,
146, 153
sleepiness in babies with, 108
treatment measures for, 105,
106–107, 107–109

K

kangaroo care, 156
Karp, Harvey, 219
Keflex, 204
Kegel exercises, 173
Kendall-Tackett, Kathleen, 213
Kleiman, Karen, 212

L

lactation professionals
adopted babies, nursing
protocols for, 141
for babies with birth
defects, 167
for babies with cleft lip and
palate, 168
for babies with tongue-tie,
122
colic relief tips of, 229
for developmental and neurological problems, 169
home visit by, 32
on hospital staff, 32, 189
hyperlactation syndrome
and, 228
for hypoplasia, 137

insurance coverage for, 47,
101, 114, 130
insurance pumping and, 258
for latch-on difficulty, 99,
101, 264
log, analyzing, 73
for milk production delay, 82
for nipple shield selection,
100, 114, 117, 118, 150, 161
nursing supplementers recommended by, 128, 137, 236
for plugged ducts, 203
for Polycystic Ovary Syn-
drome (PCOS), 138
for premature babies, nursing
assistance with, 156
pump checking by, 265
pumps recommended by, 244,
245, 248, 276
referrals and referral
services, 33
for refusal to nurse, 110, 113
reused milk and, 270–271
for sore nipples, 86
for sucking problems, 118,
169, 264
support and encouragement
from, 118, 130
for thrush nipples, 196, 197
for transgender individuals,
147
for underfeeding, 126,
128, 235
Lacti-Cups squeeze pump, 313
lactose-free formula, 152
La Leche League International
nursing support through, 366
socializing opportunities
through, 174, 378, 382
for toddler nursing, 378
volunteers in, 72
lanolin
allergic reaction to, 70, 92–93
modified, 93
obtaining, 93
before pumping, 249
sore nipples in reaction to, 70
sore nipple treatment with,
59, 88, 91
during teething, 368
lansoprazole (Prevacid), 229
Lansinoh Signature Pro,
294–295
Lansinoh Smart Pump 2.0, 295
latch-on
BAA (Breastfeeding Aversion
and Agitation), 215–216
bottle feeding and, 237, 272
after cesarean birth, 59

cleft lip and palate, babies
with, 167, 168, 169
clicking sound and, 68
Down syndrome, babies
with, 170
engorgement and, 71, 77, 78
after expressing milk, 163,
240, 251
falling asleep after, 104, 160
let-down and, 96
for multiple babies, 164
lactation professionals
and, 130
nipple problems and, 89, 90,
97–103
pacifiers and, 51
positioning, 52–56
for premature babies, 159–
160, 161
sore nipples and, 86, 88,
195, 198
sucking problems, 114–118
technique, 52–58
during teething, 358, 368
tongue-tie, 119–120, 122
underfeeding and, 66–67,
125, 234
videos demonstrating, 31, 56,
61, 127
latex nipples, 271
laxatives, 125, 173, 226, 234
lead
sources of, 178
in tap water, 6
leaking colostrum, 17
leaking milk
bags vs. bottles, 267, 269
breast pads for, 34, 71, 95
breast shells as factor in, 36,
70, 95, 329
breast size as factor in, 18
in first two months, 71, 94,
134, 191
from incisions, 207
letdown and, 94
milk collectors and, 313
overabundant milk and, 208,
346–347
overview of, 94–95
from pierced nipple sites, 28
from pumps, 286, 289,
306–309
sexual intercourse and,
334–335
at three to six months, 338
treatment for, 95, 208
at work, 329
Legendairy milk cups, 309

letdown
  aiding, 71
  delayed, 355, 375
  difficulty with, 96–97
  emotions, negative
    before, 215
  fat content of milk and, 158
  gasping and choking during,
    217, 273
  headache during, 210
  hyperlactation syndrome
    and, 228
  leaking and, 94
  low milk supply and, 254
  nipple trauma and, 90
  overabundant milk and,
    208–209
  overview of, 94
  oxytocin and, 6, 20
  pumping and, 243, 249,
    250, 278
  reflex, 20
  sensations of, 94, 96, 191, 200
  sexual activity and, 334
  stimulating, 71, 242
Limerick "Joy" Pump, 283
Limerick "PJ's Comfort"
  Pump, 283
low birth weight
  as jaundice risk factor, 106
  mothers with cytomegalovi-
    rus (CMV) and, 133
  multiple babies with, 163
  powdered formula and, 5
  pumping for babies with, 254
  underfeeding risks associated
    with, 65

M

magnesium, 199, 265, 353
malocclusion, bottle-sucking
  linked to, 7
mammogram, 207
Mammol ointment, 93
Manuka honey, 88, 90, 91
marijuana, 152
Masse breast cream, 93
mastectomy, nursing after, 138
mastitis. See also breast
  infections
  breast abscess and, 206
  methicillin-resistant
    Staphylococcus aureus (MRSA)
    and, 346
  overview, 203–205

prevention, 90, 210
risk factors, 89, 120, 370
treatment measures, 204,
  205–206
maternity leave, 319
McKenna, James, 41, 373
meconium
  bilirubin in, 50, 106
  characteristics of, 50, 69,
    104–105
  retaining of, 106
Medela Classic Electric
  Pump, 276
Medela Freestyle Flex, 288–289
Medela Harmony Pump, 310
Medela Lactina/Lactina
  Select, 280
Medela Pump in Style Max
  Flow, 286–287
Medela Sonata, 287–288
Medela Swing Maxi Double
  Electric Pump, 289–290
Medela Symphony Pump,
  276–278
Medicaid, 247
Meier, Paula, 277
melamine, 6
Melodi One Advanced
  Pump, 282
meningitis, bacterial, 5
methicillin-resistant
  Staphylococcus aureus (MRSA),
  204–205, 346
metoclopramide, 87, 229
milk. See also cow's milk;
  donated milk; expressing milk;
  foremilk; hindmilk; leaking
  milk
  appearance and characteris-
    tics of, 97, 268
  bacterial testing of, 184
  blood in, 97, 203, 208
  composition and characteris-
    tics of, 184, 187
  content during pregnancy,
    378
  defrosting and warming, 267,
    268, 270–271, 327
  digestion of, 217, 222
  discarding, 70, 132–133, 157,
    184, 318, 327
  drug content in, 20
  handling and feeding, 328
  jaundice treatment with,
    106, 107
  nutrients in, 342

overabundant, 138, 208–209,
  228, 346–347
pasteurizing, 133, 184
quality of, 9, 184
quantity of, 9
solid foods as replacement,
  342
spitting up, 68, 166, 216–217,
  218, 228
taste, change in, 374
transporting, 258, 270,
  326, 329
vitamin C levels in, 179–180
milk allergy, 364
milk banks, 183–184
milk cups, 292, 297, 302–303,
  305
milk ducts, plugged
  breast infection, 345–346
  breast lumps as sign of, 207
  breast pain accompanying, 94
  causes of, 35
  diabetic mothers and, 147
  milk oversupply and, 244
  overview of, 201–202
  preventing, 35, 165, 181,
    331, 333
  treatment measures for,
    202–203
  underwire bras and, 35
Milkies Milk Saver squeeze
  pump, 313
Milkies Milk Saver On-the-Go
  squeeze pump, 313
milk supply
  breast surgery effect on, 139
  brewer's yeast and, 179, 331
  bringing in, 144
  building, 181, 234, 235
  cereal and, 232
  decrease in, 183, 232, 254,
    255, 260, 262–263, 333,
    348, 378
  delayed letdown and, 355
  demand as factor in, 20,
    60–62, 63, 89, 103, 109, 185,
    233, 259, 329
  dietary supplements for,
    179, 331
  donating, 183–184
  ensuring, 67, 81, 84, 109,
    139, 154
  established, 143, 155, 165–
    166, 247, 261–262
  estimating, 126, 128, 145,
    235–236, 237, 245, 349
  estrogen and, 336
  evaluating, 130

in first two months, 182–183
fluctuations in, 182, 183,
192, 261
freezing, 183, 252
fussiness and, 219
herbs for, 84–85, 143, 144,
237, 348
hypothyroidism and, 149
increasing, 83, 84, 126, 157,
264–265
insufficient glandular tissue
(IGT) and, 134, 137
insurance pumping, 254–255,
258
low, 83, 96, 120, 130, 134, 139,
143–144, 152, 189, 234, 243
maintaining, 110, 116, 117,
130, 132, 157, 160, 168, 169,
190, 242, 253, 255, 260, 285,
318, 319, 324
medications for, 83, 87,
143, 348
night-waking and, 341, 357
normal, 143
one-sided nursing, 181, 350
overabundant, 244, 346–347
period and, 353
placental fragments and, 238
polycystic ovary syndrome
(PCOS) and, 138, 238
pregnancy effect on, 378
progestin and, 336
pyloric stenosis surgery
and, 217
rebuilding, 144–145, 348, 354
refusal to nurse and, 190,
192, 218, 340, 354, 374–375
requirements, 263, 338
slow weight gain and,
348–349
smoking and, 152
supplementer for, 143–144
supplementing, 63, 157–158,
182–183
tandem nursing and, 379
weight loss (mother) and, 333
work and, 319, 324, 328
Mojab, Cynthia Good, 186–187
Montgomery's tubercles, 16
Morton, Jane, 56, 82, 99, 121,
241, 259, 260, 261
mothers' groups, 12, 15–16,
174, 366
motility drugs, 229
Motif Duo pump, 300
Motif Luna pump, 300–301
Motif Twist pump, 301

N

nanny, hiring, 321–322
narcotic pain relievers, 25, 26,
60, 74, 173
narcotic dependence, 151
nasal sprays, 268
Newman-Goldfarb protocols,
141, 142–144
Newman, Jack, 61, 90, 91, 93,
141, 144, 197, 198, 199
nifedipine, 199–200
night wakings
bed-sharing vs. separate
sleeping, 341, 373
comfort objects for, 371
coping with, 150, 333, 335,
355–357, 370–373
cry-it-out method, 372
ear infections and, 371
excessive, 123–124, 341
newborns, feedings for, 67,
78, 103, 104, 127, 164,
236, 348
no-cry method, 372–373
of nursing toddlers, 377
overview of, 340–341
supplemental feedings
and, 340
teething and, 340, 356, 371
weaning and, 356–357, 381
nipples. See also sore nipples
blanching, 120, 198–120
bleeding, 53, 97, 120, 133, 203
compresses, applying to,
93, 203
compression of, 116, 198, 257
creams, 18, 70, 88, 91, 92, 93,
196, 197, 198, 200
herpes lesions on, 148
incision on or near, 65, 84,
125, 129, 138, 208, 238, 255
pierced, 28
pregnancy, changes
during, 17
preparation before breastfeeding, 28–30
preparation before
pumping, 258
relocation of, 138–139
rinsing, 91
shape of, 28–30, 70, 97–101,
110, 120
size of, 65, 110, 117, 118,
119, 255
soap and shampoo, avoiding
on, 69

spitting out, 110
tender or damaged,
treating, 59
wounds on, 90–91, 92, 370
nipple shields
appearance of, 100
emotional barriers to, 150
guidelines concerning, 100
insurance pumping and, 254
latch-on help with, 100, 111–
112, 114, 161
overview of, 100
for premature babies, 161
pumping and, 254
selecting, 117
sizing, 88, 91
sore nipples and, 88, 91
for sucking problems, 117–118
tongue-tie and, 120
underfeeding and, 125, 234
when to avoid, 88, 91
non-binary parents, 145–146
nursing bras. See also bras
convenience and comfort of,
69, 71
fitting guidelines, 34–35
pumping bustier, 260
support provided by, 71, 78
wearing at night, 78
nursing pads. See breast pads
nursing supplementation
devices
for adopted babies, 140, 141
benefits of, 238
after breast surgery, 139
cerebral palsy, babies
with, 170
cleft lip and palate, babies
with, 168
developmental and neuro-
logical problems, babies
with, 169
for donated milk, 141
insufficient glandular tissue
(IGT) and, 137
insufficient milk production,
use in event of, 129, 238
lactation professional advocacy of, 128, 236
for late-onset milk production, 82
Newman-Goldfarb protocol
role of, 143–144
overview of, 137
relactation and, 145
underfeeding and, 128,
129, 238

O

obesity, 3, 4, 7, 11, 65, 80, 138, 263, 343, 363
one-breast nursing
  benefits of, 181
  burping after, 104
  and hindmilk, 181, 228
  leaking and, 71, 94
  lopsided breasts and, 209, 350
  multiple babies, 164, 165
  overabundant milk, 347
  plugged ducts, avoiding with, 345
  preference for, 181, 338, 349–350
  reflux, treating with, 223, 228
  refusal to nurse and, 110
  sore nipples and, 88
  tongue-tie and, 112, 119
one-sided nursing, 349–350
oxytocin
  headache during let-down related to, 210
  milk release role of, 6, 20
  natural and artificial compared, 23, 24, 25

P

pacifier
  for babies with colic or reflux, 222–223, 232
  breastfeeding-as-contraception and, 337
  feeding cues and, 328, 347, 348
  fussiness and, 220, 232, 264
  latch-on difficulty after, 161
  night wakings and, 341, 356, 371
  between nursings, 150, 264
  pre-weaning introduction, 383
  pitfalls of, 51
  putting aside for nursing, 348
  refusal to nurse following, 51, 109
  sleepy babies and, 104
  sterilizing, 197
  toddler use of, 377
  tongue-tie and, 120
  underfeeding and, 337
  use guidelines, 51, 52
Palmer, Gabrielle, 3
Pantley, Elizabeth, 341, 372–373

personal-use pumps, 244, 249–251, 261, 262, 279, 280, 284
phenylpropanolamine, 226
Philips Avent bottle nipples, 272
Philips Avent Comfort Manual Breast pump, 311
Philips Avent Double Electric Breast pump, 296–297
phototherapy
  dark stools due to, 105
  nursing during, 107–108
  overview of, 107
Pitocin
  epidural combined with, 23, 25
  jaundice and, 106
  purpose of, 24
  side effects on baby, 23, 25
placental fragments in uterus
  milk supply, low due to, 66, 80–81, 238
  symptoms, 81
  underfeeding risks associated with, 66, 238
Polycystic Ovary Syndrome (PCOS)
  milk production and, 80, 84, 129, 238
  overview of, 138
  pumping in cases of, 255
  underfeeding risks associated with, 65, 125
postpartum depression
  in breastfeeding vs. bottle-feeding mothers, 11
  coping measures for, 212–215
  drug withdrawal symptoms mimicking, 74
  overview of, 210–211
  resolving, 102–103
  risk factors for, 211, 231
  in sexual abuse survivors, 151
  symptoms of, 211–212
  vitamin deficiencies, 179
premature babies. See also babies
  birth complications in, 28
  breast infections and, 205
  car seats and, 43
  cerebral palsy and, 155
  collecting milk for, 240, 269–270, 313
  colostrum for, 259
  crossover hold for, 159
  donated milk for, 158, 184

football hold for, 56, 159
formula for, 5, 158
hindmilk and, 158
infections and, 155, 205
iron supplements for, 188, 358
jaundice in, 106
kangaroo care, 156
latch-on difficulties with, 161
milk supply, establishing for, 157
of mothers with cytomegalovirus, 133
nursing of, 159–162
pumping for, 245, 247–248, 277, 282
self-feeding delayed for, 359
sleeping arrangements, 43
supplemental nutrients for, 157–158
twins, 162
underfeeding in, 126, 235
premature births
  complications of, 28
  March of Dimes and, 23
  risk of, lessening, 162
Pumpables "SuperGenie" Hospital Grade Breast Pump, 293–294
pumping. See breast pumps; clinical-grade pumps; electric pumps; expressing milk

R

Raphael, Dana, 46
Rapley, Gill, 360
Raskin, Valerie, 212
Raynaud's disease, 198
Raynaud's phenomenon, 198–200
reflux. See gastroesophageal reflux
refusal to nurse
  adopted babies, 143
  after biting episode, 369, 374
  bottle-feeding and, 109, 143, 218, 374
  after burping, 62
  cereal and, 232
  colic and, 192, 231, 232
  during illness, 218, 355
  exercise and, 174
  expressing for, 190

maternal eating as factor, 179, 217–218
before mother's period, 353
one side, refusing, 110–111, 350
pacifiers and, 109
pumping in event of, 245, 348
reflux and, 223, 350
scent and, 218
in six- to twelve-month-old babies, 355
treatment measures for, 218
Rumble Tuff Breeze, 297
Rumble Tuff Sweet Assist Manual Breast Pump, 311
Rumble Tuff Whisper Electric Breast Pump Duo, 298

S

Satter, Ellyn, 380
Sears, William, 341
sexual abuse survivors, 149–151
sick babies
breast infections and, 205
collecting milk for, 158, 258–259, 260, 269–270
expressing milk for, 155
milk pumping for, 246–247
nursing inability of, 155
nursing of, 155
pumping for, 245, 248, 258
underfeeding, 125
side-lying position
after cesarean section, 59
baby, calming in, 220, 223
one-sided nursing, treating with, 350
overview of, 58
for problem nipples, 99
for refusal to nurse, 113
for sleepy babies, 104
sucking, aiding with, 113, 117
SIDS (Sudden Infant Death Syndrome)
bed sharing role in reducing, 40, 41
risk factors for, 7, 152, 180, 220, 223
silicone nipples, 271, 272
silicone nursing pads, 71, 95, 208, 329

sore nipples
avoiding, 8, 28, 52, 96, 195
causes of, 52, 70, 195, 256, 378–379
diabetic mothers, 147
engorgement and, 70
during nursing, 378–379
overview of, 86
before period, 353
during pregnancy, 378–379
pumping for mothers with, 245, 279
struggles with, 74, 130, 240
during teething, 358, 369
treating, 70, 88–89, 91
SpecialNeeds Feeder
for babies with cerebral palsy, 170
for babies with cleft lip and palate, 168
for babies with neurological and developmental problems, 169
obtaining, 365
Spectra 9+ Pump, 293
Spectra Cara milk cups, 308–309
Spectra S1 Plus Pump, 291–292
Spectra S2 Pump, 291–292
Spectra Synergy Gold (S-G) Pump, 292–293
spitting up
in first two months, 216
in first week, 68
food allergies and, 361
hyperlactation syndrome, 228
pyloric stenosis and, 216–217
reasons for, 192, 216–217
reflux and, 166, 218
St. John's wort, 214

T

teething
coping with, 357–358
night waking due to, 340–341, 356, 371
pain, alleviating, 357, 369–370, 371
refusal to nurse due to, 355, 374
teething rings, 370

This Isn't What I Expected (Kleiman and Raskin), 212
thrush
checking for, 195
in diabetic mothers and their babies, 147
nipple irritation caused by, 92, 195, 200–201
refusal to nurse in babies with, 218
"satellite" rashes, 195–196
signs and symptoms of, 195–196, 221
treating, 196–198
tongue-tie
anesthesia for revisions, 122
crossover hold for, 113
exercises for revisions, 122
lactation professionals for, 122
latch-on problems for, 119–120, 122
nipple shield and, 120
one-breast nursing and, 112, 119
pacifier and, 120
transgender individuals, 145–146
Tommee Tippee "Made for Me" Double Electric Breast Pump, 298
Tommee Tippee "Made for Me" Single Electric Breast Pump, 309
twins
football hold for nursing of, 56
jaundice in, 106
nursing of, 162, 164–165, 259, 349
plugged ducts in mothers of, 201
premature births, 162
support groups, 162

U

Unimom Minuet Double Electric Breast Pump, 290–291
Unimom Opera Pump, 281–282
Unimom Zomee 1 and 2, 299

V

vitamin A
  cod liver oil, 187
  fluoride in combination
    with, 188
  liquid supplements, 187
  soy milk fortified with, 364
  as supplement (for baby), 187
vitamin B₆, 179, 199
vitamin B₁₂, 140, 178
vitamin B-complex sources,
  362, 374
vitamin B-complex supplements
  deficiency, 179
  first two months, 179
  for mothers of multiples, 165
  for mothers of older
    babies, 352
vitamin B deficiencies
  in babies and children, 362
  in nursing mothers, 179, 373
vitamin C (baby), 226
vitamin C (mother)
  colic symptoms caused by,
    179, 226
  fluoride with, 226
  iron absorption and, 362
  mastitis treatment with,
    206, 346
  for mothers of multiples, 165
  smoking effect of, 180
  as supplement, 226
vitamin D (baby)
  formulations with, 230
  overview of, 185–188
  soy milk fortified with, 364
  vegan diet and, 362
vitamin D (mother), 187–188
vitamin E, 70
vomiting (baby)
  as B₁₂ deficiency symptom, 140
  blood in milk as cause of, 97,
    203, 208
  as food allergy sign, 179, 361
  laryngomalacia and, 166
  maternal eating as factor in,
    97, 192, 216
  overview of, 216–217
  pyloric stenosis and, 216
  reflux and, 216
vomiting (mother), 74, 173, 189

W

Walker, Marsha, 5, 356
weaning
  antidepressants and, 214
  baby-led weaning, 360
  bloody stools and, 224
  bone density changes
    after, 178
  breast biopsies and, 208
  breast changes after, 9
  breast lumps and, 207–208
  cereal and, 232
  cholesterol and, 334
  considerations, 365–366
  defined, 365
  for diabetic mothers, 147
  early, 51, 106, 185, 232, 254,
    336, 342
  hospitalization and, 318
  "lactation headaches"
    and, 210
  medication, unsafe as reason
    for, 318
  during mother's pregnancy,
    379
  nursing, resuming after, 144
  older babies, 365–366
  pacifiers and early weaning,
    51
  refusal to nurse compared
    to, 350
  relactation after, 144
  self-weaning, 192, 217, 354
  sleeping patterns and,
    356–357
  temporary, 189, 225, 318
  toddlers, 216
WIC (Women, Infants, and Children Supplemental Nutrition)
  Affordable Care Act and, 247
  breastfeeding classes spon-
    sored by, 15–16
  breastfeeding support and
    guidance offered by, 47
  breast pumps, obtaining
    through, 8, 247, 248, 262,
    279, 280
  vegetarian diet guidelines
    from, 362
Willow Gen 3 Breast Pump,
  304–306

Y

yeast infection
  in diabetic mothers, 147
  fussiness and, 221
  signs of, 221
  sore and traumatized
    nipples, 92
  treatment, 222

Z

zinc (baby)
  at six months, 359
  solid-food sources of, 358–
    359, 361, 362
zinc (mother), 140
zinc oxide ointment, 221